Radiologic Physics

THE ESSENTIALS

Radiologic Physics

THE ESSENTIALS

Zhihua Qi, PhD

Department of Radiology
Henry Ford Hospital
Detroit, Michigan

Robert D. Wissman, MD

Department of Radiology
University of Missouri
Columbia, Missouri

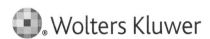 Wolters Kluwer

Philadelphia • Baltimore • New York • London
Buenos Aires • Hong Kong • Sydney • Tokyo

Acquisitions Editor: Sharon Zinner
Development Editor: Eric McDermott
Editorial Coordinator: John Larkin
Marketing Manager: Phyllis Hitner
Production Project Manager: Barton Dudlick
Design Coordinator: Elaine Kasmer
Manufacturing Coordinator: Beth Welsh
Prepress Vendor: S4Carlisle Publishing Services

9 8 7 6 5 4 3 2 1

Printed in China

Library of Congress Cataloging-in-Publication Data

ISBN-13: 978-1-4963-8629-8

ISBN-10: 1-4963-8629-9

Library of Congress Control Number: 2019910449

---

shop.lww.com

To my wife, Huimin, and my daughters, Blair and Allison

—ZQ

To my wife Carole, daughters Aimee and Abby, and grand-daughter Alivia. To my fathers both here and in heaven.

—RW

CONTRIBUTORS

Michael Burch, MD
Department of Radiology
University of Cincinnati College of Medicine
Cincinnati, Ohio

Eric England, MD
Associate Professor
Department of Radiology
University of Cincinnati
Cincinnati, Ohio

Bruce Mahoney, MD
Assistant Professor
Department of Radiology
University of Cincinnati
Cincinnati, Ohio

Kaushal Mehta, MD
Assistant Professor
Department of Radiology
University of Cincinnati
Cincinnati, Ohio

Nabeel Porbandarwala, MD
Department of Radiology
Beth Israel Deaconess Medical Center
Boston, Massachusetts

Jennifer L. Scheler, MD
Assistant Professor
Department of Radiology
University of Cincinnati
Cincinnati, Ohio

Ryan Christopher Sieve, MD
Department of Radiology
University of Wisconsin-Madison
Madison, Wisconsin

Joshua Adam Tarrence, DO
Department of Radiology
University of Cincinnati
Cincinnati, Ohio

Huimin Wu, PhD
Diagnostic Radiology and Molecular Imaging
Beaumont Hospital
Royal Oak, Michigan

Sammy Abid Yacob, DO
Department of Radiology
Duke University
Durham, North Carolina

Vineeth Yeluru, MBBS
Research Analyst
Department of Radiology
University of Cincinnati
Cincinnati, OH

SERIES FOREWORD

T he Essentials series is a collection of radiology textbooks following a standardized format. Each book in the Essentials series is a practical tool for those wanting to quickly acquire a broad base of knowledge in a specialty area. The content is limited to the essentials of that specialty so as not to overwhelm the novice, yet provides enough detail that it can serve as a quick review for residents or practicing radiologists, a guide for those who teach the specialty, and a reference for specialty physicians and other healthcare professionals whose patients are referred for imaging in that specialty area. What sets Essentials texts apart from other similar texts is that they (a) are compact and of practical size for a resident to read during an initial 4-week rotational experience, (b) include learning objectives at the beginning of each chapter, and (c) provide an exercise for self-assessment. Each book includes citations from the most recent literature that are called out in the text.

Self-assessment is a key component of the Essentials texts. Multiple-choice items are included at the end of every chapter, and a self-assessment examination is included at the end of each text. This should be of particular benefit to those who are preparing for the new image-rich computer-based examinations that are a component of professional certification and maintenance of certification.

The series includes not only texts related to clinical specialties that are rich in radiologic images and illustrations but also texts related to noninterpretive subjects such as radiologic physics and quality and safety in medical imaging. The goal of the Essentials series is to provide a collection of practical references to accompany a well-rounded education in diagnostic imaging and imaging-guided therapy.

Jannette Collins

PREFACE

Radiologic physics, in a broad sense, is concerned with all technical aspects involved in the clinical use of imaging technologies in making diagnosis, guiding interventional procedures, and others. In becoming an expert clinician in radiology, the importance of a solid understanding of radiologic physics should never be understated.

As part of the Essentials series, this book aims to help readers grasp the essence of modern medical imaging technologies from the perspective of physics. Although there have been a larger number of books on radiologic physics, this book may be best suited for radiologists who intend to know more than is required to pass their board exams but do not want to get overwhelmed by extensive details that go in depth.

The contents of the book are organized into 10 chapters, described as follows:

- The book opens with an overview of basic concepts in Chapter 1, including the origin of radiation, its interaction mechanisms with matter, the assessment of image quality, and basic informatics pertaining to medical imaging.
- Chapters 2 to 5 cover diagnostic X-ray imaging. With fundamentals about X-ray imaging covered in Chapter 2, different X-ray imaging modalities are discussed in the next three chapters (radiography and fluoroscopy in Chapter 3, mammography in Chapter 4, and computed tomography in Chapter 5).
- Chapters 6 and 7 discuss magnetic resonance imaging and ultrasound imaging, two modalities that do not use ionizing radiation.
- Chapters 8 and 9 focus on nuclear medicine, which uses radiation more energetic than X-ray for imaging and therapeutic applications. Fundamentals about nuclear medicine are reviewed in Chapter 8 before discussion of radiation detection and imaging in Chapter 9.
- The last chapter discusses radiation biology and radiation safety.

Radiology constantly and rapidly evolves with newly acquired knowledge and newly developed technologies. Although this book may seem inevitably limited in covering the breadth and the depth of knowledge in radiologic physics, it is the very intention of the book that readers, with the essential principles and understandings presented in this book, may develop rational approaches of their own for a lifelong learning process.

ACKNOWLEDGMENT

e thank Dr. Jannette Collins for the opportunity to participate in this project and all the contributing authors for their time and effort in writing the chapters amid their busy schedules. The editors also express their thanks to the editorial team from Wolters Kluwer, led by Sharon Zinner, whose work is much appreciated in the process of bringing this book to life.

CONTENTS

Basic Concepts

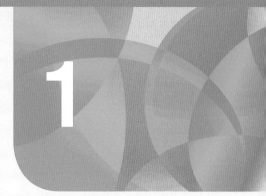

Sammy Abid Yacob, DO and Kaushal Mehta, MD

LEARNING OBJECTIVES

1. Understand the principles of radiation and X-ray production.
2. Describe the different forms of photon and charged particle interactions.
3. Define the concepts of exposure, absorbed dose, equivalent dose, and effective dose.
4. Describe the main aspects of image quality.
5. Understand the basic principles of digital imaging.
6. Explain the structure and functions of picture archiving and communication system (PACS).

This chapter reviews physics-related basic concepts in medical imaging and prepares the readers for a more detailed discussions of modality specific topics in the following chapters.

RADIATION AND ATOM

Radiation

Radiation is energy in the form of waves or particles that travels through space or matter. In a broad sense, three types of radiation are used in diagnostic imaging: acoustic radiation, electromagnetic (EM) radiation, and particulate radiation. According to wave-particle duality in quantum mechanics, all three types of radiation have both wave characteristics and particle characteristics. A wave is often described by wavelength, frequency, speed, and amplitude, and a particle by mass, momentum, and energy; any quantum entity, according to wave-particle duality, may be characterized by a combination of these characteristics. Often in medical imaging, a certain type of radiation may demonstrate more pronounced characteristics in one of the two, wave or particle, dependent on the type of object it interacts with. Generally speaking, acoustic radiation and nonionizing EM radiation (like radiofrequency waves used in magnetic resonance imaging [MRI]) are more often treated as waves, and particulate radiation and ionizing radiation (including X-rays and gamma rays) are more often considered as particles.

Acoustic radiation

Ultrasound, sound wave at frequencies higher than the upper audible limit of human hearing, is the mainly used acoustic radiation in medical imaging. Other than its higher frequencies, ultrasound is not particularly different from audible sound in physical properties; frequencies of audible sound to humans are typically between 20 and 20 000 Hz (20 kHz), whereas ultrasound imaging devices operate at frequencies from 20 kHz up to a few gigahertz (10^9 Hz).

Like all other types of waves, the speed (c), wavelength (λ), and frequency (f) of the ultrasound wave are related by the following equation:

$$c = \lambda \cdot f$$

The frequency of ultrasound in imaging is determined by the transducer, which is used to generate the wave. The speed is closely related to the physical properties of the medium in which the ultrasound wave travels. The average speed of ultrasound in soft tissues is about 1540 m/s. If a 5 MHz frequency beam is used for imaging, it can be easily derived that the wavelength of the ultrasound wave is about 0.3 mm (Figure 1.1).

Electromagnetic radiation

EM radiation is a form of energy that is all around us and takes on many forms. EM radiation encompasses a broad spectrum of energies that comprise the EM spectrum. Categories of EM radiation include radiant heat, radio, TV, microwaves, infrared, visible light, TV light, X-rays, and gamma rays (Figures 1.2 and 1.3).

EM radiations have no mass, are unaffected by either electric or magnetic disturbances, and travel at a constant speed in a given medium. The speed of EM radiations is a function of the medium transport characteristics. In a vacuum, EM radiation travels at its maximum speed, the speed of light (2.998×10^8 m/s). EM radiation travels in straight lines; however, this trajectory can be altered by interaction with matter. Interactions can occur either by absorption (removal of radiation) or scattering (change in trajectory).

The types of EM radiation utilized in diagnostic imaging include X-rays, gamma rays, visible light, and radiofrequency EM radiation. X-rays are used in radiography and computed tomographic (CT) imaging. Gamma rays are used in nuclear imaging to image the distribution of radiopharmaceuticals. Visible light, which is produced in detecting X- and gamma rays, is used for the observation and interpretations of images. EM radiation at

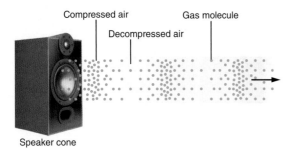

A The nature of sound waves

FIG. 1.1 ● **Ultrasound, as a type of acoustic radiation used in diagnostic imaging, mostly exhibits wave characteristics.** Ultrasound is a special kind of sound wave whose frequencies are beyond the audible limit of the human being. Sound waves are pressure waves originated from a vibrating source (A). The air pressure at any point on its path undergoes periodic changes and can be measured and plotted as a sinusoidal function of time (B). Reprinted with permission from McConnell TH, Hull KL. *Human Form, Human Function.* 1st ed. Philadelphia, PA: Wolters Kluwer Health/Lippincott Williams & Wilkins; 2010.

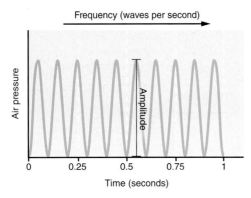

B Sound wave characteristics

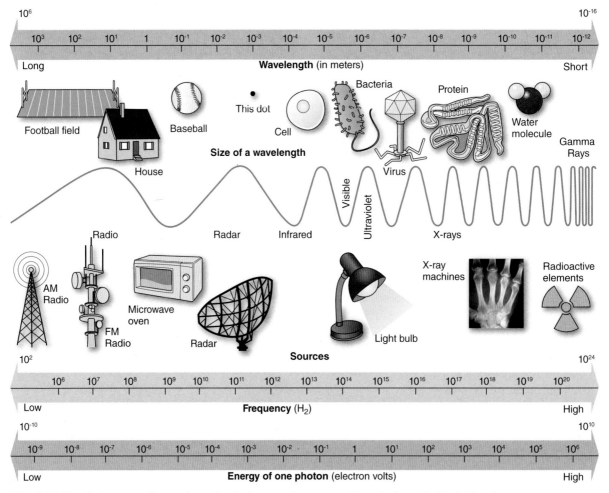

FIG. 1.2 ● **The electromagnetic spectrum.** An electromagnetic wave must have both an electric field and a magnetic field component. Electromagnetic radiation propagates as oscillating electric and magnetic fields perpendicular to each other and perpendicular to the direction the wave travels. Reprinted with permission from Orth D. *Essentials of Radiologic Science.* 2nd ed. Philadelphia, PA: Wolters Kluwer; 2017.

FIG. 1.3 ● The oscillating electric and magnetic fields associated with electromagnetic radiation. The oscillating directions of the electric field and the magnetic field are perpendicular to each other, and they are both perpendicular to the direction of the propagation of the electro-magnetic wave (A). The oscillation of electric field (or magnetic field) is typically characterized as a sinusoidal function of timer or distance (B). Reprinted with permission from Sinko P. *Martin's Physical Pharmacy and Pharmaceutical Sciences.* 7th ed. Philadelphia, PA: Wolters Kluwer; 2016.

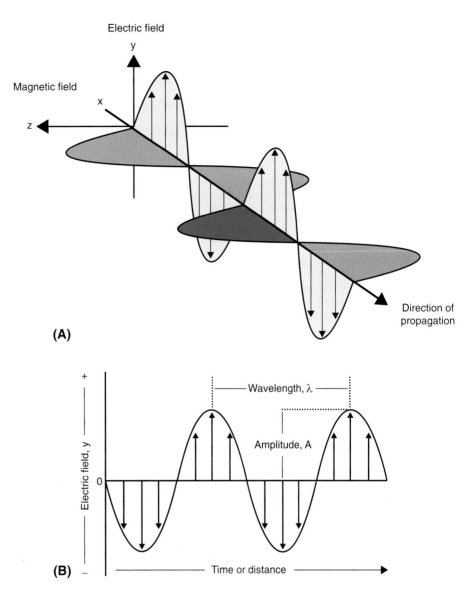

radio frequencies is used as the transmission and reception signal for MRI.

Like the ultrasound wave, the EM wave follows the same relation that its speed is equal to the product of the frequency and the wavelength. Because, in air, all EM waves travel at the same speed (~3.0×10^8 m/s), their frequency varies linearly with the reverse of the wavelength. In the air, wavelengths of X-rays and gamma rays are typically measured in nanometers (nm), where 1 nm = 10^{-9} m, whereas wavelengths of radio frequency waves used in MRI are typically on the order of meters.

EM radiation can also exhibit particle-like behavior when interacting with matter. It is particularly true for X-rays and gamma rays; they can be viewed as particle-like energy packets, often called photons. Photons are discrete quantities in which EM radiation can be quantified. Photon energy is directly proportional to frequency and inversely proportional to wavelength. The energy of a photon is given by the following equation:

$$E = hf = hc/\lambda$$

where h = Plank's constant = 6.62×10^{-34} J·s. For X- and gamma-ray photons, energy (E) is often expressed in keV and wavelength (λ) in nanometers (nm). The energies of photons are commonly expressed in electron volts (eV). One electron volt is the amount of energy gained by an electron when accelerated through an electrical potential difference of one volt in vacuum. Multiples of electron volts (eV) commonly used in medical imaging are the keV (1000 eV) and the MeV (1 000 000 eV).

Ionizing radiation refers to types of radiation where the radiation carries sufficient energy to ionize atoms. In terms of the EM spectrum, radiations of higher frequency, near-UV region of the spectrum, typically carry enough energy per photon to remove bound electrons from atomic shells, thus producing ionized atoms. Ionizing radiation on the EM spectrum includes UV radiation, X-rays, and gamma rays. Nonionizing radiation, or radiations with lower energies, on the EM spectrum includes visible light, infrared, and radio waves.

The threshold energy for ionization depends on the type of matter. Ionization potential is the minimum energy necessary to

Table 1.1 FUNDAMENTAL PROPERTIES OF PARTICULATE RADIATION

Particle	Symbol	Relative Charge	Mass (amu)	Energy Equivalent (MeV)
Alpha	α, ^{4}He^{2+}	+2	4.0028	3727
Proton	ρ, ^{1}H$^+$	+1	1.007593	938
Electron (beta minus)	e$^-$, β^-	−1	0.000548	0.511
Positron (beta plus)	e$^+$, β^+	+1	0.000548	0.511
Neutron	n^0	0	1.008982	940

Adapted with permission from Bushberg JT, Seibert JA, Leidholdt EM, Boone JM. *Essential Physics of Medical Imaging*. 3rd ed. Philadelphia, PA: Wolters Kluwer Health/Lippincott Williams & Wilkins; 2012.

remove an electron. For example, the minimum energy necessary to remove an electron (ie, the *ionization potential*) from water is 12.6 eV.

Particulate radiation

Table 1.1 summarizes the physical properties of particulate radiations associated with medical imaging. They include the following:
- Electron
  - It is the most commonly utilized particulate radiation in diagnostic imaging. An electron has a rest mass of 9.109×10^{-31} kg and a rest energy of 511 keV. Electrons carry a negative charge and exist in atomic orbits. Electrons may also be emitted by the nuclei of some radioactive atoms. In such a case, they are referred to as beta-minus particles (β^-), negatrons or "beta particles."
- Positron
  - Positrons are positively charged electrons. It is the antiparticle or the antimatter particle of electrons.
  - During radioactive decay, positrons may be emitted from some nuclei.
- Proton
  - Protons are found in the nuclei of all atoms. A proton has a single positive charge and is the nucleus of a hydrogen-1 atom.
- Neutrons
  - Neutrons are uncharged nuclear particles that have a mass slightly greater than a proton. Neutrons are released by nuclear fission and are used for radionuclide production.
- Alpha particle
  - An alpha particle (α^{2+}) consists of two protons and two neutrons; therefore, it carries a net charge of +2 and is identical to the nucleus of a helium atom (^{4}He^{2+}). Certain naturally occurring radioactive materials emit alpha particles, such as uranium, thorium, and radium. In such emissions, the α^{2+} particle will eventually acquire two electrons from the surrounding medium and become a neutral helium atom (^{4}He).

Mass energy equivalence

According to Einstein's theory of relativity, mass and energy are interchangeable and the sum of the mass and energy must be conserved. This is true of objects moving at high speeds such as the speeds associated with some nuclear processes, which approach the speed of light. Einstein showed that at these speeds, mass and energy are equivalent according to the expression:

$$E = mc^2$$

where E represents the energy equivalent to mass (m) at rest and c is the speed of light in a vacuum (2.98×10^8 m/s). For example, the energy equivalent of an electron (mass of 9.109×10^{-31} kg)

can be calculated using Einstein's equation, which turns out to be 0.511 MeV or 511 keV.

A common unit of mass used in atomic and nuclear physics is the atomic mass unit (amu), defined as 1/12th of the mass of an atom of ^{12}C. One amu is equivalent to 931.5 MeV of energy.

Atom

An atom is the smallest constituent unit of matter in which the element's chemical identity is maintained. The atom is composed of three types of particles: protons, neutrons, and electrons. Protons and neutrons make up the nucleus of an atom, whereas electrons are extranuclear in location.

Protons have a positive charge. Neutrons are electrically neutral. Protons and neutrons are essentially the same mass and together make up the extremely dense atomic nucleus. Electrons are negatively charged and make up the largely unoccupied extranuclear space (Figure 1.4).

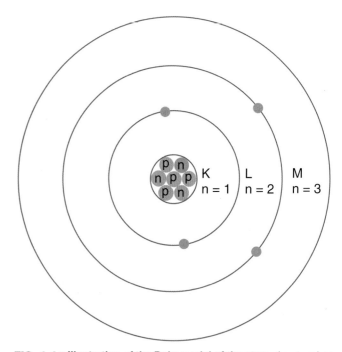

FIG. 1.4 ● Illustration of the Bohr model of the atom. An atom has a nucleus in the center composed of protons and neutrons. Electrons revolve around the nucleus in specific orbits, which are at discrete energy levels. Depending on their energy levels, the orbits are often denoted by letters K, L, M, ... Reprinted with permission from Halperin EC, Brady LW, Perez CA, et al. *Perez & Brady's Principles and Practice of Radiation Oncology*. 6th ed. Philadelphia, PA: Wolters Kluwer Health/Lippincott Williams & Wilkins; 2013.

Electronic structure

Electron Orbits and Electron Binding Energy

According to the Bohr model of an atom, electrons orbit the dense positively charged nucleus at fixed distances called electron shells. Each electron shell corresponds to a discrete energy state. These electron shells are assigned the letters K, L, M, N, . . ., with K signifying the innermost shell. Quantum numbers are also assigned, with the quantum number 1 designating the K shell, 2 designating the L shell, and so on.

Each shell can hold a maximum number of electrons, as given by this equation ($2n^2$), where n is the quantum number of the shell. For example, the K shell ($n = 1$) can only hold two electrons, whereas the L shell ($n = 2$) can hold 2×2^2 or eight electrons (Figure 1.5).

Electrons are held in place by the electrostatic pull of the positively charged nucleus. Electron binding energy is the energy required to remove an electron completely from the atom (Figure 1.6). The binding energy of a particular electron in orbit increases with the number of protons in the nucleus (ie, the atomic number). Therefore, atoms with more positively charged protons have a greater electrostatic pull on the orbiting electrons, which equates to the higher energy required to remove an electron from the atom. Electron binding energies of inner shell electrons are higher than those of more outer-shell electrons because of the decreased electrostatic pull from the positively charged nucleus. The energy required to move an electron from the innermost electron orbit (K shell) to the next orbit (L shell) is the difference between the binding energies of the two orbits. The outermost electron shell of an atom is known as the valence shell. The valence shell determines the chemical properties of the element.

Furthermore, the energy required to move an electron from the innermost electron orbit (K shell) to the next orbit (L shell) is the difference between the binding energies of the two orbits (ie, $E_{bK} - E_{bL}$) or the transition energy. The K- to L-shell transition energies for hydrogen and tungsten are as follows:

Hydrogen: $13.5 \text{ eV} - 3.4 \text{ eV} = 10.1 \text{ eV}$
Tungsten: $69\,500 \text{ eV} - 11\,000 \text{ eV} = 58\,500 \text{ eV (58.5 keV)}$

Radiation from Electron Transitions

When an electron is removed from its shell through any interaction, a vacancy is created in that shell. An electron from an outer shell fills this vacancy, subsequently leaving a vacancy that again will be filled by an electron transition from a more distant shell. This series of transitions is called an *electron cascade*. Each transition releases energy equal to the difference in binding energy between the original and final shells of the electron. The atom may release this energy through emission of either characteristic X-rays or Auger electrons.

- Characteristic X-rays
  The radiation emitted when an outer-shell electron fills a vacancy in an inner shell of an atom is characteristic of each atom, because the electron binding energies depend on atomic number (Z). Radiation emissions from electron transitions exceeding 100 eV are called characteristic X-rays.
- Auger electrons
  Characteristic X-rays are not always the product of an electron cascade. Auger electron emission is a competing process that predominates in low Z elements. In Auger electron emission, the energy released is transferred to an orbital electron, typically in the same shell as the cascading electron. The ejected Auger electron possesses kinetic energy equal to the difference between the transition energy and the binding energy of the ejected electron.

The atomic nucleus

Protons and neutrons make up the atomic nucleus and they are collectively known as nucleons. The atomic number (Z) is the number of protons in the nucleus. The mass number (A) is the total number of protons and neutrons (N) within the nucleus, that is, $A = N + Z$. Note that mass number is different from atomic mass. For example, the mass number of fluorine-19 is 19 (9 protons and 10 neutrons), whereas its atomic mass is 18.9984 amu.

Standard nuclear notation shows the chemical symbol, the mass number, and the atomic number of the isotope. For example, an atom with the chemical symbol X is ($_Z^A X_N$). In this notation, Z and N are redundant because the chemical symbol identifies the element and thus the numbers of protons and neutrons. For example, the symbol Tc refers to the technetium atom, which has a $Z = 43$. Therefore, $_{43}^{98}\text{Tc}_{55}$ is usually simply written as ^{98}Tc or as Tc-98.

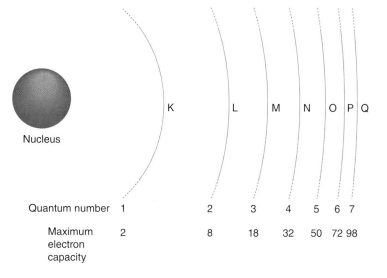

FIG. 1.5 ● **Illustration of rules governing the filling of electron shells.** If the quantum number of the electron shell is *n*, then the maximum number of electrons the electron shell may have is $2n^2$. Reprinted with permission from Bushberg JT, Seibert JA, Leidholdt EM, Boone JM. *Essential Physics of Medical Imaging.* 3rd ed. Philadelphia, PA: Wolters Kluwer Health/ Lippincott Williams & Wilkins; 2012.

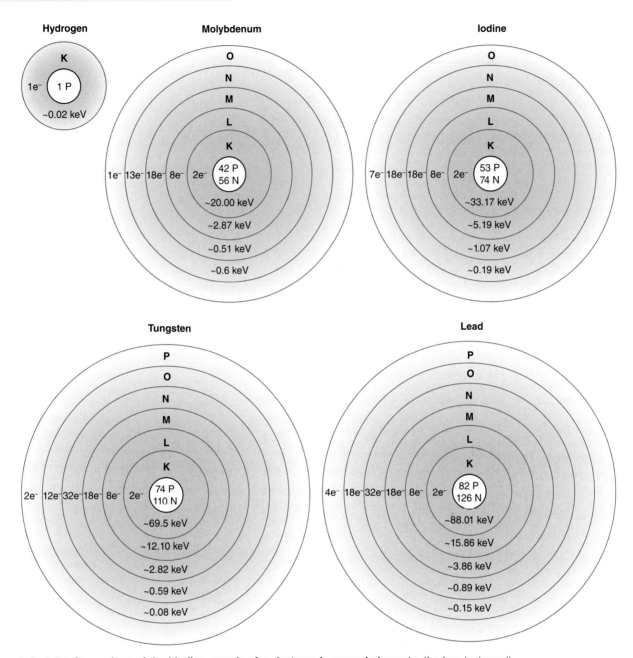

FIG. 1.6 ● Comparison of the binding energies for electrons in several elements. If a free (unbound) electron is assumed to have a total energy of zero, then the total energy of a bound electron is zero minus its binding energy. Since tungsten has a much higher atomic number (*Z* = 74) compared to hydrogen (*Z* = 1), a K-shell electron of tungsten will have a much higher binding energy (−69 500 eV) than the K-shell electron of hydrogen (−13.5 eV). Reprinted with permission from Fosbinder RA, Orth D. *Essentials of Radiologic Science.* 1st ed. Philadelphia, PA: Wolters Kluwer Health; 2012.

The charge of an atom is indicated by a superscript to the right of the chemical symbol. For example, Al^{3+} indicates that the aluminum atom has lost three electrons.

Nuclear Forces and Energy Levels

Nuclear forces are the forces that act between the nucleons and bind protons and neutrons ("nucleons") into atomic nuclei. Nuclear forces are millions of times stronger than chemical binding forces that hold atoms together in molecules. This is why nuclear reactors produce million times more energy per mass unit as compared to chemical fuels like oil or coal.

In the nucleus, there are two main forces that act in opposite directions on particles: the coulombic forces and the exchange forces (aka strong forces). The coulombic forces between protons in the nucleus are repulsive. These forces are countered by the exchange forces which is the exchange of pions (subnuclear particles) among all nucleons. It is the exchange or strong forces that hold the nucleus together, but they only operate over very short nuclear distances ($<10^{-14}$ m).

Although comparable, the energy levels in the nucleus are often much higher than those in the orbital electron shells. The lowest energy state is called the ground state of an atom. When nuclei have energy in excess of the ground state, they are said to be in an excited state. Atoms in the excited state have lifetimes with a vast range. Excited states can last from 10^{-16} s to more than 100 years. Excited states that exist longer than 10^{-12} s are referred to as metastable or isometric states. These excited nuclei can be denoted by the letter m after the mass number of the atom (ie, Tc-99m).

Nuclear Binding Energy and Mass Defect

When two subatomic particles approach each other under the influence of this strong nuclear force, their total energy will decrease and the lost energy is emitted in the form of radiation. Therefore, the total energy of the bound particles will be less than the energy of the separated free particles at the expense of the emitted radiation. *Atomic binding energy* is the energy required to separate an atom into its constituent parts. As such, it is the sum of the *electron binding energy* and the *nuclear binding energy*; atomic binding energy is dominated by the much higher nuclear binding energy.

The binding energy can be calculated by subtracting the mass of the atom from the total mass of its constituent protons, neutrons, and electrons; this mass difference is called the *mass defect*.

For example, an O-16 atom is composed of 8 electrons, 8 protons, and 8 neutrons. Therefore, the total mass of its constituent particles in the unbound state is

Mass of 8 protons + Mass of 8 neutrons + Mass of 8 electrons

$= 8 \,(1.00727 \text{ amu}) + 8 \,(1.00866 \text{ amu}) + 8 \,(0.00055 \text{ amu})$

$= 16.11591 \text{ amu}$

and the mass of an O-16 atom is 15.99491 amu. Thus, the mass defect of the O-16 atom is

$16.11591 \text{ amu} - 15.99491 \text{ amu} = 0.12100 \text{ amu}$

Using the mass energy equivalence formula, this mass defect is equal to

$(0.121 \text{ amu}) \,(931 \text{ MeV/amu}) = 112.6 \text{ MeV}$

Taking this equation a step further, the *binding energy per nucleon* can be simply calculated by dividing the total binding energy of the nucleus by the mass number A. Figure 1.7 shows the average binding energy per nucleon as a function of mass number. An extremely important observation to make from this graph is that the curve reaches its maximum near the middle elements and decreases at either end. This predicts that the energy contained in matter can be released. The two processes by which this can occur are called *nuclear fission* and *nuclear fusion*.

Nuclides

Nuclides are species of atoms that are characterized by the number of protons, neutrons, and the energy content of the atomic nucleus. Isotopes, isotones, isomers, and isobars are all families of nuclides that share specific properties. Isotopes are nuclides with the same atomic number (Z). Isotones are nuclides with the same number of neutrons (A-Z). Isomers are nuclides with the same atomic and mass numbers *but* with different energy states. Isobars are nuclides with the same mass number (A).

Nuclear Stability

For a nucleus to be stable there needs to be a certain ratio of neutrons and protons. For nuclides with low atomic number, the ratio of neutrons to protons is approximately 1. However, for nuclides with a high atomic number, the ratio of neutrons to protons is closer to 1.5. In heavier elements, a higher neutron-to-proton ratio is required to offset the coulombic repulsive forces between protons. This ratio can be plotted with Z on the x-axis and N on the y-axis and a nuclide "line of stability" can be plotted, as shown in Figure 1.8.

Radioactivity

Unstable combinations of neutrons and protons do exist. Over time, however, these unstable combinations will transform into nuclei that are stable. Nuclear instability can be classified into two types: neutron excess and neutron deficiency (ie, proton excess).

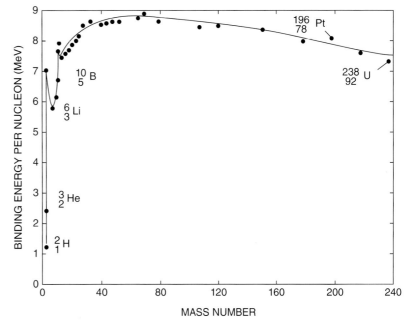

FIG. 1.7 ● **Plot of the binding energy per nucleon for a nucleus as a function of its mass number (total number of protons and neutrons).** Reprinted with permission from Johnson TE, Birky BK. *Health Physics and Radiological Health.* 4th ed. Philadelphia, PA: Wolters Kluwer Health/Lippincott Williams & Wilkins; 2011.

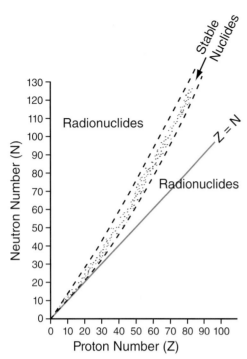

FIG. 1.8 ● **Plot of the number of neutrons (*N*) versus the number of protons (*Z*) for all stable nuclides (points in *pink*).** The line corresponding to equal number of protons and neutron (*N = Z*) is also shown. When the proton number is low, the ratio *N/Z* is close to 1 for stable nuclides; when the proton number is high, that ratio approaches approximately 1.5. Radionuclides lie on both sides of the stability curve, with those above for neutron-rich radionuclides and those below for proton-rich ones. Reprinted with permission from Chandra R, Rahmim A. *Nuclear Medicine Physics: The Basics.* 8th ed. Philadelphia, PA: Wolters Kluwer; 2017.

Unstable nuclei have a surplus of internal energy compared with a stable arrangement of neutrons and protons. The transformation from unstable nuclei to stable nuclei is achieved through the conversion of a neutron to a proton or vice versa, and these events are accompanied by the emission of energy. Nuclides that transform (ie, decay) to more stable nuclei are said to be *radioactive* and the transformation process is called *radioactive decay.* The radionuclide at the beginning of a particular decay sequence is called the *parent*, and the nuclide produced by the decay is called the *daughter.* Several decays may occur before a stable configuration is achieved. Therefore, the daughter nuclide may be either stable or radioactive.

Gamma Rays

The daughter nucleus formed as a result of radioactive decay is often in an excited state. When the nucleus in the excited state decays to a lower (more stable) energy state, a gamma ray is emitted. This transfer of energy is analogous to the emission of characteristic X-rays, which occurs following electron transition. However, the fundamental difference is that, by definition, gamma rays emanate from the nucleus. Since the energy states within the nucleus are often considerably larger than those associated with electron transitions, gamma rays are much more energetic than are characteristic X-rays. *Isometric transition* is when this nuclear de-excitation process takes place in a metastable isomer (eg, Tc-99m) and the nuclear energy state is reduced with no change in A or Z.

INTERACTIONS OF RADIATION WITH MATTER

Particle interactions

Particles of ionizing radiation may be charged particles or uncharged particles. Charged particles include alpha particles, protons, electrons, beta particles, and positrons. Uncharged particles include neutrons. Heavy charged particles such as alpha particles and protons behave differently than do lighter charged particles such as electrons and positrons.

Interactions of charged particles

As charged particles pass through and interact with matter, they are subject to the coulombic forces from the material and, as a result, lose kinetic energy by excitation, ionization, and radiative interaction. Positron-electron annihilation may also occur for positrons while they slow down while traversing matter.

Excitation and Ionization

The mechanism of energy transfer in excitation and ionization can both be characterized by collisional energy loss, as a result of the columbic forces between them and the orbital electrons in the medium. In excitation, an electron is displaced to a higher energy shell of the atom, whereas, in ionization, an electron is completely removed from the atom.

In excitation, energy from the incident particle is transferred to electrons in the absorbing material, promoting them to electron orbitals farther from the nucleus. Therefore, in excitation, the energy transferred to an electron does not exceed its binding energy. After excitation, in a process known as de-excitation, the electron will return to a lower energy level emitting the excitation energy in the form of EM radiation or Auger electron.

Ionization occurs when the transferred energy exceeds the binding energy of the electron; therefore, the electron is ejected from the atom. As a result, an ion pair is formed consisting of the ejected "free" electron and the positively charged atom from which the electron was removed. At times, the ejected electrons may possess sufficient energy to produce further ionizations called *secondary ionization.* These electrons are called *delta rays* (Figure 1.9).

Radiative Interaction—Bremsstrahlung

Ionization and excitation occur when charged particles interact with atomic electrons in the medium. Charged particles may also interact with the atomic nuclei; although most of these interactions are elastic, inelastic interactions occur in which the charged particle changes the direction of its path and lose part of its energy while emitting EM radiation. The emitted radiation is called bremsstrahlung, a German word meaning "braking radiation." The energy of the emitted radiation is equal to the energy lost by the charged particle, as required by the conservation of energy, and it can be any value up to the entire kinetic energy of the charged particle. Therefore, when a large number of charged particles undergo bremsstrahlung interactions, the result is a continuous spectrum of EM radiation (often as X-rays if electrons are the charged particles). This principle is widely used by X-ray tubes in diagnostic imaging for X-ray beam production (Figure 1.10).

The probability of bremsstrahlung emission is proportional to the value of Z^2/m^2, where Z is the atomic number of the absorber (or the target) of incident charged particle and m is the mass of the incident charged particle. Clearly, owing to the strong influence of the particle's mass, bremsstrahlung production by electrons is

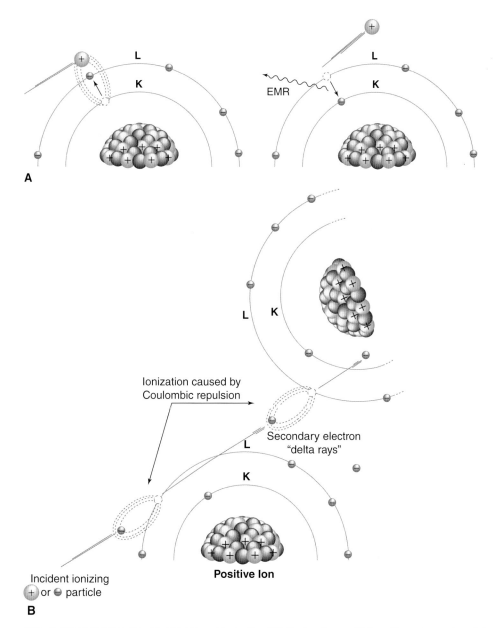

FIG. 1.9 ● Illustration of excitation (A) and ionization (B), the two types of interactions charged particles have with the medium they travel within and lose their kinetic energy. During excitation, an atom within the medium is first excited by having an orbital electron elevated to an outer orbit, and later is de-excited when the orbital electron returns to its original orbit, emitting a photon with energy equal to the difference in the energy levels of the two involved orbits. During ionization, an atom within the medium is ionized by having an orbital electron knocked out of the atom by coulombic repulsion and the free electron may undergo further interactions with the medium while traveling. Reprinted with permission from Bushberg JT, Seibert JA, Leidholdt EM, Boone JM. *Essential Physics of Medical Imaging*. 3rd ed. Philadelphia, PA: Wolters Kluwer Health/Lippincott Williams & Wilkins; 2012.

at a much higher efficiency ($>10^6$) than that by heavier charged particles such as protons and alpha particles. Also, materials with a high atomic number, such as tungsten ($Z = 74$), are suitable as targets, because of their higher probability of bremsstrahlung radiation production than are materials with lower atomic numbers. However, one has to realize that the absolute efficiency of bremsstrahlung production is still extremely low, even with the use of electrons, as the incident particles, and tungsten, as the target material. For example, bremsstrahlung X-ray productions account for approximately 1% of energy loss when electrons are accelerated to an energy of 100 keV and collide with a tungsten

target in an X-ray tube. Heat accounts for the majority of the energy loss in other forms, which implies the importance of heat management in X-ray production systems.

Positron Annihilation

In addition to the interactions described (ionization, excitation, and radiative loss), positrons may also get involved in a unique type of interaction called positron-electron annihilation. A positron, as it decelerates and comes to rest, may interact with a negatively charged electron, which results in the annihilation of the electron-positron pair. The rest mass of the two particles converts

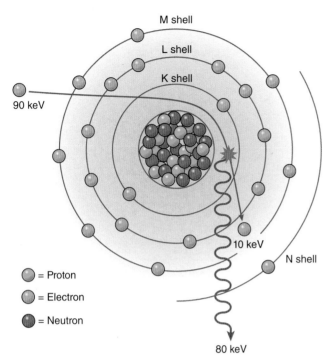

FIG. 1.10 ● Illustration of the production of bremsstrahlung radiation by projectile electrons through interaction with the nucleus. In this example, the kinetic energy of an electron reduces from 90 to 10 keV, while at the same time, an X-ray photon equal to the energy loss of the electron is produced. Reprinted with permission from Fosbinder RA, Orth D. *Essentials of Radiologic Science.* 1st ed. Philadelphia, PA: Wolters Kluwer Health; 2012.

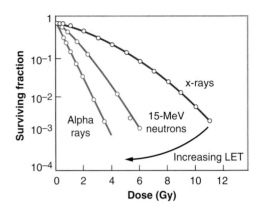

FIG. 1.11 ● **The relationship between the radiobiologic effect of radiation and its linear energy transfer (LET), as demonstrated by survival curves for cultured cells of human origin exposed to different types of radiation, including X-rays, neutrons, and alpha particles.** Different LETs lead to different surviving fractions of cells, indicating their different radiobiologic effects and the need for considering such effects in their use on human subjects. From Broerse JJ, Barendsen GW, van Kersen GR. Survival of cultured human cells after irradiation with fast neutrons of different energies in hypoxic and oxygenated conditions. *Int J Radiat Biol Relat Stud Phys Chem Med.* 1968;13:559-572. Reprinted by permission of Taylor & Francis Ltd, www.tandfonline.com; and Reprinted from Barendsen GW. Responses of cultured cells, tumors, and normal tissues to radiation of different linear energy transfer. *Curr Top Radiat Res Q.* 1968;4:293-356. Copyright © 1968 Elsevier with permission.

to energy in the form of two 0.511 MeV annihilation photons emitting in nearly opposite directions. Positron-electron annihilation, or simply positron annihilation, involves the conversion of mass into energy and forms the basis for positron emission tomography.

Specific Ionization and Linear Energy Transfer

Specific ionization (SI) is a quantity used to describe particle energy loss in charged particle interactions. SI is the number of ion pairs produced per unit track length of the charged particle's path; it increases with the electrical charge of the particle and decreases with particle velocity. Larger particles interact with a greater coulombic field. As a particle loses energy, it slows down, which allows the coulombic field to interact at a given location for a longer period of time. Therefore, the SI of an alpha particle is higher than that of a proton. The SI of an alpha particle can be as high as approximately 7000 ion pair per mm path length in air.

The amount of energy deposited per unit path length is called the linear energy transfer (LET). LET is the product of SI (ion pairs per mm) and the average energy deposited per ion pair (eV per ion pair). The LET of a charged particle is proportional to the square of the charge and inversely proportional to the particle's kinetic energies. The LET of a particular type of radiation portrays the energy deposition density, which largely determines the radiobiologic effect of radiation. High LET radiations such as alpha particles and protons cause much damage to a biologic system than do low LET radiations such as electrons and ionizing EM (gamma and X-rays) (Figure 1.11).

Scattering and Charged Particle Tracks

Scattering refers to an interaction that results in the deflection of a particle or photon from its original trajectory. A scattering event can

be characterized as elastic or inelastic depending on the change in kinetic energy. An elastic scattering event is when the total kinetic energy of the colliding particles is unchanged. When there is a net loss of the total kinetic energy, the interaction is said to be inelastic.

The path in matter is an important distinction between heavy charged particles and electrons. As a result of multiple scattering events caused by coulombic deflections (repulsion and/or attraction), electrons follow tortuous paths in matter. The sparse non-uniform ionization track of an electron is shown in Figure 1.12A. The larger mass of a heavy charged particle, on the other hand, results in a dense and usually linear ionization track as the particle travels in a medium (Figure 1.12B).

The *path length* of a particle is defined as the actual distance the particle travels in a medium. The *range* of a particle is defined as the actual depth of penetration of the particle in matter. The path length of the electron almost always exceeds its range. However, the straight ionization track of a heavy charged particle results in the path and range being nearly equal, as demonstrated in Figure 1.12.

Interactions of neutrons

Neutrons are uncharged particles that do not interact with electrons and therefore do not directly cause excitation and ionization. However, neutrons do interact with atomic nuclei, and, therefore, may liberate charged particles or nuclear fragments that can directly cause excitation and ionization. The use of neutrons in medical imaging is very limited. One of the applications of neutron interactions is the production of radiopharmaceuticals for nuclear medicine imaging, which is discussed later in the book.

X-ray and gamma-ray interactions

When radiation passes through matter, photons will penetrate, scatter, or be absorbed. The major types of interactions involving X-ray and gamma-ray photons include Rayleigh scattering,

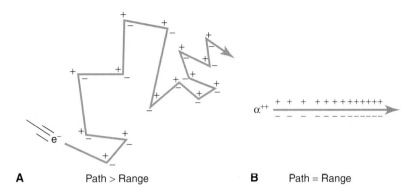

FIG. 1.12 ● **Different tracks produced by different types of charged particles when they interact with tissues and gradually lose energy.** An electron goes through multiple scattering events and typically has a very tortuous track before it completely slows down (A). By comparison, an alpha particle, as an example of heavy charged particles, produces a nearly linear track (B). For the former, the path length of an electron's track is longer than its range; for the latter, however, the path length of an alpha particle is basically equal to its range. Reprinted with permission from Bushberg JT, Seibert JA, Leidholdt EM, Boone JM. *Essential Physics of Medical Imaging.* 3rd ed. Philadelphia, PA. Wolters Kluwer Health/Lippincott Williams & Wilkins; 2012.

Compton scattering, photoelectric absorption, and pair production. Compton scattering and photoelectric absorption are two most important interactions in diagnostic imaging. Pair production only occurs when photon energy is at least 1.22 MeV, which is not used by medical imaging. Rayleigh scattering has a very small effect for most diagnostic imaging applications, unless the used photon energy is very low (like in mammography).

Details regarding the different types of X-ray interactions can be found in the next chapter, whose focus is on X-rays.

Absorption of energy from X- and gamma rays

Fluence, flux, and energy fluence

Fluence is the number of photons passing through a unit cross-sectional area, expressed in square centimeters. The fluence is given the symbol Φ:

$$\Phi = \text{Photons/Area}$$

Flux is the fluence rate or the rate at which photons or particles pass through a unit area per unit time. It is often expressed in $cm^{-2}s^{-1}$. Flux is useful when a photon beam is on for an extended period of time, such as in fluoroscopy.

Energy fluence is the amount of energy passing through a unit cross-sectional area. For a monoenergetic beam of X-rays, the energy fluence (Ψ) is the product of the fluence (Φ) and the energy per photon (E):

$$\Psi = (\text{photon/area}) \times (\text{energy/photon}) = \Phi E$$

Exposure

Exposure (X) is the total electrical charges (ΔQ) produced by ionizing EM per unit mass of air (Δm).

$$X = (\Delta Q)/(\Delta m)$$

Exposure is measured in coulombs per kilogram (C/kg). The historic unit of exposure is the roentgen (abbreviated R).

Absorbed dose

When there is exposure to radiation, energy is transferred from radiation to the interacting medium (kerma). The transferred energy may be absorbed in the medium or may partly radiate out in the form of bremsstrahlung. Therefore, absorbed dose is equal to the difference between kerma and the bremsstrahlung loss.

Absorbed dose is defined as the energy (ΔE) deposited by ionizing radiation per unit mass of material (Δm).

$$\text{Dose} = \Delta E / \Delta m$$

The SI unit for absorbed dose (D) is gray (Gy); 1 gray = 1 J/kg. The traditional unit for absorbed dose is the rad. One rad is equal to 0.01 J/kg. Therefore, 100 rad = 1 gray and 1 rad = 10 mGy.

Equivalent dose

All types of radiation do not cause the same biologic damage per unite dose. To account for the relative effectiveness of the type of radiation in producing biologic damage, the International Commission of Radiological Protection (ICRP) established radiation weighting factors (w_R). High LET radiations produce more biologic damage per unit dose than do low LET radiations and thus have higher radiation weighting factors. The equivalent dose (H) can be calculated by multiplying the absorbed dose (D) to the radiation weighting factor:

$$H = D \star (w_R)$$

The SI unit for equivalent dose is the sievert (Sv). The weighting factor (w_R) for radiations used in diagnostic imaging (X-rays, gamma rays, and electrons) is 1; therefore 1 mGy = 1 mSv. Heavy charged particles, such as alpha particles, have a much higher LET radiation and therefore the biologic damage and associated w_R is much greater (Table 1.2).

Effective dose

The radiosensitivity of different tissues to ionization radiation is variable. The ICRP publication 60 has established tissue weighting factors (w_T) to account for the variations in radiosensitivity among different tissues. The tissue weighting factor of a particular tissue is the proportion of the stochastic effect (cancer and genetic effects) resulting from irradiation of that tissue or organ compared to the whole-body irradiation. The effective dose (E) can be calculated as the sum of the products of the equivalent dose of each tissue or organ irradiated (H_T) and the corresponding weighting factor of tissue (w_T) for that tissue or organ. The effective dose is expressed in sievert or rem (roentgen equivalent man), the same unit used for the equivalent dose.

$$E \text{ (Sv)} = \Sigma(w_T) \star (H_T)$$

Tissue weighting factors are shown in Table 1.3.

IMAGE QUALITY

Evaluation of the quality of medical images is not about how aesthetically appealing they are; it is focused on how much value these images add to the understanding of the underlying anatomy and physiology. To meet the requirements in image quality is a major consideration in setting up optimal acquisition protocols

Table 1.2 RADIATION WEIGHTING FACTORS (W_R) FOR VARIOUS TYPES OF RADIATION

Type of Radiation	Radiation Weighting Factor (w_R)
X-rays, gamma rays, beta particles, and electrons	1
Protons (>2 MeV)	5
Neutrons (energy dependent)	5-20
Alpha particles and other multiple-charged particles	20

For radiations primarily used in medical imaging (X-rays, gamma rays, beta particles, etc) the $w_R = 1$; therefore, the absorbed dose and equivalent dose are equal in value.

Adapted with permission from Bushberg JT, Seibert JA, Leidholdt EM, Boone JM. *Essential Physics of Medical Imaging*. 3rd ed. Philadelphia, PA: Wolters Kluwer Health/Lippincott Williams & Wilkins; 2012. Data from ICRP Publication 103, *The 2007 Recommendations of the International Commission on Radiological Protection. Ann. ICRP 37 (2–4)*:1-332.

Table 1.3 TISSUE WEIGHTING FACTORS ASSIGNED BY THE INTERNATIONAL COMMISSION ON RADIOLOGICAL PROTECTION

Tissue or Organ	Tissue Weighting Factor, w_T
Gonads	0.20
Bone marrow (red)	0.12
Colon	0.12
Lung	0.12
Stomach	0.12
Bladder	0.05
Breast	0.05
Liver	0.05
Esophagus	0.05
Thyroid	0.05
Skin	0.01
Bone surface	0.01
Other	0.05
Total	**1.00**

Adapted with permission from Bushberg JT, Seibert JA, Leidholdt EM, Boone JM. *Essential Physics of Medical Imaging*. 3rd ed. Philadelphia, PA: Wolters Kluwer Health/Lippincott Williams & Wilkins; 2012. Data from ICRP Publication 103, *The 2007 Recommendations of the International Commission on Radiological Protection. Ann. ICRP 37 (2–4)*:1-332.

for any medical imaging modality, although the tradeoff between image quality and other factors, in particular those related to patient risks, has to be considered. A general overview of image quality aspects pertaining to medical imaging is provided here.

Contrast

Contrast refers to difference in signal. An imaging process is typically a chain of many steps, and each step could affect the contrast.

Depending on its sources, contrast can be classified into subject contrast, detected contrast, and displayed contrast.

- **Subject contrast**

Subject contrast comes from the differences in the interaction of tissues with the type of radiation used for imaging. In X-ray imaging modalities, subject contrast primarily comes from the different attenuation coefficients for different tissues (Figure 1.13). In MRI, subject contrast could come from differences in T1, T2, proton density, and many other clinically relevant parameters among tissues. In nuclear medicine, it is the different

concentrations of the injected radiopharmaceutical within different tissues that leads to subject contrast. Ultrasound utilizes differences in tissues' interactions with the ultrasound wave to produce subject contrast.

Contrast medium is often used in medical imaging to bring subject contrast to the desired level. Examples include the use of iodine-based contrast media in CT because of the X-ray attenuation characteristics of iodine, and the use of gadolinium-based contrast media in MR primarily because of its T1 shortening effect. Nuclear medicine is another interesting example, because the use of radiopharmaceutical is a definite requirement for tissue differentiation.

For the same type of imaging technology, three-dimensional imaging typically offers improved contrast over two-dimensional imaging, because tissue overlapping is eliminated.

- **Detected contrast**

Detected contrast refers to the difference in the detected signal, as is affected by the characteristics of the detector and its ancillaries.

The use of collimators in nuclear medicine for imaging of gamma ray photons is an example of considerations made for detected contrast. Without collimators, a point source of radioactivity in air, despite a high subject contrast with respect to its background, would result in a uniform image with minimal contrast in it; collimators are essential to ensure detected contrast in this example (Figure 1.14).

- **Displayed contrast**

When medical images are read by human, it is ultimately the perceived contrast from the displayed image that determines how well different tissues may be differentiated.

On display monitors, lookup tables (LUTs) are used to transform pixel values in images to gray levels to be displayed. LUT becomes necessary primarily due to the mismatch between the range of the pixel values and the maximum number of gray levels display monitors support. Nowadays, most display monitors are able to display up to 1000 gray levels; digital imaging systems, however, often use more than 10 bits for storing pixel values, meaning that a few thousand different pixel values may need to be displayed with much fewer gray levels. It is therefore important to adjust the LUT such that certain anatomic areas of interest may fully utilize the entire range of gray levels for best displayed contrast.

The WW/WL method is commonly used for defining the LUT; WW stands for window width, and WL for window level. This method essentially uses a piece-wise linear function in

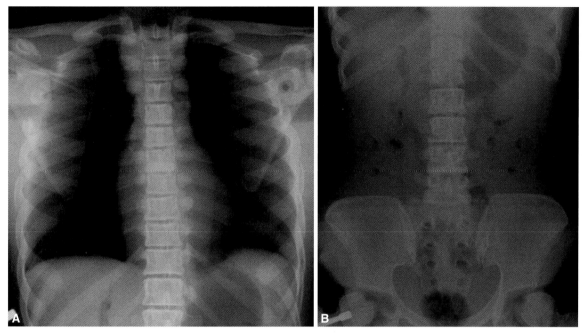

FIG. 1.13 ● Different subject contrast on chest X-ray (A) and abdominal X-ray (B) images. Subject contrast on a chest image is generally higher than that on abdominal X-ray images. Reprinted with permission from Orth D. *Essentials of Radiologic Science.* 2nd ed. Philadelphia, PA: Wolters Kluwer; 2017.

transforming pixel value to gray level. If a pixel value is less than WL − WW/2, it will be displayed as black, the lowest gray level the display supports. If a pixel value is more than WL + WW/2, it will be displayed as white, the highest gray level the system supports. If a pixel value falls somewhere between WL − WW/2 and WL + WW/2, its gray level for display will be determined following a linear function of the pixel value. It is typical that a list of WW/WL settings is made available in viewing software for user selection depending on the application (Figure 1.15).

Noise

Noise causes fluctuations in measured signal, and, as a result, negatively impacts precision of measurement and conspicuity of areas of interest from the images. Noise, although random, typically follows a statistical distribution, so the understanding of the behavior of noise is often through the understanding of the underlying distribution. The normal distribution, or the Gaussian distribution, is the most widely used statistical distribution

FIG. 1.14 ● **Different detected contrast mostly related to the use of different imaging techniques.** Within the span of a year, the patient had two mammographic studies, one with screen-film technique and (A) the other with digital technique (B). On the screen-film image, breast tissues appear dense and little intrinsic contrast is observed; on the digital image, however, greater tissue contrast is observed, mostly due to a much-improved dynamic range. Reprinted with permission from Harris JR, Lippman ME, Osborne CK, et al. *Diseases of the Breast.* 4th ed. Philadelphia, PA: Wolters Kluwer Health/ Lippincott Williams & Wilkins; 2009.

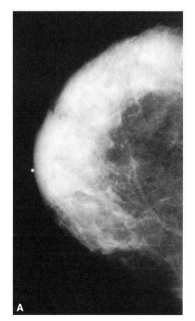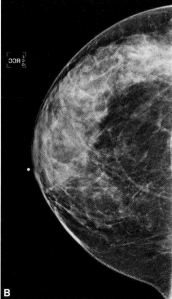

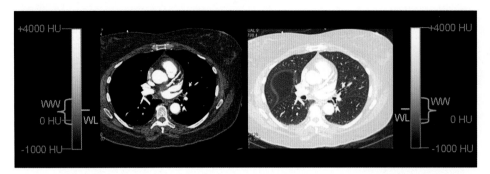

FIG. 1.15 ● **Different displayed contrast from the same computed tomography data set due to the use of two different display settings.** The display with cardiac window (left) uses a window width (WW) of 600 HU and a window level (WL) of 70 HU. By comparison, the display with lung window (right) uses a WW of 1500 HU and a WL of −600 HU. Reprinted with permission from Garcia MJ. *Noninvasive Cardiovascular Imaging: A Multimodality Approach.* 1st ed. Philadelphia, PA: Wolters Kluwer Health/Lippincott Williams & Wilkins; 2011.

in characterizing a lot of statistical processes. The normal distribution, when plotted, follows a bell-shaped curve that is characterized by two parameters, the mean value and the standard deviation.

There are multiple sources of noise within the imaging process; for electronic imaging, noise primarily comes from two sources:

- **Quantum noise**

  Quantum noise refers to signal fluctuations related to the number of particles, aka, quanta, collected during data acquisition. Although all types of radiation exhibit particle-like behaviors more or less, due to the wave-particle duality, X-ray photons and gamma ray photons demonstrate more quantum effects than do others because of their very short wavelengths.

  Quantum noise of X-ray photons and gamma-ray photons follows the Poisson distribution, which can be viewed as a special type of Gaussian distribution with its standard deviation equal to the square root of its mean value. In images of X-ray photons and gamma-ray photons when no additional processing is applied, the perception of the noisy level of images is largely affected by the ratio between the standard deviation and the mean value of signal; in other words, the noisy level of an image is inversely proportional to the square root of the mean signal, that is, the number of detected photons. One may derive from here a simple but true rule of thumb in adjusting radiation dose for image quality: the more radiation, the less noisy images.

- **Electronic noise**

  Any electronic imaging system may be affected by electronic noise arising from its measurement of electronic signals. There is a variety of sources of electronic noise, including thermal noise (temperature dependent), flicker noise (related to semiconductor defects), and others.

  Electronic noise typically has a more complicated relationship with quite a few factors, compared to quantum noise, and therefore is more difficult to characterize and deal with. It is preferred that imaging systems for detecting X-rays or gamma rays work at a level that quantum noise is the stronger source of noise.

The amplitude of noise is often used as a simple quantity to describe its effect on visual perception of an image. Studies have shown that, however, visual perception of images is affected by not only the amplitude but also by the spatial correlation of noise, aka, noise texture; detailed discussions can be found in later chapters.

Contrast resolution

Contrast resolution refers to the ability of an imaging system to resolve contrast between different tissues. It is affected by both the contrast itself and by the effect of noise. Contrast to noise ratio, defined as the ratio between the contrast (between the tissue of interest and the background tissue) and the standard deviation of the noise (often in the background tissue), is often used as a simple metric to evaluate contrast resolution, although it is known to be inadequate in capturing the effect of noise texture on contrast resolution.

Spatial resolution

Spatial resolution describes the level of details one can resolve from an image. The level of details is related to how rapid changes in signal occur; the smaller the details, the more rapid the change in signal intensity. A practical imaging system cannot resolve all details that come with the object; therefore, when the size of details is below a certain level, one cannot separate one from another in the proximity. Spatial resolution may be characterized in either the spatial domain or the frequency domain, as described in the following.

In the spatial domain, the spatial resolution of an imaging system is typically characterized by the point spread function (PSF). PSF is the output of an imaging system when the object being imaged is an infinitesimal point (its integral signal over the entire spatial domain is unity). In practice, a few variants of PSF are also used in evaluating spatial resolution, including line spread function, edge response function, and others.

Alternatively, spatial resolution can also be characterized by the modulation transfer function in the frequency domain. The rationale for such a characterization is as follows. Any spatially varying signal is viewed as the summation of many sinusoidal functions, each with its frequency and representative of details at a certain level; the spatial resolution of an imaging system can therefore be broken down to how the system preserves the intensity of the input sinusoidal signal for each different frequency. Typically, an imaging system is able to preserve 100% of the input signal when its spatial frequency is at or near zero (zero frequency means that the object is the same everywhere); the preserved percentage often decreases with the frequency of the input signal until it reaches zero at a certain frequency (the system is not able to resolve details at or higher than the frequency).

For any imaging modality, spatial resolution is affected by a number of factors; these factors may be system dependent, or operation dependent, or patient dependent, or any combination of them. In radiographic and mammographic imaging, spatial resolution is often affected by the focal spot size, the detector pixel size, and the location of the object of interest (magnification effect). Spatial resolution of CT is affected by these factors as well; in addition, reconstruction algorithms have major impacts on spatial resolution. In imaging of gamma photon emitting radionuclides, collimator selection is a major factor impacting spatial resolution. In MRI, technical factors affecting spatial resolution include the gradient field strength, the receiver coil characteristics, the sampling bandwidth, the reconstruction settings (algorithm, matrix), and others. Spatial resolution of ultrasound images is affected by

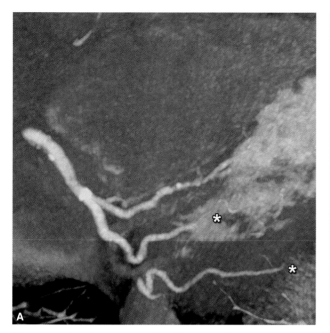 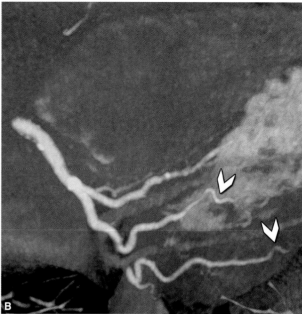

FIG. 1.16 ● For the same cardiac CT scan, different reconstruction techniques (half-scan reconstruction used by [A], and multisegment reconstruction by [B]) result in different temporal resolution of the reconstructed images and, therefore, visualized differences of distal right coronary artery on these maximum intensity projection images. The discontinuous vessels in the left image (asterisks) become continuous in the right image (arrowheads), due to improvement in temporal resolution. Reprinted with permission from Higgins CB, de Roos A. *MRI and CT of the Cardiovascular System.* 3rd ed. Philadelphia, PA: Wolters Kluwer Health/Lippincott Williams & Wilkins; 2012.

the frequency of the ultrasound, the dimensions of the transducer aperture, the beam focusing mechanism, the object location, and so on.

Temporal resolution

Temporal resolution refers to the ability of an imaging system to resolve moving objects and dynamic processes. Limited temporal resolution potentially results in blurs on images and inaccuracy in quantitative measurements. When an image includes a single frame, temporal resolution is determined by the acquisition duration. Using radiography as an example, temporal resolution is essentially the exposure time. When an image involves contributions from multiple acquired frames (each has its own acquisition time), temporal resolution becomes less straightforward, dependent on how the contribution of each frame to the final image varies from one another. As an example, fluoroscopy usually applies weighted time averaging over a few consecutive raw frames in creating the displayed frames, and the temporal resolution of the displayed frames is often not simply the total time in acquiring the multiple frames used for weighted averaging. The quantitative evaluation of temporal resolution based on images is a very involved process; instead of directly measuring the effective time window for data acquisition, one often measures the spatial resolution over the boundaries of moving structures and derives from it the blur caused by residual motion only (Figure 1.16).

INFORMATICS IN MEDICAL IMAGING
Digital images

On analog images, signals are represented by a physical quantity that varies continuously within a certain range and are typically displayed on a continuous physical medium, like film or screen.

On digital images, signals are represented by a physical quantity that has only a limited number of discrete levels and are distributed on a matrix with finite size for each dimension.

In medical imaging, the initial measurement of signals always produces analog values, and the display of the final images also always involves an output of analog signals. All the steps in between within this process, however, can be either analog or digital. Film-based radiography is an example of a completely analog imaging process. CT, on the other hand, is inherently digital since its inception; once signals are measured and converted into digital data, all the ensuing steps in handling the data are nearly all in the digital nature. With the numerous benefits of digital data over analog data, radiology practices today have largely gone digital, with very limited uses of analog means in handling radiology-related data.

The handling of digital data often requires conversion of data between their digital and analog forms. The conversion of analog signal into digital data is often referred to as digitization and performed by devices named analog-to-digital converters (ADCs). Similarly, digital-to-analog converters (DACs) convert digital data into analog data (Figure 1.17).

A digital image is essentially a matrix of individual elements named pixels, each of which has its pixel value. A digital image is typically two-dimensional without special mention, but images of three or more dimensions can certainly be formed by stacking multiple two-dimensional ones along certain dimensions. Each pixel value is best described as a numerical value in the binary form, consisting of a number of bits, whose value is either 0 or 1. Such a binary form is adopted because each bit can be easily set to one of the two stable states by semiconductor-based electronics. Bits can be grouped into bytes, each consisting of 8 bits. Therefore, the amount of data associated with a digital image is the product of the number of bytes used by each pixel and the number of pixels in the matrix.

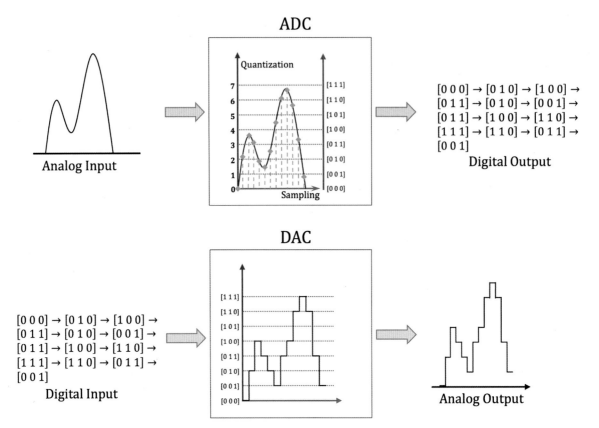

FIG. 1.17 ● Illustration of the working principles of analog-to-digital converter (ADC) and digital-to-analog converter (DAC). ADC converts an analog signal to digital signal (top), and a DAC converts a digital signal into an analog signal (bottom). In this example, a 3-bit digital signal output (quantization) is shown ($2^3 = 8$ discrete levels; ie, 0-7). The analog input has been sampled 13 times (thus 13 digital outputs are shown in binary system). At the bottom, to demonstrate the concept of a DAC, the 13 digital measurements are converted back to analog output. The result is not an exact replica of the original analog signal shown in (top). To achieve that, a much higher sampling rate is required. Reprinted with permission from Chandra R, Rahmim A. *Nuclear Medicine Physics: The Basics.* 8th ed. Philadelphia, PA: Wolters Kluwer; 2017.

A major advantage that digital images have over analog images is their robustness to electronic noise in their transmission. The signals of analog images vary continuously; when electronic noise is inevitably present, it is often superimposed on the signal and causes distortion. The signals of digital images, at discrete levels, are transmitted in bits; unless the noise is so high in its amplitude that it causes drastic change larger than the difference between a 0 bit and a 1 bit, no signal distortion is expected. In addition, additional safeguard measures can be introduced in the transmission of digital signals to further reduce data distortion.

Image storage

The handling of a tremendous amount of clinical data, especially clinical images, by radiology practice demands mass storage devices of high performance. The following storage media have been used, including magnetic disk (or hard drive), optical disk, solid state drive, magnetic tape, and others.

Image compression is an effective means of addressing the challenge of storing massive clinical data. Images are compressed to reduce storage space and decompressed to reveal all information while being displayed. The compression ratio is the number of bytes of the original image divided by the number of bytes of the compressed image. There are two categories of compression algorithms: lossless and lossy algorithms. Lossless algorithms typically rely on the redundancy inherent to the original images; the more the redundancy (like in dynamic series where images contain the same anatomic structures changing their locations as time varies), the more compression to be achieved. Lossy algorithms, on the other hand, often result in more aggressive size reduction at the expense of some information loss. The use of lossy compression for mammography is not allowed by the U.S. Food and Drug Administration; there is no restriction, however, on its use in other imaging modalities. It is recommended that, if lossy compression is used, the algorithms included in the DICOM (Digital Imaging and Communications in Medicine) standard should be considered first.

Image display

Through the use of a computer monitor, any image, essentially a matrix of numerical values, can be displayed in pictorial form for its visual assessment. Although some monitors can only display grayscale images, others are capable of displaying images both in grayscale and in color depending on the needs. For viewing of medical images, cathode ray tube (CRT) monitors had been used for several decades as electronic display devices before they were replaced by flat panel monitors. Among various technologies for flat panel display, liquid crystal displays (LCDs) have been most often used because of their overall superior performance.

A CRT monitor produces light signal by directing high-speed electrons toward a screen that converts the kinetic energy of the electrons to visible light photons. Its major component is a vacuum tube that encloses one or more electron guns, a fluorescent screen, and other components inside glass housing. The tube has a pair of electrodes at its two ends, with high voltage (about 10-30 kV) applied between them. The negative electrode (cathode) is located at the rear end of the tube, whereas the positive electrode (anode) is at the front. In a grayscale CRT, an electron gun is attached to the cathode; when heated by electrical current, it emits a flow of electrons, whose intensity is modulated by a set of grid electrodes. The electrons emitted by the electron gun are directed toward the anode by the electric field created by the voltage applied between the cathode and anode. These electrons are further manipulated by a set of focusing coils and deflection coils to have precise control on where they land on the screen in contact with the anode. The interactions of the incident electrons with the screen produce visible light signals proportional to the intensity of the electron flow. The display of an image is achieved by fast scanning of the electron beam across the screen. A color CRT shares the same basic principles with a grayscale CRT, as described earlier. Different from a grayscale CRT, a color CRT has three electron guns. Each produces its own flow of electrons and modulates the intensity independently. Also, the fluorescent screen consists of triads of tiny dot-emitting lights of different base colors (red, green, and blue), and each of the three incident electron beams is only able to interact with dots of a single color. The mix of light signals of the three base colors eventually creates the visual perception of many colors (Figure 1.18).

LCDs utilize the unique optical properties of liquid crystal materials in the presence or absence of an electric field. Inside an LCD, a thin layer of liquid crystal is positioned between two polarization filters that are perpendicular to each other, with a uniform planar light source sitting in the back of the display. Like polarized sunglasses, a polarization filter only allows light with the same polarization angle to pass through while blocking light polarized in the perpendicular orientation. The liquid layer

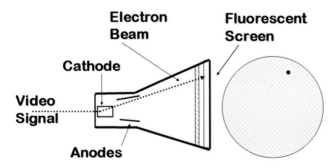

FIG. 1.18 • Illustration of the traditional cathode ray tube (CRT). The CRT has rows of phosphor dots that glow when struck by electrons. The incoming video signal provides the location and intensity that each dot needs to be struck to correspond to the image that was acquired. Reprinted with permission from Kern MJ, Berger PB, Block PC, et al. *SCAI Interventional Cardiology Board Review Book*. Philadelphia, PA: Lippincott Williams & Wilkins; 2006.

is divided into a large matrix of tiny square areas called pixels, and each pixel has a pair of electrodes attached to it. With no voltage between the electrodes, each crystal pixel has all of its molecules in the same orientation as that of the first polarization filter (the one close to the light source); therefore, all light arriving at the second polarization filter gets completely blocked because of their orientations, and the pixel appears dark. With the right amount of voltage applied between the electrode, the orientation of the molecules gradually changes from that of the first filter to the second, causing the light traveling through the pixel to gradually "twist" its orientation until in complete alignment with the second filter while arriving at it; therefore, all light gets through completely, and the pixel appears the most bright. In short, each liquid crystal pixel is electrically controlled to modulate the amount of light that passes through it, eventually producing the appearance of an image (Figures 1.19 and 1.20).

The performance of a display monitor significantly impacts the readers' interpretation of images. The evaluation of a display monitor's performance typically includes contrast resolution, spatial resolution, dynamic range, uniformity, distortion, and others.

The brightness levels of a display monitor at certain conditions have direct impacts on visual perception of contrast in images. Luminance is a physical quantity to describe the brightness of a light source; it measures, in a certain direction, the amount of traveling light per unit area. The SI unit for luminance is candela per square meter (cd/m^2). The contrast resolution of a display monitor is primarily determined by the luminance ratio, namely, the ratio of the maximum luminance and the minimum luminance. The minimum luminance is affected by both the luminance when the driving signal of the display is zero (also called black level) and the level of ambient light. The maximum luminance is primarily affected by the luminance given by the highest level of driving signal and minimally affected by the ambient light. Note that dynamic range, often defined as the ratio of the luminance of the highest signal to that of the lowest signal, differs from the luminance ratio by excluding the effect of ambient light, despite their correlation. The ACR–AAPM–SIIM Technical Standard for Electronic Practice of Medical Imaging, in its latest version of 2017, recommends that the luminance ratio be at 350 for optimal contrast perception based on its equivalence to the film's optical density range of 0.20 to 0.75 and be greater than 250 for acceptable contrast. On the basis of this principle, diagnostic displays with a minimum luminance of $1.0 \, cd/m^2$ should have a maximum luminance greater than $350 \, cd/m^2$ and mammographic displays with a minimum luminance of $1.2 \, cd/m^2$ should have a maximum luminance greater than $420 \, cd/m^2$.

The pixel pitch of a display monitor affects how well fine details are revealed on images. Assuming a pixel pitch of p millimeter, the limiting spatial frequency of a display made with such pixels is $1/(2p) \, mm^{-1}$. At a typical viewing distance of 60 cm, studies have found that the highest spatial frequency people with good vision can perceive is between 2 and 4 mm^{-1}. As a result, ACR–AAPM–SIIM Technical Standard for Electronic Practice of Medical Imaging (2017) recommends that the pixel pitch of monitors used in diagnostic interpretation be about 0.2 mm and not larger than 0.21 mm. Considering the matrix sizes of typical diagnostic images and the comfortable view area without much movement of the reader's head, a display monitor used for diagnostic interpretation commonly has thousands of pixels in both dimensions (a few megapixels in total) and a diagonal size around 50 cm.

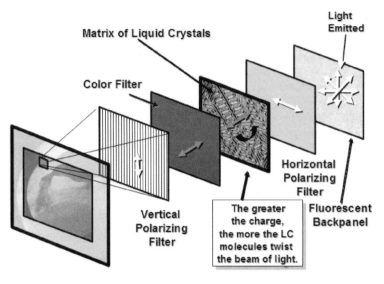

FIG. 1.19 ● Illustration of the functional elements of a liquid crystal display (LCD) monitor. The flat LCD monitor is made up of a series of panels. A matrix of thin-film transistors is located on polarizing and color filters. Each pixel has its own transistors. Light vibrating in all directions is produced by the fluorescent back panel. This light passes through a horizontal polarizing panel. These light waves then travel through the liquid crystal panel, where the liquid crystals twist the light in proportion to the amount of voltage applied by the incoming video signal. The greater the signal intensity, the more the light is twisted. This twisted light is sent through a color filter to another polarizing panel that only allows mostly vertical light to pass. If the light is not twisted by the LCD panel, it will not pass through this polarizing panel, and the pixel will appear black. If it is twisted to 90° (maximally), the pixel will appear white. Any twisting between 0° and 90° results in various shades of gray. In this manner, the image is formed on the monitor. Reprinted with permission from Kern MJ, Berger PB, Block PC, et al. *SCAI Interventional Cardiology Board Review Book*. Philadelphia, PA: Lippincott Williams & Wilkins; 2006.

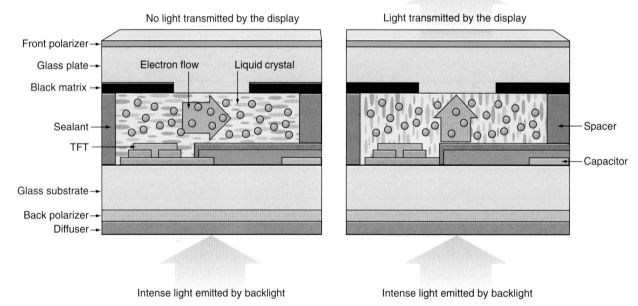

FIG. 1.20 ● Cross-sectional illustration of one pixel in an active matrix liquid crystal display. Reprinted with permission from Orth D. *Essentials of Radiologic Science*. 2nd ed. Philadelphia, PA: Wolters Kluwer; 2017.

A display monitor uses LUTs in its process of mapping from pixel value to light intensity to adjust the perceived image contrast. Proper selection of LUTs improves the conspicuity of certain anatomy or features within the images. A commonly used method of adjusting the LUT is named windowing and leveling. This method assumes the use of a three-part piece-wise linear function as the LUT and allows the user to make a selection of two parameters, the window level and the window width, for the exact shape of the LUT. In this method, a lower level is defined as the pixel value below which any pixel is displayed with the lowest light intensity, and an upper level is defined as the pixel value above which any pixel is displayed with the highest light intensity. For any pixel with values in between the two levels, the light intensity varies between the lowest and the highest, with its exact gray level determined as a function of where the pixel values is between the lower level and the upper level. Users may adjust the lower level and the higher level by adjusting the window level and the window width, because the window level is the average of the two levels, whereas the window width is the difference between them.

Picture Archiving and Communication System (PACS)

PACS has become the technological core of a modern radiology department. Its functions, at the basic level, include the storage, transfer, and display of radiologic images. Through integration with other IT infrastructures within enterprise, like radiology information system (RIS), hospital information system (HIS), electronic medical record (EMR), and others, PACS also supports efficient and robust exchange of patient information in their care and facilitates workflow management among the entire clinical team. A recent trend of PACS is the extension of the access to radiologic images, reports, and other relevant information to referring physicians and patients through web-based interface by utilizing the Internet's capabilities (Figure 1.21).

PACS performs its core functions with an image archive connected to a multitude of devices, including acquisition devices, diagnostic workstations, and other supporting components. Acquisition devices acquire patient images and send the desired series over to the archive for storage; these series may first go through a quality assurance server to verify patient information and study attributes before being sent. Diagnostic workstations query and transfer from the archive active studies to be interpreted, and display the images for radiologists' review and diagnosis. In addition to various tools for image processing and analysis, these workstations may be also equipped with reporting software to support radiologists' dictation of reports.

Reports along with other information (measurements, key images) generated on these workstations can be updated to the archive. The image archive, being the central component of PACS, utilizes modern storage technologies to meet requirements in both capacity and performance. RAID (Redundant Array of Independent Disks), as an example, is commonly used by enterprise storage systems to provide both high availability and protection against failures. In addition, it is important that image data recovery mechanisms are in place for the prevention of error and disaster, as is mandated by HIPAA (Health Insurance Portability and Accountability Act of 1996); this often requires the setup of a data backup infrastructure.

Storage and transfer of image data (and some other nonimage data) within PACS typically follows the standard of DICOM. The standard includes the definition of a file format and a network communication protocol for files using the format. It allows images and related information to be exchanged between devices from multiple vendors. A DICOM object, whether it is an image or a nonimage object (work list, radiation dose record, etc),

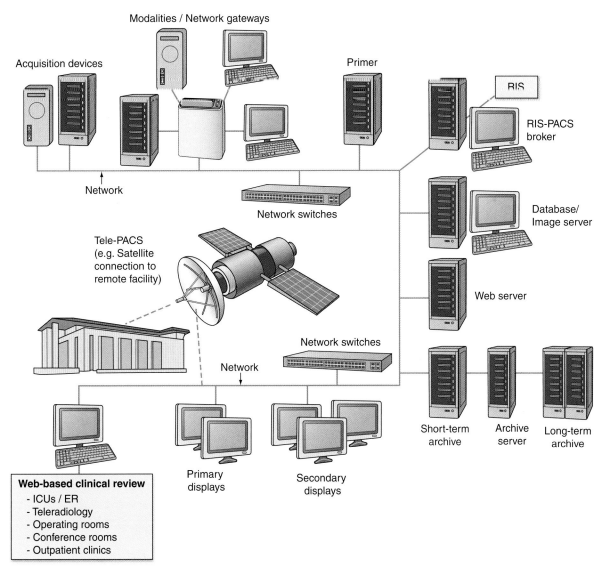

FIG. 1.21 • Illustration of the setup of a typical picture archiving and communication system (PACS) network. Reprinted with permission from Orth D. *Essentials of Radiologic Science.* 2nd ed. Philadelphia, PA: Wolters Kluwer; 2017.

consists of a large number of data elements, or attributes. The main attribute of a DICOM object is the pixel data, where all pixel values are stored. Services to be performed on DICOM objects, as defined by the standard, include store, storage commitment, query/retrieve, modality worklist, modality performed procedure step, print, and off-line media.

PACS integration with RIS, HIS, EMR, and other IT systems across the enterprise introduces more automation in the workflow, leading to numerous benefits for patient care, including, but not limited to (1) examination orders can be electronically sent and their status updated and monitored; (2) risks from entering incorrect patient identification are minimized; (3) patient history and prior studies can be prefetched to facilitate study interpretation; (4) images and diagnostic reports can be made accessible within patient records shortly after the examination; (5) performance management can be monitored and reported automatically, and so on.

 ## CHAPTER SELF-ASSESSMENT QUESTIONS

1. Which of the following is NOT true regarding radiation?
   A. When there is a vacancy created in one of the inner shells of an atom, an outer-shell electron may fill the vacancy accompanied by the release of energy in the form of either characteristic x-rays or Auger electrons.
   B. For the same amount of radiation dose, protons cause more biologic damage to tissue than do x-ray photons because of their higher LET (linear energy transfer).
   C. All stable nuclei have equal numbers of protons and neutrons; otherwise they would undergo radioactive decay.
   D. When electrons interact with a certain material, the probability of Bremsstrahlung x-ray emission increases with the atomic number of the material.

2. For a tungsten atom with the following binding energies, K-shell = 70 keV, L-shell = 12 keV, and M-shell = 3 keV, characteristic x-rays of which of the following different energies (in keV) could be emitted by a 100-keV electron striking a tungsten target?
   A. 100, 70, 30
   B. 97, 88, 30
   C. 70, 12, 3
   D. 67, 58, 9
   E. 30, 18, 15

3. The contrast in an image as perceived by the observer is determined by:
   A. Subject contrast
   B. Displayed contrast
   C. Detected contrast
   D. All of the above

Answers to Chapter Self-Assessment Questions

1. C   When the atomic number is low, the ratio between the numbers of neutrons and protons of a nucleus is close to 1. But as the atomic number increases, the ratio begins to increase until it approaches about 1.5 for the heaviest nuclei.

2. D   After the 100-keV electron knocks a K-shell electron out of its orbit, filling of the K-shell vacancy by an M-shell electron, filling of the K-shell vacancy by an L-shell electron, and filling of the L-shell vacancy by an M-shell electron lead to emitted x-ray photons at 70 keV − 3 keV = 67 keV, 70 keV − 12 keV = 58 keV, and 12 keV − 3 keV = 9 keV, respectively.

3. D   All the three factors from A to C affect the perceived image contrast.

X-Ray Imaging: Fundamentals

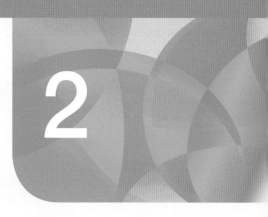

2

Michael Burch, MD, Eric England, MD, Sammy Abid Yacob, DO, and Kaushal Mehta, MD

LEARNING OBJECTIVES

1. Name the four major types of interactions for X-ray photons.
2. Define half-value layer (HVL) and describe its relationship with the linear attenuation coefficient (LAC).
3. Explain the beam hardening effect.
4. Name the main components of an X-ray tube and describe their roles in X-ray production.
5. Explain the anode heel effect.
6. Explain the importance of low-voltage rippler for X-ray generators.
7. Explain how automatic exposure control (AEC) works.

X-RAY INTERACTION

Types of interactions

When radiation passes through matter, photons will penetrate, scatter, or be absorbed. X-ray interactions with matter include Rayleigh scattering, Compton scattering, photoelectric absorption, and pair production. Compton scattering and photoelectric absorption are the two most important interactions in diagnostic imaging. Pair production only occurs when photon energy is at least 1.02 MeV, which is not used by medical imaging. Rayleigh scattering, for the photon energies used in diagnostic x-ray imaging applications, is never more than a minor contributor compared to other interaction mechanisms.

Rayleigh scattering

Rayleigh scattering (also called coherent or classical scattering) is an interaction in which the incident photon interacts with an electron of an atom and sets the total atom in the excited state.

The excited atom immediately radiates this energy as an emitting photon of the same energy but in a different direction. As a result, no ionization occurs and no electrons are ejected. The emitted photon undergoes a change in direction without a change in wavelength, and as the X-ray energy decreases, the scattering angle increases (Figure 2.1).

In medical imaging, the image quality is negatively affected by the detection of scattered X-ray. However, in the energy range used in diagnostic imaging the probability of this type of interaction is low. For example, in soft tissues, Rayleigh scattering accounts for less than 5% of X-ray interaction above 70 keV, whereas it accounts for about 12% of interactions at 30 keV.

Compton scattering

In the diagnostic imaging energy range, Compton scattering is the predominate type of interaction of X-ray and gamma-ray photons. In Compton scattering, a photon interacts with an outer shell (valence) electron of an atom. The electron is ejected from the atom and the photon is scattered with some reduction in energy. The energy of the incident photon (E_0) is equal to the sum of the energy of the scattered photon (E_{SC}) and the kinetic energy of the ejected electron (E_{e-}) as

$$E_0 = E_{SC} + E_{e-}$$

The binding energy of the electron that was ejected is comparatively small and often ignored (Figure 2.2).

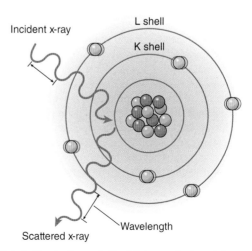

FIG. 2.1 ● Illustration of Rayleigh scattering (aka coherent scattering). The scattered photon has the same wavelength and energy as the incident photon. Reprinted with permission from Fosbinder RA, Orth D. *Essentials of Radiologic Science.* 1st ed. Philadelphia, PA: Wolters Kluwer Health; 2012.

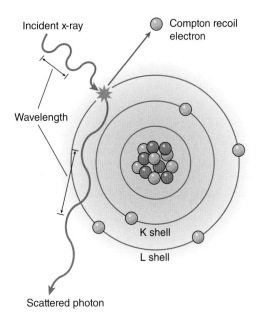

FIG. 2.2 ● **Illustration of Compton scattering.** The incident photon interacts with one of the atom's outer electrons, resulting in the scattered photon and the ejection of the electron. Reprinted with permission from Fosbinder RA, Orth D. *Essentials of Radiologic Science.* 1st ed. Philadelphia, PA: Wolters Kluwer Health; 2012.

Compton scattering results in the ionization of the atom and the energy of the incident photon is divided between the scattered photon and the ejected electron. The ejected electron will lose its kinetic energy by excitation and ionization of atoms in the surrounding tissues, thereby contributing to the patient's radiation dose. The Compton scattered photon may travel through the medium without further interactions or may undergo one or more subsequent interactions.

The energy of the incident photon and the angle of the scattered photon can be used to calculate the energy of the scattered photon. This relationship is expressed by the following equation:

$$E_{SC} = E_0/[1 + (E_0/511 \text{ keV}) * (1 - \cos\theta)]$$

where E_{SC} is the energy of the scatter photon, E_0 is the incident photon energy, and θ is the angle of the scattered photon relative to the incident one. According to the equation, the maximal energy transfer to the Compton electron (the scattered photons goes to its minimum energy at the same time) occurs when the incident photon is scattered back at $\theta = 180°$.

Compared to Rayleigh scattering, the relative probability of a Compton interaction increases as the incident photon energy increases. The probability of a Compton interaction is also dependent on the electron density. With the exception of hydrogen, the total number of electrons per unit mass is fairly constant in tissue; therefore, the probability of Compton scattering per unit mass is essentially independent of Z, and the probability of Compton scattering per unit volume is approximately proportional to the density of the material. Hydrogenous materials have a higher probability of Compton scattering because the absence of neutrons in the hydrogen atom results in increased electron density.

Scattered X-rays provide no useful information for imaging and deteriorate image contrast and quality. Scattered X-rays also provide radiation hazards, particularly in fluoroscopy, in which radiation is scattered from the patient contributing to occupational radiation exposure.

The photoelectric effect

In the photoelectric effect, the incident photon collides with an atom transferring all of its energy to an electron, which is subsequently ejected from the atom. The energy of the ejected electron, called the photoelectron (Ee), is equal to the incident photon energy ($E0$) minus the binding energy of the orbital electron (Eb) (Figure 2.3).

$$E_e = E_0 - E_b$$

The probability of photoelectric absorption, by approximation, is considered proportional to Z^3/E^3, where Z is the atomic number and E is the energy of the incident photon. Therefore, as the atomic number increases, the photoelectric absorption effect becomes more pronounced. This is why barium ($Z = 56$) and iodine ($Z = 53$), which have high atomic numbers, are used as contrast agents in X-ray imaging. Also, the probability of photoelectric absorption generally decreases with the increase in photon energy. However, there are sharp discontinuities to be observed at certain photon energies. As the incident photon energy increases to just above the binding energy of the K shell, the absorption of the photon markedly increases. This is known as the K-edge absorption. Every element has one or a few sharp "absorption edges" in which the probability of a photoelectric interaction dramatically increases for photons of energies just above the absorption edge relative to energies just below the edge. For example, an iodine atom which has a K-edge of 33.2 keV is six times more likely to have a photoelectric interaction with a 33.2 keV X-ray photon than with a 33.1 keV photon (Figure 2.4).

The photon energy of an absorption edge is the binding energy of the electrons in a particular shell or subshell. Each different shell or subshell has its own absorption edge. For example, K-edge refers to the absorption edge of the K shell, the closest shell to the nucleus in an atom. The absorption edge corresponding to the same shell typically increases with the atomic number (Z). The absorption edges of the primary elements that comprise soft tissue (H, C, N, and O) are below 1 keV. Iodine ($Z = 53$) and barium ($Z = 56$), on the other hand, have K-edges of 33.2 and 37.4 keV, respectively, which provide enhanced X-ray attenuation.

The photoelectric effect plays an important role in soft-tissue imaging, for photon energies below 50 keV. Attenuation differences between tissues with slightly different atomic numbers are amplified by the photoelectric absorption process, which turns into image contrast. This differential absorption is exploited to improve image contrast in various applications. Examples include the selection of X-ray tube target material and fillers in mammography, and the use of phosphors containing rare earth elements (lanthanum and gadolinium) in intensifying screens.

The photoelectric process predominates when lower energy photons interact with high Z materials. Photoelectric absorption serves as the primary mode of interaction of diagnostic X-rays with high Z materials like screen phosphors, radiographic contrast media, and bone. Conversely, Compton scattering predominates at most diagnostic photon energies in materials of lower atomic numbers such as soft tissue and air (Figure 2.5).

Pair production

Pair production is not significant in diagnostic X-ray imaging and requires extremely high energies for it to occur. Pair production can only occur when the energies of X-rays exceed 1.02 MeV. In pair production, an X-ray photon interacts with the electric field of the nucleus of an atom and the photon energy is transformed

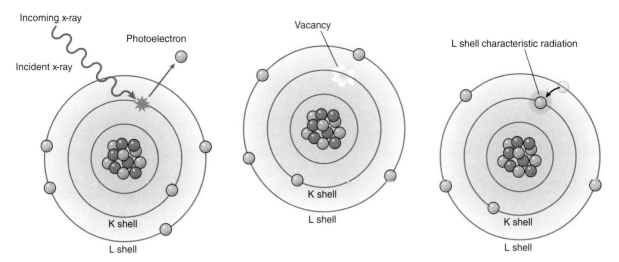

FIG. 2.3 ● **Illustration of the photoelectric effect.** For a photoelectric effect to occur, the incident photon energy must be equal to or greater than the binding energy of the ejected electron. For example, photons whose energies exceed the K-shell binding energies will most likely result in photoelectric interactions with the K-shell electrons. As a result of a photoelectric interaction, atoms are ionized with a vacancy of an inner shell electron. An electron from a more outer shell, with a lower binding energy, will fill this vacancy. This will, in turn, create another vacancy, which is filled from an even lower binding energy shell, creating an electron cascade from outer to inner shells. The difference in binding energy is released as either characteristic X-rays or Auger electrons. As the atomic number of the absorber decreases, the probability of characteristic X-ray emission decreases. Reprinted with permission from Fosbinder RA, Orth D. *Essentials of Radiologic Science.* 1st ed. Philadelphia, PA: Wolters Kluwer Health; 2012.

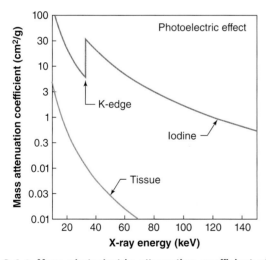

FIG. 2.4 ● **Mass photoelectric attenuation coefficient plotted against photon energy for iodine and tissue.** Reprinted with permission from Bushberg JT, Seibert JA, Leidholdt EM, Boone JM. *Essential Physics of Medical Imaging.* 3rd ed. Philadelphia, PA: Wolters Kluwer Health/Lippincott Williams & Wilkins; 2012.

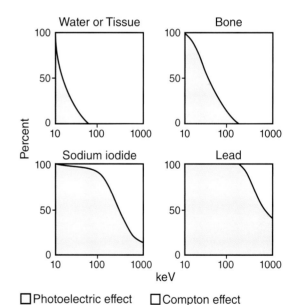

FIG. 2.5 ● **Relative contributions of photoelectric and Compton interaction to the total attenuation of four types of materials, including water, bone, sodium iodide, and lead, as a function of photon energy.** Reprinted with permission from Chandra R, Rahmim A. *Nuclear Medicine Physics: The Basics.* 8th ed. Philadelphia, PA: Wolters Kluwer; 2017.

into an electron–positron pair. Each electron has a rest mass energy equivalent of 0.511 MeV, hence the energy threshold for this reaction to occur is 1.02 MeV. When photon energy is greater than the threshold, the excess is transferred to the electrons as kinetic energy. In turn, the electron and positron lose their kinetic energy via excitation and ionization. A positron may interact with a negatively charged electron as it comes to rest, resulting in the formation of two oppositely directed 0.511 MeV annihilation photons (Figure 2.6).

X-ray attenuation

Attenuation is the removal of photons from a beam of X-rays as it passes through matter because of the various types of interactions that may occur (Figure 2.7).

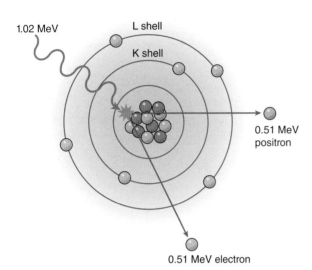

FIG. 2.6 ● **Illustration of pair production, in which photons with energy equal to or above 1.02 MeV concerts to two oppositely charged electrons (one positron and one electron) upon interaction with the nucleus of an atom.** Reprinted with permission from Fosbinder RA, Orth D. *Essentials of Radiologic Science*. 1st ed. Philadelphia, PA: Wolters Kluwer Health; 2012.

Linear attenuation coefficient

LAC (μ) is the reduction in radiation intensity per unit length. In other words, it is the fraction of photons removed from a monoenergetic beam of X-rays per unit thickness of material. LAC is often expressed in units of inverse centimeters (cm^{-1}). The exponential relationship between the number of incident photons (N_0) and those that are transmitted (N) through a thickness x without interaction can be expressed by the following equation:

$$N = N_0 e^{-\mu x}$$

The LAC is the sum of the individual LACs for each type of interaction:

$$\mu = \mu_{\text{Rayleigh}} + \mu_{\text{photoelectric}} + \mu_{\text{Compton scatter}} + \mu_{\text{pair production}}$$

In the diagnostic energy range (30-100 keV), the LAC decreases with increasing energy except at absorption edges or the "k-edge". The LAC for soft tissue ranges from approximately 0.35 to 0.16 cm^{-1} for photon energies ranging from 30 to 100 keV.

The density of the material also affects the probability of an interaction to occur. For a given thickness of material, the probability of interaction will depend on the number of atoms the X- or gamma rays encounter. Photons will encounter more atoms per unit distance through materials with higher densities.

Half-value layer

The HVL quantifies the tissue penetrability of X-ray photons. It is defined as the thickness of material required to attenuate the intensity of an X-ray beam to half (50%) of its original value. It is important to understand the relationship between the LAC and the HVL. The HVL can be easily calculated from the LAC (μ), and vice versa by the following equation:

$$\text{HVL} = 0.693/\mu$$

HVL is a function of photon energy and attenuating material, and it increases with increasing photon energy and decreases with increasing atomic number of the material.

Effective energy

In radiology, X-ray beams are typically composed of a spectrum of energies; they are often referred to as poly-energetic beams. The HVL, which is usually measured in millimeters of aluminum (mm Al) in diagnostic radiology, can be converted to a quantity called the *effective energy*. The effective energy of a poly-energetic X-ray beam is essentially an estimate of the penetrating power of the X-ray beam (as if it were a monoenergetic beam).

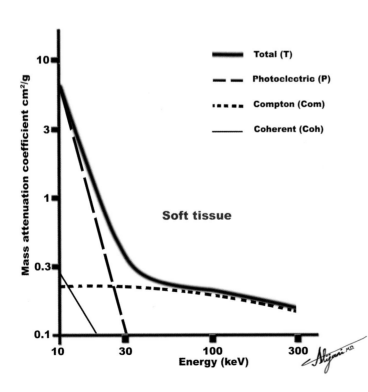

FIG. 2.7 ● **Tissue mass attenuation coefficient as a function of energy.** Individual contributions of coherent scattering (or Rayleigh scattering), Compton scattering and the photoelectric effects are also plotted. There is no contribution of pair production within the energy range of the plot because pair production occurs only for photons at or above 511 keV. Reprinted with permission from Huda W. *Review of Radiologic Physics*. 4th ed. Philadelphia, PA: Wolters Kluwer; 2016.

Beam hardening

In poly-energetic X-ray beams, the lower energy photons will be preferentially removed from the beam as they pass through matter. Beam hardening refers to the shift of the X-ray spectrum towards higher effective energies as the beam transverses matter (Figure 2.8).

Beam hardening may have implications on image quality. Using computed tomography (CT) as an example, the beam hardening effect, if unaccounted for, is known to cause nonuniformity in the reconstructed images of a homogeneous object. To reduce the beam hardening effect, one may insert additional filters in the X-ray beam before it passes through the image object. The added filter not only narrows the X-ray energy spectrum, resulting in less pronounced beam hardening effect, but also removes a larger amount of lower energy X-rays that make little contribution to the image because of their poor tissue penetration.

X-RAY PRODUCTION

An X-ray beam is produced through the interaction of highly energetic electrons with matter. This conversion of kinetic energy into electromagnetic energy from the deceleration of these highly energetic electrons after interacting with a metal target generates X-rays. This interaction occurs in a highly controlled environment, the X-ray tube. The components of the X-ray tube are optimized in medical imaging for the generation of X-rays to visualize the anatomic structure of interest. The following is to review the important aspects of the creation of X-rays, equipment needed to generate these X-rays, and the important characteristics of the X-ray beam.

Bremsstrahlung radiation

X-ray tubes rely on the conversion of electron kinetic energy into electromagnetic radiation for X-ray production. A simplified understanding of the X-ray production process within an X-ray tube is as follows. An X-ray tube can be viewed as a pair of electrodes, enclosed in a vacuum tube, with the negatively charged cathode as the source of the electrons and the positively charged anode as the target. When a large potential difference (voltage) is applied between two electrodes, electrons are accelerated between these electrodes and attain kinetic energy while traveling from the cathode to the anode. The kinetic energy gained by an accelerated electron is measured in electron volts (eV) and is proportional to the potential difference between the cathode and the anode. For example, the energies of electrons accelerated by a potential difference of 20 and 100 kilovolt peak (kVp) are 20 and 100 keV, respectively.

Electrons can be accelerated to different energy levels. When electrons impact the anode, the vast majority of energy is converted to heat through collisional energy exchanges; however, a small fraction of the electrons (about 0.5%) travel close enough to an atomic nucleus within the target that the nucleus slows down and alters the path of the electron. The nucleus is positively charged, and as these electrons near the nucleus, it exerts coulombic attractive forces which decelerate and alter the trajectory of the electron. This process produces an X-ray photon with energy equal to the kinetic energy lost through deceleration. "Bremsstrahlung" is a German word meaning "braking radiation", which can be understood from the deceleration of the electron. This radiative energy loss is responsible for the majority of the X-rays produced by X-ray tubes (see Figure 2.2).

The distance between the incident electron and the nucleus determines the amount of energy lost by each electron during the bremsstrahlung interaction because the coulombic force of attraction increases with the inverse square of the interaction distance. The coulombic attraction is weak at relatively long distances from the nucleus, and these interactions produce low-energy X-rays. Conversely, for encounters that occur closer to the nucleus, the coulombic forces acting on the electron are greater, the change in the electron's speed and trajectory are more profound, and the X-rays produced have higher energy. Rarely will the electron collide with the nucleus and lose all of its energy. When this occurs, the maximum X-ray energy is produced (equal to E_{max}) (Figure 2.9).

The probability of a low-energy interaction is greater than that of a high-energy interaction because on an atomic scale, the atom is mainly empty space and the volume occupied by the atomic nucleus is very small. In fact, the nucleus accounts for about 1/100 000th of the total volume of the atom. As a result, lower X-ray energies are produced in greater numbers, and the quantity of higher energy X-rays decreases with energy up to and including the maximum energy of the incident electrons.

Because the bremsstrahlung process depends on the positive charge of protons in the nucleus, anode elements with a greater atomic number (and thus more protons) are more likely to produce bremsstrahlung radiation. The probability of this interaction occurring for a particular atom is proportional to Z^2. Tungsten serves as the anode material for most medical imaging, in part due to its high atomic number ($Z = 74$) and high melting point.

For completeness sake, it should be noted that particles other than electrons (such as protons and alpha particles) can produce

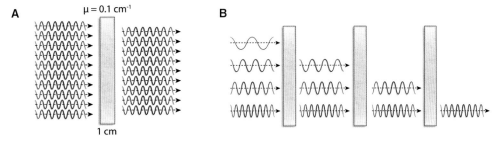

FIG. 2.8 ● Illustration of the attenuation of monochromatic (A) and polychromatic (B) X-ray beams. Attenuation of a monochromatic X-ray beam means reduction in its beam intensity (or the number of photons). Attenuation of a polychromatic X-ray beam is more complicated because of the difference in the attenuation of photons of different energies; lower energy photons have a higher attenuation coefficient than higher energy photons, so there will be relatively more high-energy photons and fewer low-energy photons as the beam traverses the object. Reprinted with permission from Huda W. *Review of Radiologic Physics*. 4th ed. Philadelphia, PA: Wolters Kluwer; 2016.

bremsstrahlung radiation; however, the amount of energy emitted varies inversely with the square of the mass of the incident particle. Because protons and alpha particles are orders of magnitude more massive than are electrons, they produce less than one-millionth the amount of bremsstrahlung radiation as do electrons of the same energy.

Bremsstrahlung spectrum

A bremsstrahlung spectrum illustrates the distribution of all X-ray photons produced as a function of energy. The unfiltered bremsstrahlung spectrum demonstrates a linearly decreasing relationship between the number and the energy of the X-rays produced, with the maximum X-ray energy determined by the voltage (kVp) applied across the X-ray tube.

Photons at the lower end of the bremsstrahlung spectrum are of little value in diagnostic imaging and are removed by filtration. This process involves passing the photons through a thin layer of material that preferentially attenuates lower energy X-rays (filtration is discussed in detail later in this chapter). After filtration, a typical bremsstrahlung spectrum shows a distribution with minimal X-rays below 10 keV (Figure 2.10). The average X-ray energy in the filtered spectrum is typically about one-half of the highest X-ray energy (E_{max}), and the peak of the curve is approximately one-third of E_{max}. For example, a filtered spectrum with E_{max} of 120 keV will generally have a peak around 40 keV.

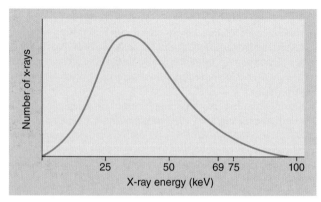

FIG. 2.10 ● The continuous spectrum of Bremsstrahlung radiation from a tungsten or tungsten-rhenium target. Reprinted with permission from Orth D. *Essentials of Radiologic Science.* 2nd ed. Philadelphia, PA: Wolters Kluwer; 2017.

Bremsstrahlung production efficiency

The most important factors affecting X-ray production efficiency are the atomic number of the target material and the kinetic energy of the incident electrons (determined by the voltage potential of the X-ray tube). The ratio of radiative energy loss caused by bremsstrahlung production to collisional (excitation and ionization) energy loss can be approximated with the following equation:

$$\text{Radiative energy loss/Collisional energy loss} = E_k \times Z/820\,000$$

where E_k is the kinetic energy of the incident electrons in keV and Z is the atomic number of the target material.

For energy levels used in diagnostic medical imaging, the vast majority of incident energy is converted to heat. As an example, for 100 keV electrons colliding with tungsten ($Z = 74$), the approximate ratio of radiative to collisional losses is $(100 \times 74)/820\,000 = 0.009$ or 0.9%. Therefore, about 99.1% of the incident energy will be released as heat.

Note that as the energy of the incident electrons increases, the efficiency of X-ray production increases proportionately. Thus, at an energy level of 6 MeV electrons (typical for radiation oncology), the ratio of radiative to collisional losses is $(6000 \times 74)/820\,000 = 0.54$ or 54%. Therefore, under these conditions heat production is less of a problem.

Characteristic radiation

Each electron in an atom of the anode has a binding energy that is specific to the shell in which it is located. When the energy of an incident electron exceeds the binding energy of an electron of a target atom, it is possible for a collision to eject the electron and ionize the atom (a previously neutral atom would lose 1 electron and acquire a +1 charge). The partially unfilled shell is now unstable, and an outer shell electron with less binding energy will drop down to fill the vacancy. As the outer shell electron transitions to a lower energy state, the excess energy can be converted to a so-called characteristic X-ray. The energy of the X-ray photon will be equal to the difference between the binding energies of the electron shells (Figure 2.11).

Each element has specific binding energies for each shell, so the X-rays produced have distinct energies characteristic of the

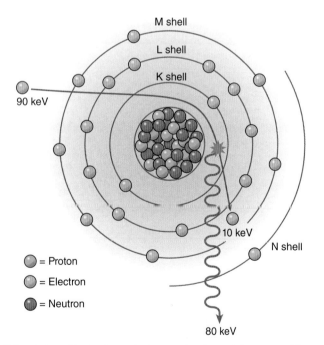

FIG. 2.9 ● Illustration of the production of bremsstrahlung radiation. In this figure, the incoming electron decelerates from 90 keV down to 10 keV; at the same time, an X-ray photon of 80 keV is produced. When a large number of electrons of the same energy have these interactions, the energies of the produced photons are continuously distributed within a range, the upper limit of which is equal to the kinetic energy of the incoming electron. The closer the electron is to the atomic nucleus, the higher energy the released X-ray photon has. Reprinted with permission from Fosbinder RA, Orth D. *Essentials of Radiologic Science.* 1st ed. Philadelphia, PA: Wolters Kluwer Health; 2012.

anode. For tungsten, when a K-shell vacancy is filled by an electron in the L shell, the energy of the emitted electron can be determined as follows:

$$E_{\text{K-shell}} - E_{\text{L-shell}} = 69.5 \text{ keV} - 10.2 \text{ keV} = 59.3 \text{ keV}$$

Characteristic X-rays can be produced by transitions between adjacent and nonadjacent electron shells (eg, an M → K transition or L → K transition). Occasionally, even an unbound electron from outside the atom can fill the vacancy. As a result, several distinct energy peaks are produced (Figure 2.12). These are superimposed on the continuous spectrum of X-rays produced by the bremsstrahlung process (Figure 2.13).

The most common characteristic X-rays produced for the purposes of diagnostic imaging result from K-shell vacancies that are filled by electrons from the L, M, and N shells. The shell capturing the electron designates the characteristic X-ray transition, and a subscript of α or β indicates whether the transition is from an adjacent shell (α) or a nonadjacent shell (β). For example, K_α refers to an electron transition from the L to the K shell, and K_β refers to an electron transition from M, N, O shell (or an electron outside

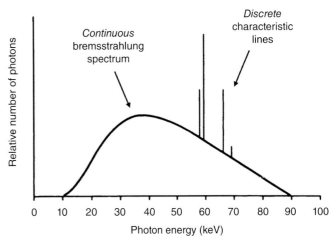

FIG. 2.13 ● **A typical energy spectrum of X-rays produced by applying 90 kV to an X-ray tube using a tungsten target.** The energy spectrum is composed of two parts: the continuous bremsstrahlung spectrum (after being filtered by materials on the beam path like tube envelope, oil, etc) and the discrete characteristic energy peaks. Reprinted with permission from Garcia MJ. *NonInvasive Cardiovascular Imaging: A Multimodality Approach.* 1st ed. Philadelphia, PA: Wolters Kluwer Health/Lippincott Williams & Wilkins; 2011.

the nucleus) to the K shell. Not surprisingly, K_β X-rays will have more energy than do K_α X-rays because the transition difference is greater.

As discussed in the previous chapter, each shell other than the K shell comprises discrete energy subshells. Consequently, there is subtle splitting of the energy levels for characteristic X-rays produced from the same shell transitions. By convention, these are designated with an additional subscript 1, 2, etc. For tungsten, the three tallest peaks on the combined bremsstrahlung/characteristic spectrum result from the $K_{\alpha 1}$, $K_{\alpha 2}$, and $K_{\beta 1}$ transitions.

Only characteristic X-rays produced by K-shell transitions are relevant for the purposes of medical imaging. Characteristic X-rays from transitions to the L shell, M shell, etc are of relatively low energy and almost entirely attenuated by the X-ray tube filter.

For a characteristic K X-rays to be emitted, the energy of the incident electron must exceed the binding energy of a K-shell electron. Therefore, voltage potential must be at least 69.5 kVp for tungsten anodes or 20 kVp for molybdenum targets (primarily used in mammography) to produce K characteristic X-rays. The proportion of characteristic X-ray emission relative to bremsstrahlung X-ray emission increases with kVp above the minimum energy for characteristic X-ray production. For example, with a tungsten anode, about 5% of the total X-ray photons will be characteristic radiation at 80 kVp; at 100 kVp, it increases to about 10%.

Characteristic X-ray production in an X-ray tube is mostly the result of electron–electron collisions; however, collisions between bremsstrahlung X-ray photons and electrons (the photoelectric effect) also make a small contribution to the total characteristic X-ray production.

Auger electrons and fluorescent yield

It is important to realize that electron collisions creating vacancies in electron shells do not always result in the production of a characteristic X-ray. There is a separate process called the Auger effect in which the energy released is transferred to an orbital electron instead of creating an X-ray photon. The electron that receives the

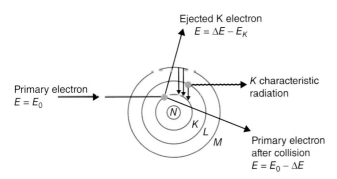

FIG. 2.11 ● **Illustration of the production of characteristic X-ray.** When an electron from outer shells fills the vacancy on an inner shell, a characteristic X-ray is produced with energy equal to the difference in binding energy between the two shells. Reprinted with permission from Halperin EC, Brady LW, Perez CA, et al. *Perez & Brady's Principles and Practice of Radiation Oncology.* 6th ed. Philadelphia, PA: Wolters Kluwer Health/Lippincott Williams & Wilkins; 2013.

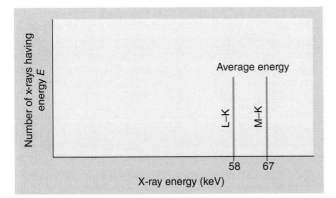

FIG. 2.12 ● **The discrete energy peaks on the energy spectrum of characteristic X-rays produced from a tungsten anode.** Reprinted with permission from Fosbinder RA, Orth D. *Essentials of Radiologic Science.* 1st ed. Philadelphia, PA: Wolters Kluwer Health; 2012.

energy transfer, called an Auger electron, is generally located in the same shell as the cascading electron and is ejected from the atom. The Auger electron will have kinetic energy equal to the difference between the transition energy and its binding energy (Figure 2.14).

The chance that the electron transition will generate a characteristic X-ray is called the fluorescent yield (ω). Therefore, (1 − ω) is the probability that the transition will result in the ejection of an Auger electron. Auger emission is more likely in target elements with a low atomic number. Consequently, the fluorescent yield will be greater in higher Z elements. The fluorescent yield for tungsten is about 80%.

X-RAY TUBES

X-ray tubes are designed to provide an optimal environment for the production of bremsstrahlung and characteristic radiation. The most basic components are the cathode, anode, rotor, stator, envelope, and tube housing (Figure 2.15).

The three major factors controlling the X-ray beam characteristics (quality and quantity) are as follows:

1. The **peak voltage** that accelerates electrons from the cathode to the anode is measured in kilovolt peak (kVp). For diagnostic medical imaging, the peak voltage ranges from 20 to 150 kVp.
2. The **tube current**, or the rate of electron flow from the cathode to the anode, measured in milliamperes (mA). 1 mA is equal to 6.24×10^{15} electrons per second. Continuous fluoroscopy generally utilizes tube currents in the range of 1 to 5 mA. Projection radiography uses tube currents from 100 to 1000 mA.
3. **Exposure time**, or the (ms), which is the amount of time X-ray photons are produced for a particular examination.

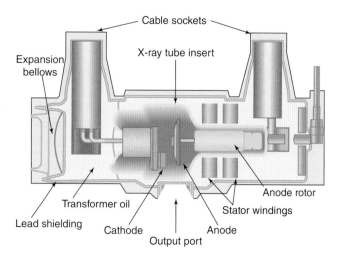

FIG. 2.15 ● **Diagram of a modern X-ray tube and its housing assembly.** Reprinted with permission from Bushberg JT, Seibert JA, Leidholdt EM, Boone JM. *Essential Physics of Medical Imaging.* 3rd ed. Philadelphia, PA: Wolters Kluwer Health/Lippincott Williams & Wilkins; 2012.

Cathode

The cathode is the source of electrons in the X-ray tube. It is composed of a helical tungsten filament surrounded by a focusing cup. Both of these are connected electronically to the filament circuit. Electric current directed through the filament creates heat. At very high temperatures, electrons on the surface of the anode essentially "boil" off and are released into the evacuated tube. This process is called "thermionic emission" or the "Edison effect." Increasing the filament current will lead to greater heating of the filament and therefore the release of more electrons. Tungsten filaments typically operate in the range of 2000 to 2500 kelvin (K). As previously described, the electrons released from the filament are then accelerated through the vacuum of the X-ray tube when a voltage potential is applied between the anode and the cathode.

Most tungsten anodes contain a trace amount of thorium (Th, $Z = 90$), which diffuses to the surface when the filament is heated. The thorium layer protects the metal against ion bombardment at high voltages, increasing the efficiency of electron emission and prolonging filament life.

Because electrons are negatively charged, they repel each other and tend to spread out once they are liberated from the filament. This tendency is disadvantageous because the electrons must be directed toward the anode to create X-rays. The focusing cup (also called the cathode block) surrounds the filament and helps counteract this process, shaping the electrons into a concentrated beam. Usually, the voltage applied to the cathode block is the same as that applied to the filament. This creates a negative charge on the block, effectively acting as an electron "lens" and producing a narrow area of interaction (focal spot) on the anode. Some X-ray tubes (called "grid-biased" tubes) utilize an insulated focusing cup which is more negatively charged (about 100 V less) than the filament. This creates an even stronger electric field around the filament, further reducing the spread of the beam and resulting in an even narrower focal spot.

Although the width of the focal spot is determined by the focusing cup, its length is proportional to the length of the cathode filament. X-ray tubes used in diagnostic imaging usually have two filaments of different lengths with a slot in the focusing cup for

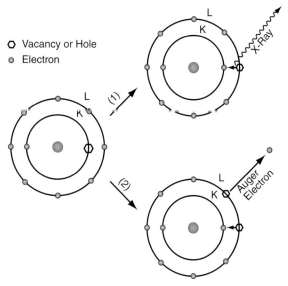

○ Vacancy or Hole
● Electron

FIG. 2.14 ● **Illustration of the Auger effect.** When there is a vacancy or a hole on the inner orbit, an electron from an outer orbit may fill the vacancy/hole and release the energy in excess in one of the two forms, an X-ray photon characteristic of the energy difference between the two orbits, or the emission of an electron (called Auger electron), so that the atom may return to a stable state. Reprinted with permission from Chandra R, Rahmim A. *Nuclear Medicine Physics: The Basics.* 8th ed. Philadelphia, PA: Wolters Kluwer; 2017.

each. The length of the focal spot can be controlled by selecting one filament or the other (Figure 2.16).

Tube and filament current

The rate of thermionic electron emission is controlled by the temperature of the filament, which is determined by the amount of heat generated from the filament current. As the electrical resistance to the filament current heats the filament, electrons are emitted from its surface. If there is no voltage potential between the cathode and the anode, an electron cloud accumulates around the filament. This is called a "space charge cloud." The number of electrons in the space charge will remain constant. Applying a positive high voltage to the anode with respect to the cathode accelerates the electrons from the space charge cloud toward the anode. The number of electrons traveling from the cathode to the anode at any given time is called the tube current. Small changes in the filament current can produce relatively large changes in the tube current.

At low tube potentials (40 kVp and below), the space charge cloud insulates the electric field, and only electrons along the periphery of the cloud are available to be accelerated toward the anode. Under these circumstances, the operation of the X-ray tube is said to be "space charge limited," meaning that increases in the filament current will not produce additional tube current. Above 40 kVp, the space charge cloud insulation is outweighed by the greater potential difference; thus, the tube current is limited only by the emission of electrons from the filament (called "emission limited.")

Under emission-limited conditions, the filament current controls the tube current in a predictable manner; the tube current will be about 5 to 10 times less than the filament current. Higher kVp produces slightly higher tube current for the same filament current. For example, if the filament current is 5 amps (A), 80 kVp produces about 800 mA tube current and 120 kVp produces about 1100 mA tube current. This relationship does not continue indefinitely. Over a certain kVp, all of the electrons emitted from the filament are immediately accelerated toward the anode and a further increase in kVp has essentially no effect on tube current (Figure 2.17).

Anode

The anode is the target of the electrons produced by the cathode and accelerated by the X-ray tube voltage potential. Electrons colliding with the anode release the vast majority of their energy as heat, with a small fraction converted to X-ray photons. Accordingly, the production of X-rays in quantities required for diagnostic imaging results in significant heating of the anode. To avoid heat damage to the X-ray tube, the rate of X-ray production must be limited. Tungsten ($Z = 74$) is the most popular anode material because of its high melting point and high atomic number. A tungsten anode can withstand significant heat deposition without cracking or pitting of its surface. Generally, 10% rhenium (Re, $Z = 75$) is added, providing additional heat resistance and protection against surface damage. As previously mentioned, the high atomic number of tungsten provides better bremsstrahlung production efficiency compared with elements of lower atomic number.

Molybdenum (Mo, $Z = 42$) and rhodium (Rh, $Z = 45$) are used as anode materials in mammographic X-ray tubes. These materials provide lower energy characteristic X-rays that are useful in breast imaging.

Anode configurations

X-ray tubes can have either fixed or rotating anodes. The simplest type of X-ray tube, used in many dental X-ray units and portable X-ray machines, has a fixed anode. The anode comprises a tungsten insert embedded in a copper block. The copper both supports

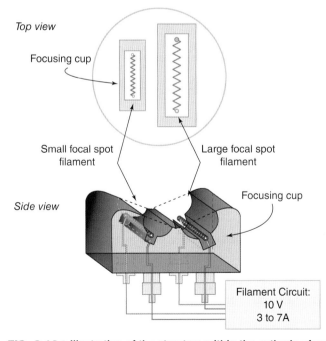

FIG. 2.16 ● Illustration of the structure within the cathode of an X-ray tube. Typically, more than one filament are placed inside a focusing cup. Electric current from the filament circuit heats one of the filaments and results in thermionic emission of electrons. Reprinted with permission from Bushberg JT, Seibert JA, Leidholdt EM, Boone JM. *Essential Physics of Medical Imaging.* 3rd ed. Philadelphia, PA: Wolters Kluwer Health/Lippincott Williams & Wilkins; 2012.

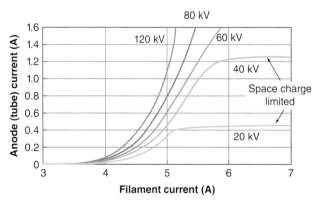

FIG. 2.17 ● The relationship between the tube current and the filament current. This relationship demonstrates a dependence on the tube voltage. When the tube voltage is low and the filament current is high, the space charge cloud near the cathode surface shields the electric field and therefore makes it impossible for further increase in tube current. When tube voltage is high, the filament current becomes the major limiting factor of the tube current. Reprinted with permission from Bushberg JT, Seibert JA, Leidholdt EM, Boone JM. *Essential Physics of Medical Imaging.* 3rd ed. Philadelphia, PA: Wolters Kluwer Health/Lippincott Williams & Wilkins; 2012.

the tungsten target and removes heat. The main disadvantage of a fixed anode is that the small target area results in a relatively low rate of heat dissipation. This limits the maximum tube current and thus the rate of X-ray production.

Rotating anodes are more technically complex, but they allow for much more effective heat loading and X-ray output and are therefore more common in diagnostic imaging. The rotating anode consists of a disk with a ring of tungsten along its edge. The anode disk is connected to a rotor comprised of copper bars surrounding a central iron cylinder. This entire apparatus is mounted on bearings and contained within the vacuum X-ray tube. Just outside the tube, a series of electromagnets called the stator surround the rotor. When alternating current (AC) is applied to the stator, it creates a rotating magnetic field which induces a small electric current within the copper bars of the rotor. This current creates an opposing magnetic field that applies force to the rotor, causing the entire rotor/anode assembly to spin. As the anode rotates, electrons collide with a target that is continuously moving, spreading the generated heat over a large area.

X-ray machines with rotating anodes are designed such that X-rays will not be produced until the anode reaches its full rotating speed. This explains the short delay (1–2 seconds) that occurs between the X-ray tube exposure button being pushed and the exposure being taken.

Rotor bearings are heat sensitive and are often the cause of X-ray tube failure. Bearings located within the vacuum environment of the X-ray tube require special heat-resistant metallic-based lubricants. The anode is attached to the rotor by a molybdenum stem. Molybdenum has a high melting point (2600°C) and is a very poor heat conductor, providing a thermal barrier between the anode disk and rotor assembly. Thus, the anode is thermally insulated and must be cooled by radiation of heat into the oil bath surrounding the X-ray tube.

The maximum allowable heat load depends on the anode rotation speed and the focal spot area. Faster rotation speeds allow for greater heat capacity because a particular location on the anode will be exposed to the electron beam for a shorter period of time per rotation. Typical anode rotation speeds range between 3000 and 10 000 rpm. These and other factors described later in this chapter determine the maximum possible heat load for an X-ray tube.

Anode angle and focal spot size

The anode angle is defined as the angle of the target relative to the incoming electron beam. Most diagnostic X-ray tubes (other than some mammography tubes) utilize anode angles in the range of 12° to 15°.

Focal spot size is defined in two ways: actual and effective. The actual focal spot size is the area on the anode where the electrons collide. Its length is determined by the length of the cathode filament, and its width is controlled by the focusing cup. Actual focal spot sizes range from 0.1 to 1.2 mm.

The effective focal spot size is the cross-sectional area of the emitted X-ray beam. The effective focal spot width is equal to the actual focal spot width under all conditions. The length, however, is affected by the anode angle which effectively shortens the X-ray beam, causing the effective focal spot length to be smaller than the actual focal spot length. This process is called the line focus principle. The effective focal spot length can be calculated as follows:

$$\text{Effective focal length} = \text{Actual focal length} \times \sin(\theta)$$

where θ is the anode angle. (Theoretically, an anode angle of 45° would result in an effective focal length equal to the actual focal length, although such an angle is never used in practice.) (Figure 2.18).

The optimal anode angle for a particular imaging application depends on several factors. A small anode angle produces a smaller effective focal spot relative to the actual focal area. This results in better spatial resolution but limits the size of the X-ray field, particularly at short spot-to-image distances. X-ray tubes with small anode angles (7°–9°) are commonly utilized in angiography, where the size of the X-ray field is already limited by the small diameter of the image intensifier. General radiographic imaging requires larger anode angles (in the range of 12°–15°) to achieve a larger field of coverage.

The length of the effective focal spot also varies depending on the position in the image plane. Toward the anode side of the X-ray field, the projected length of the focal spot is shorter. Conversely, it lengthens on the cathode side of the field. Effective focal spot width is the same regardless of position. The nominal focal spot size (width and length) is specified at the central ray of the X-ray beam. The central ray is a line from the focal spot to the image receptor that is perpendicular to both the anode-cathode axis and the plane of the image receptor (Figure 2.19).

Anode heel effect

The anode heel effect refers to variation in the intensity of X-rays along the anode-cathode axis. X-ray photons are produced inside the anode material and therefore they must pass through a portion of the anode before leaving the X-ray tube. Tungsten

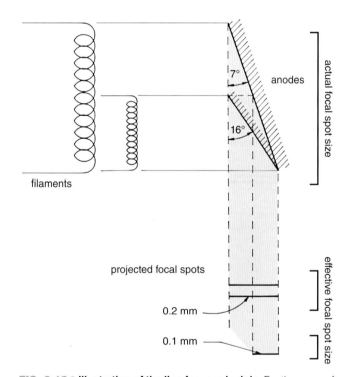

FIG. 2.18 ● Illustration of the line focus principle. For the same effective focal spot size, a smaller anode angle allows for a larger actual focal spot size and a larger area of target face for heat dissipation; its disadvantages, however, are smaller field size and more pronounced anode-heel effect. Reprinted with permission from Lille S, Marshall W. *Mammographic Imaging.* 4th ed. Philadelphia, PA: Wolters Kluwer; 2018.

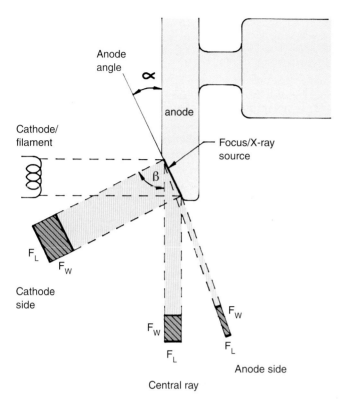

FIG. 2.19 ● **The size of the effective focal spot as a function of the central ray.** Reprinted with permission from Andolina VF, Lille SL. *Mammographic Imaging.* 3rd ed. Philadelphia, PA: Wolters Kluwer Health/Lippincott Williams & Wilkins; 2010.

attenuates X-rays significantly, almost as much as lead. Photons traveling on the anode side of the X-ray field must traverse more of the anode and will be attenuated more than those directed toward the cathode side of the X-ray field.

Major factors that can lessen the heel effect are (1) increasing anode angle, (2) increasing source to image distance (SID), and (3) decreasing the size of the X-ray field.

In some circumstances, the heel effect can be exploited to improve image quality. For example, in chest radiography, the anode side of the field should be oriented at the upper chest and the cathode should be oriented toward the abdomen. Because the abdomen is generally denser and attenuates more than the chest, the heel effect will result in more balanced attenuation across the X-ray field (Figure 2.20).

Off-focus radiation

Off-focus radiation is produced by electrons in the X-ray tube that strike the anode outside the focal spot area. As the incident electrons collide with the anode, a small number scatter from the target and are accelerated back toward the anode, striking it outside the focal spot. These electrons create a low-intensity X-ray source over the face of the anode. In general, rotating anodes create more off-focus radiation than do stationary anodes because there is a greater total volume of anode material.

Off-focus radiation is undesirable because it increases patient dose and reduces image quality. It can be mitigated by a small lead collimator located near the X-ray tube output window. Some X-ray tubes include a metal casing with the same voltage charge as the anode. This can further reduce off-focus radiation because scattered electrons are attracted to the positively charged casing.

X-ray tube insert

The X-ray tube insert refers to the glass or metal envelope and its contents: the cathode, anode, rotor assembly, and support structures. The entire insert is sealed under high vacuum, which prevents electrons from colliding with gas molecules. No X-ray tube can maintain a perfect vacuum over time. Gas molecules that leak into the envelope are eliminated by an active ion trap, also called a "getter circuit."

The tube insert includes a small window through which the X-ray beam passes, called the "tube port." X-rays are emitted in all directions from the focal spot, but only X-rays that exit through the tube port contribute to the X-ray beam. In most X-ray tubes, the port is composed of the same material as the tube envelope. An exception is mammography tubes, which use beryllium ($Z = 4$) in the port to minimize attenuation of low-energy X-rays that are important for breast imaging.

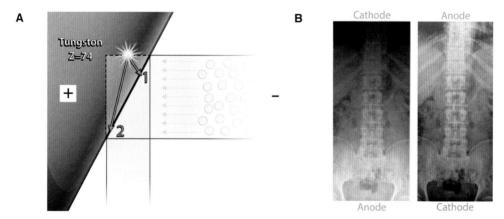

FIG. 2.20 ● The anode-heel effect (A) and its implications on the orientation of X-ray tubes in radiographic exams (B). The anode-heel effect occurs because X-ray photons emitting in the directions parallel to the anode surface are much more likely to be absorbed than those in other directions, causing a reduction in X-ray intensity across the generated radiation field from the cathode to the anode. One may utilize the anode-heel effect to produce more uniform images in chest X-ray imaging, by pointing anodes toward the less attenuating, upper chest region. Reprinted with permission from Huda W. *Review of Radiologic Physics.* 4th ed. Philadelphia, PA: Wolters Kluwer; 2016.

X-ray tube housing

The X-ray tube housing surrounds the insert. Its major functions are to insulate and protect the X-ray tube insert from the environment. The space between the housing and insert is filled with dielectric oil that provides both electrical insulation and heat conduction. During operation, the oil expands as the X-ray tube heats. A sensor monitors oil expansion and shuts off the X-ray tube in the event of excessive heating.

Heavy lead shielding within the housing is designed to attenuate all X-rays other than those that exit via the X-ray tube port. A small fraction of very high-energy X-ray photons will penetrate the shielding. In the United States, federal regulations require that radiation leakage not exceed 100 mR/h, measured at 1 m from the focal spot when the tube is operating at its maximum mA and kVp.

Grid-biased tubes

Grid-biased tubes contain a focusing cup that is electrically insulated from the cathode filament and maintained at a more negative voltage. When the voltage difference is sufficiently large (about −2000 V), the resulting electric field is strong enough to cut off the tube current. This allows the focusing cup to be used as a control switch, with the ability to turn the anode voltage on and off quickly. This configuration is used in applications where rapid pulsing of the X-ray beam is required, such as pulsed fluoroscopy. The increased voltage and technical complexity demanded by biased X-ray tubes make them substantially more expensive than nonbiased tubes.

Filtration

As previously discussed, filtration is the partial removal of X-rays as the beam passes through a layer of material. X-rays are attenuated both by the filtration properties of the tube itself (inherent filtration) and by a dedicated filter located near the X-ray port (added filtration). The sum of these equals total filtration.

Tube inserts are typically composed of glass (silicon oxide) or aluminum, both of which have similar filtration properties. A thin layer of either material at the tube port will attenuate nearly all photons below 15 keV. The oil bath surrounding the tube insert also contributes to inherent filtration.

Added filtration is achieved by placing a thin sheet of metal in the path of the X-ray beam. In most diagnostic radiology applications (with the exception of mammography), low-energy photons have very little chance of penetrating the patient and therefore contribute nothing to image quality. Filtering these photons reduces the absorbed radiation dose without sacrificing image quality. Aluminum (Al, $Z = 13$), copper (Cu, $Z = 29$), and acrylic are the most common added filter materials.

Compensation filters are a special type of added filter than can be used to alter the spatial pattern of the X-ray beam for specific applications. They are typically placed over the X-ray port external to the collimator. Examples include the following:

1. **Trough filters**, used in chest radiography, contain a vertical band of reduced thickness to compensate for the relatively high attenuation of the mediastinum.
2. **Wedge filters**, used in the lateral projection of cervicothoracic spine imaging, can compensate for the increased soft-tissue density of the chest and shoulders.
3. **Bow-tie filters** are used in CT to attenuate the periphery of the X-ray beam because it passes through less of the patient.

Filtration always decreases the X-ray tube output but increases the beam penetration. Because low-energy photons are preferentially removed, the remaining X-ray beam has a higher mean energy.

Collimators

Collimators adjust the size and shape of the X-ray beam as it emerges from the tube port. They contain two sets of lead shutters (one vertical and one horizontal) that completely attenuate X-ray photons and can be adjusted to define the dimensions of the X-ray field. Inside the collimator housing, there is a beam of light which is reflected by a mirror onto the patient and serves to simulate the size and shape of the X-ray field. Collimators must be checked periodically to verify that the X-ray field and collimator light are properly aligned.

Positive beam limitation collimators feature a safety mechanism to ensure that the field size never exceeds the size of the detector.

X-RAY GENERATORS

Electromagnetic induction and voltage transformation

The purpose of the X-ray generator is to provide electric current at a high voltage to the X-ray tube. Electrical power available to most medical facilities provides up to about 480 V, much lower than the 20 000 to 150 000 V at which X-ray tubes require to operate. The conversion of low voltage into high voltage is accomplished by an electrical apparatus called a transformer.

A basic transformer comprises two electrically insulated wires wrapped around an iron core. One insulated wire wrapping, called the "primary winding," carries the input voltage and current. The other insulated wire or "secondary winding" carries the output voltage and current. The primary and secondary windings are electrically isolated by insulation, but they are magnetically linked by the iron core. When AC is passed through the primary winding, it creates an oscillating magnetic field. The secondary windings are bathed in the oscillating magnetic field, and an alternating voltage is induced in the secondary windings as a result. The law of transformers states that the ratio of the number of coil turns in the primary winding to the number of coil turns in the secondary winding is equal to the ratio of the primary voltage to the secondary voltage:

$$V_p/V_s = N_p/N_s$$

where N_p is the number of turns of the primary coil, N_s is the number of turns of the secondary coil, V_p is the amplitude of the alternating input voltage on the primary side of the transformer, and V_s is the amplitude of the alternating output voltage on the secondary side.

Transformers can increase, decrease, or isolate voltage, depending on the ratio of the numbers of turns in the two coils. For $N_s > N_p$, a "step-up" transformer increases the secondary voltage; for $N_s < N_p$, a "step-down" transformer decreases the secondary voltage; and for $N_s = N_p$, an "isolation" transformer produces a secondary voltage equal to the primary voltage. Because transformers depend on the oscillating nature of AC, they cannot function with direct current.

Power is the rate of energy production or expenditure per unit time. The SI unit of power is the watt (W), which is defined as 1 joule (J) of energy per second. For electrical devices, power is equal to the product of voltage and current:

$$P = I \cdot V$$

Because a volt is defined as 1 joule per coulomb and an ampere is 1 coulomb per second:

$$1 \text{ watt (W)} = 1 \text{ volt (V)} \times 1 \text{ ampere (A)}$$

Because the power output is equal to the power input (for an ideal transformer), the product of voltage and current in the primary winding is equal to that in the secondary winding:

$$V_p I_p = V_s I_s$$

Thus, a decrease in current must correspond to an increase in voltage, and vice versa.

The high-voltage section of an X-ray generator contains a step-up transformer, typically with a primary-to-secondary turns ratio of 1:500 to 1:1000. Within this range, a tube voltage of 100 kVp requires an input peak voltage of 200 to 100 V, respectively.

Autotransformers

An autotransformer consists of only one winding. It has a fixed number of turns, two lines on the input side and two lines on the output side. When an alternating voltage is applied to the pair of input lines, an alternating voltage is produced across the pair of output lines. The law of transformers applies to the autotransformer, just as it does to the standard transformer.

A switching autotransformer has several taps on the input and output sides, which allow small incremental increases or decreases in the output voltage. Most X-ray generators use switched autotransformers to adjust the kVp (Figure 2.21).

Other components

Other components of the X-ray generator include the high-voltage power circuit, the stator circuit, the filament circuit, the focal spot selector, and AEC circuits. In modern systems, microprocessor control and closed-loop feedback circuits help ensure proper exposures.

Most modern generators used for radiography have AEC circuits, whereby the technologist selects the kVp and mA, and the AEC system determines the correct exposure time. The AEC (also called a phototimer) measures the exposure with the use of radiation detectors located near the image receptor, which provide feedback to the generator to stop the exposure when the proper exposure to the image receptor has been reached. AECs are discussed in more detail later in this chapter.

Many generators have circuitry that is designed to protect the X-ray tubes from potentially damaging overload conditions. Combinations of kVp, mA, and exposure time delivering excessive power to the anode are identified by this circuitry, and such exposures are prohibited. Heat load monitors calculate the thermal loading on the X-ray tube anode, based on kVp, mA, and exposure time, and take into account the time required for cooling. Some modern X-ray systems are equipped with sensors that measure the temperature of the anode, protecting the X-ray tube and housing from excessive heat by prohibiting exposures that would damage them.

Operator console

At the operator console, the operator selects the tube potential (kVp), tube current (mA), exposure time, and focal spot size. The peak kilovoltage (kVp) determines the X-ray beam quality (penetrability), which is important in determining image contrast. The X-ray tube current (mA) determines the X-ray flux (number of photons per square centimeter) emitted by the X-ray tube at a given kVp. The product of tube current (mA) and exposure time

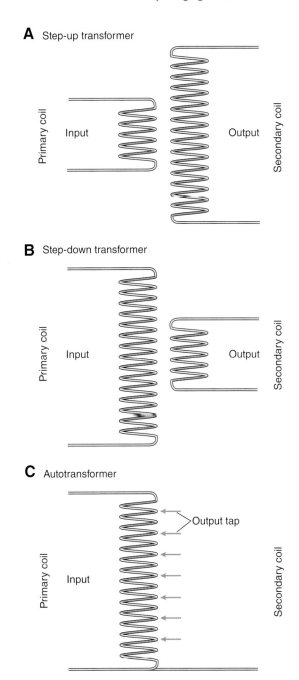

FIG. 2.21 • Three types of transformers are shown, including a step-up transformer (A), a step-down transformer (B), and an autotransformer (C). Reprinted with permission from Fosbinder RA, Orth D. *Essentials of Radiologic Science*. 1st ed. Philadelphia, PA: Wolters Kluwer Health; 2012.

(seconds) is expressed as milliampere-seconds (mAs). Some generators used in radiography allow the selection of a "three-knob" technique (individual selection of kVp, mA, and exposure time), whereas others only allow a "two-knob" technique (individual selection of kVp and mAs). The selection of focal spot size (large or small) is usually determined by the mA setting. Low mA selections allow the small focus to be used. Larger mA requires a larger focal spot to provide greater surface area for heat dissipation. Most X-ray generators have preprogrammed settings for various radiographic examinations (chest, spine, KUB [kidneys, ureters, and bladder], etc).

Generator power supply

Most household appliances are powered by a single-phase AC. In contrast, the electrical power for the X-ray generator is most commonly provided by a three-phase AC power supply (Figure 2.22). Three voltage sources, each with a single-phase AC waveform, are oriented one-third of a cycle (120°) apart from each other (in other words, at 0°, 120°, and 240°). Step-up transformers are utilized to increase voltage.

AC must be converted to direct current to apply a constant voltage potential across the X-ray tube. This is achieved through a rectifier circuit. The circuit is composed of multiple diodes, electrical components that allow current to flow only in one direction. Because alternating continuously reverses direction, a single diode will only allow current during half of the cycle for a particular AC waveform. Full-wave rectifiers use a series of diodes to reverse the flow of electrons when the waveform is negative.

When three of these rectified voltage waveforms are combined, the result is an almost constant voltage with the effective (average) voltage (kV) being nearly equal to the peak voltage (kVp). Small variations referred to as "ripple," which is defined as follows:

$$\% \text{ voltage ripple} = ([V_{max} - V_{min}]/V_{max}) \times 100$$

Lower ripple means less variability in current, producing a superior X-ray beam both in terms of the quantity of photons and the average energy. Ripple for three-phase generators is generally between 4% and 13%.

FACTORS AFFECTING X-RAY PRODUCTION

The output of an X-ray tube can be characterized in terms of quality, quantity, and exposure.

Quality describes the penetrability of an X-ray beam, with higher energy X-ray photons having higher quality.

HVL refers to the thickness of a particular material required to reduce the X-ray beam to half its original intensity. HVL provides an objective measure of X-ray beam quality, because a higher energy beam will require a greater thickness of material to attenuate half its intensity. X-rays used in diagnostic imaging typically have HVL values in the range of 2.3 to 5 mm for aluminum.

Quantity refers to the number of photons in an X-ray beam. Exposure is proportional to the energy flow of the X-ray beam and therefore has quality- and quantity-associated characteristics. X-ray production efficiency, exposure, quality, and quantity are determined by six major factors: X-ray tube target material, voltage, current, exposure time, beam filtration, and generator waveform.

The anode material affects the efficiency of bremsstrahlung radiation production, with output exposure roughly proportional to atomic number. Incident electrons are more likely to have bremsstrahlung interactions in materials with higher atomic number. The energies of characteristic X-rays produced are unique to each element and depend on the target material. Therefore, the anode material affects the quantity of bremsstrahlung photons and the quality of the characteristic radiation.

Tube voltage (kVp) determines the maximum energy in the bremsstrahlung spectrum and affects the quality of the output spectrum. In addition, the efficiency of X-ray production is directly related to tube voltage. Exposure is approximately proportional to kVp^2 in the diagnostic energy range. For example, the relative exposure of a beam generated with 80 kVp compared with that of 60 kVp for the same tube current and exposure time would be equal to $(80/60)^2 = 1.78$ (meaning that output exposure increases by ~78%). An increase in kVp increases the efficiency of X-ray production and the quantity and quality of the X-ray beam.

Changes in the kVp must be compensated for by corresponding changes in mAs to maintain the same exposure. At 80 kVp, 1.78 units of exposure occur for every 1 unit of exposure at 60 kVp. To achieve the original 1 unit of exposure, the mAs must be adjusted to 1/1.78 = 0.56 times the original mAs, a reduction of 44%. An additional consideration of technique adjustment concerns the X-ray attenuation characteristics of the patient. To achieve equal transmitted exposure through a typical patient (eg, 20 cm tissue), the mAs varies with the fifth power of the kVp ratio:

$$(kVp_1/kVp_2)^5 \times mAs_1 = mAs_2$$

Accordingly, if a 60 kVp exposure requires 40 mAs for a proper exposure through a typical adult patient, at 80 kVp the proper mAs is approximately $(60/80)^5 \times 40$ mAs = 9.5 mAs or about one-fourth of the original current. The value of the exponent (between four and five) depends on the thickness and attenuation characteristics of the patient.

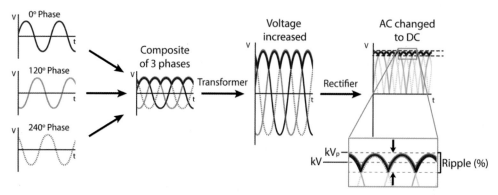

FIG. 2.22 ● **Illustration of steps involved in generating nearly constant voltages for an X-ray tube by a generator.** The three-phase alternate current power supply works together with transformers and rectifiers to produce a nearly constant voltage to apply to the X-ray tube; the fluctuations in the voltage is often characterized by percentage voltage ripple. DC, direct current. Reprinted with permission from Huda W. *Review of Radiologic Physics.* 4th ed. Philadelphia, PA: Wolters Kluwer; 2016.

FIG. 2.23 ● **The differences in the generated X-ray spectrum using generators of different percentage voltage ripple factors while the tube voltage, the tube current, and the exposure time are kept constant.** Lower percentage of voltage ripple leads to higher effective energy and greater output of X-ray photons. Reprinted with permission from Bushberg JT, Seibert JA, Leidholdt EM, Boone JM. *Essential Physics of Medical Imaging.* 3rd ed. Philadelphia, PA: Wolters Kluwer Health/Lippincott Williams & Wilkins; 2012.

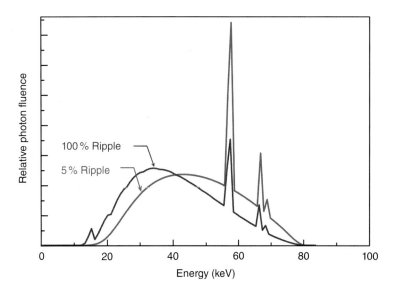

The tube current (mA) is equal to the number of electrons flowing from the cathode to the anode per unit time. The exposure of the beam for a given kVp and filtration is proportional to the tube current.

The exposure time is the duration of X-ray production. The quantity of X rays is directly proportional to the product of tube current and exposure time (mAs).

Beam filtration preferentially removes the low-energy photons in the spectrum. This decreases the number of photos (quantity) and shifts the average energy to higher values, increasing the quality.

The generator waveform affects the quality of the emitted X-ray spectrum. For the same kVp, a single-phase generator provides a lower average potential difference than does a three-phase or high-frequency generator. Both the quality and quantity of the X-ray spectrum are affected (Figure 2.23).

In summary, the X-ray quantity is approximately proportional to

$$Z_{anode} \times kVp^2 \times mAs$$

The X-ray quality depends on the kVp, the generator waveform (ie, ripple), and beam filtration. Exposure depends on both the quantity and quality of the X-ray beam. A change in kVp requires adjustment of mAs on the order of the fifth power of the kVp ratio, because kVp determines quantity, quality, and transmission through the object, whereas mAs determines quantity only.

Automatic exposure control

AEC is often used instead of fixed exposure times in radiography. AEC depends on a phototimer circuit, which measures the amount of radiation reaching the image receptor and stops X-ray production once a specified amount is obtained. The phototimer ensures a more consistent exposure to the receptor by accounting for differences in patient thickness and attenuation (Figure 2.24).

A typical chest or table cassette stand has three phototimer sensors. The technologist can select which sensors are used for a particular examination, depending on the configuration of the anatomic region being imaged. For example, for a chest radiograph, the two outside sensors are activated; thus, the transmitted X-ray beam through the lungs determines the exposure time. This prevents overpenetration of the lungs, which can occur due to

the highly attenuating mediastinum. In some cases, particularly examinations that involve nonstandard patient positioning, the sensors cannot be adjusted to adequately represent the region of interest. If this occurs, the technologist can use a "density switch" to manually adjust the exposure time up or down as needed. In the event of phototimer failure, a backup timer terminates the exposure after a preset time (Figure 2.25).

SYSTEM RATINGS

Power ratings

The power rating is the maximum energy per unit time that can be supplied by an X-ray generator or received by an X-ray tube. The power rating for a generator or focal spot is defined as the

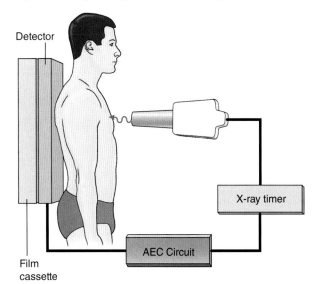

FIG. 2.24 ● **Illustration of how automatic exposure control (AEC) works.** The film-cassette image receptor is used here as an example. A detector or phototimer is placed at the entrance surface of the image receptor; when its received signal is above a predefined threshold value, it sends control signals to the timer of the X-ray tube to terminate the exposure. Reprinted with permission from Fosbinder RA, Orth D. *Essentials of Radiologic Science.* 1st ed. Philadelphia, PA: Wolters Kluwer Health; 2012.

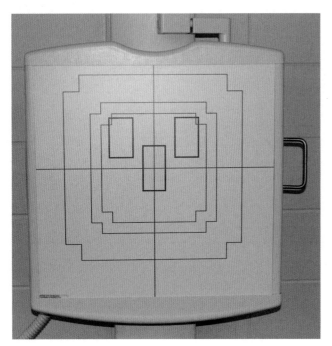

FIG. 2.25 ● **A typical configuration of the automatic exposure control (AEC) phototimers (indicated by the three rectangular marks) for chest X-ray imaging.** Reprinted with permission from Orth D. *Essentials of Radiologic Science.* 2nd ed. Philadelphia, PA: Wolters Kluwer; 2017.

average power delivered by the maximum tube current (A_{max}) at 100 kVp with an exposure time of 0.1 seconds.

$$\text{Power} = 100 \text{ kVp} \times A_{max} \text{ for 0.1 second exposure}$$

Factors that contribute to higher power ratings include (1) large focal spots, (2) high anode rotation speed, (3) large anodes (greater heat dissipation), and (4) small anode angle.

Heat loading

The amount of heat being deposited in or dissipated from the anode is typically measured in heat units (HUs). For X-ray tubes with single-phase generators, the heat load can be calculated as follows:

$$\text{HU} = \text{kVp} \times \text{mA} \times \text{exposure time}$$

For three-phase generators, this value must be multiplied by 1.35 to account for the near-constant potential waveform.

The joule (J) is the SI unit of energy which is equal to 1 watt per second. Because 1 W = 1 A × 1 V, the amount of heat energy deposited on the anode (assuming constant voltage potential) can be calculated as follows:

$$\text{Energy (J)} = \text{kVp} \times \text{mA} \times \text{exposure time}$$

Thus, for a three-phase generator, heat input in HU is approximately equal to 1.35 times heat input in joules.

Exposure rating charts

Rating charts describe the maximum heat load that a particular X-ray tube can withstand at various kVp, mA, and exposure times without causing damage. Factors that influence the operational limits of a tube include its design (focal spot size, anode rotation speed, etc) and the type of generator (single-phase, three-phase, etc).

A single-exposure rating chart reports the maximum heat load for a single exposure. An X-ray tube typically has four single-exposure charts, each for a specific focal spot size and anode rotation speed.

The exposure time is graphed on the *x*-axis (typically in a logarithmic scale), the kVp is graphed on the *y*-axis, and series of curves represent the maximum allowable mA. Curves toward the lower left of the graph indicate greater mA values and smaller values are toward the upper right. Because low kVp and short exposure time will produce less heat, the maximum mA will be greater for these combinations.

To determine whether a particular exposure is feasible, one may (1) find the correct graph (this will depend on focal spot size and anode rotation speed), (2) locate the point on the graph corresponding to the desired exposure time and kVp, and (3) by finding the nearest mA curve, make an estimate of the maximum allowable mA. If the desired mA is larger than this value, the may result in damage to the X-ray tube.

Rating charts for multiple exposures exist for X-ray tubes used in applications such as angiography where continuous or sequential imaging is required. In practice, these charts are rarely used and have largely been replaced by computerized systems that continuously monitor heat loading and determine whether a particular series of exposures is safe. Similarly, modern CT scanners utilize software that automatically prevents exposure beyond the heat limitations of the X-ray tube.

Anode cooling chart and house cooling chart

Multiple exposures deliver a cumulative heat load to the anode. Thus, a one-time exposure that is within operating limits may cause damage if there is significant heat remaining from prior exposures. An anode cooling chart shows how long a wait is necessary before the anode can safely handle a particular heat load. HUs are represented on the *y*-axis and time on the *x*-axis. The anode cooling curve shows how much heat remains in the anode as a function of time. Note that the slope of the curve is steeper at greater heat loads because the anode cools faster at higher temperatures.

As previously discussed, the X-ray tube insert is filled with dielectric oil that allows for heat dissipation. During normal tube operation, heat causes the oil to expand. Most X-ray tubes are equipped with a bellows that monitors the volume of oil expansion. If the oil heats beyond design limits, the bellows will activate a switch that shuts off the X-ray tube. Heat removal can be enhanced by a heat exchanger. This involves either circulating the oil through a radiator or by pumping water through the housing. The housing cooling chart graphs the housing heat load as a function of cooling time. The largest value on the *y*-axis indicates the maximum heat load that the housing can withstand.

CHAPTER SELF-ASSESSMENT QUESTIONS

1. Which of the following is NOT true regarding x-ray interactions?

   A. Compton scattering and the photoelectric effect are two primary interactions for diagnostic x-rays.

   B. The photoelectric effect is more pronounced with materials of low effective atomic number.

   C. The energy of the x-ray photon remains unchanged in Rayleigh scattering.

   D. The probability of the photoelectric effect generally decreases with the energy of the x-ray photons, but sharply increases right at the K-edge.

2. The photon interaction most responsible for the high soft tissue contrast in mammography with 15–30-keV x-rays is:

   A. Compton scattering
   B. Coherent scattering
   C. Photoelectric effect
   D. Pair production
   E. Photonuclear disintegration

3. Which of the following is true regarding x-ray production?

   A. The discrete energy peaks of characteristic x-ray photons are the same for different anode materials.

   B. The closer a high-speed electron gets to the atomic nucleus, the lower energy the resulting bremsstrahlung radiation has.

   C. Materials with higher atomic numbers are preferred for the anode because of their high attenuation coefficients.

   D. When high-speed electrons interact with the anode, the majority of the kinetic energy of these electrons is lost via heat.

4. Which of the following is NOT true regarding x-ray tubes?

   A. The anode heel effect becomes more pronounced with a smaller anode angle.

   B. X-ray tubes typically can operate at higher power when the large focal spot is selected.

   C. The effective focal spot size is constant across the radiation field.

   D. Thicker filter results in higher effective energy of the produced x-ray beam.

Answers to Chapter Self-Assessment Questions

1. B The photoelectric effect is more pronounced for higher-Z elements.

2. C Interactions of 15–30-keV x-ray photons are dominated by photoelectric effect. Both Compton scattering and coherent scattering have substantially fewer interactions within the range. Pair production and photonuclear disintegration occur only at much higher photon energies.

3. D Photon energies of characteristic x-ray are strongly dependent on the type of anode material. When the high-speed electron gets closer to the nucleus, there is more energy loss from the electron and therefore the resulting bremsstrahlung radiation has higher energy.

4. C The effective focal spot size varies across the radiation field. Along the cathode–anode direction, the effective focal spot size is typically larger on the cathode side.

X-ray Imaging: Radiography and Fluoroscopy

3

Zhihua Qi, PhD

LEARNING OBJECTIVES

1. Describe the functions of the main components of an X-ray tube, including the cathode, the anode, the collimator, and the filters.
2. Describe the roles of an X-ray generator and its desired characteristics for medical imaging.
3. Explain the working principles of the image receptors used by three types of X-ray imaging technologies: screen-film radiography, computed radiography, and digital radiography.
4. State the differences between indirect conversion and direct conversion in digital radiography.
5. Describe both the effects of scatter on image quality and the main techniques used for scatter reduction in radiography.
6. Explain how technical parameters of a radiographic acquisition affect image quality.
7. Describe the differences between image intensifier–based and flat panel detector–based fluoroscopic systems.
8. Explain the benefits of the pulsed mode in fluoroscopy compared to the continuous mode.

RADIOGRAPHY

X-ray radiography is the most commonly performed X-ray imaging examination. It produces one or more planar views of the anatomy of interest for quick diagnosis of many common conditions.

Radiographic technologies

Radiographic technologies are featured by the image receptor technologies for image acquisition. Screen-film radiography was the mainstream technology before the digital trend in radiography. Computed radiography and digital radiography are both radiographic technologies with digital capabilities.

Screen-film radiography

Before the digital era of radiology, screen-film cassettes were the majorly used X-ray image receptor. A screen-film cassette encapsulates intensifying screens inside a light-tight cassette and is loaded with a sheet of film during the exposure for imaging.

Film

The film inside a screen-film cassette converts incident light photons into varying levels of darkness as a function of light flux. It is composed of a thin plastic base coated on one or both sides with a light-sensitive emulsion layer, which consists of silver halide (AgBr and AgI) crystals held inside water-soluble gelatin (Figure 3.1). Each silver halide crystal has on its surface specks of Ag^+ ions because of artificially introduced defects to the crystal lattice. When a grain of silver halide crystal is exposed to visible

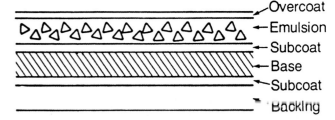

FIG. 3.1 ● **Cross-section view of X-ray film.** Reprinted with permission from Christman R. *Foot and Ankle Radiology.* 2nd ed. Philadelphia, PA: Wolters Kluwer; 2015.

light, a small number of Ag^+ ions on the crystal surface gain electrons and get reduced to metallic Ag atoms, and, as a result, the crystal grain forms a stable latent center locally. The opacities introduced by these Ag atoms are still too weak to form a visible image; hence a developing process is needed to amplify the signal by converting all Ag^+ ions at each latent center to Ag atoms (Figure 3.2). After film development, the film then has its residual silver halide crystals in unexposed areas dissolved by a bath of an aqueous oxidizing solution called fixer before it is rinsed and dried for image presentation.

A developed film is viewed in front of a light box. The local darkness of the film is caused by the presence of Ag atoms after they are converted from ions and reflects local X-ray exposure made during image acquisition; the higher the exposure, the darker the area. Film images are therefore considered as negative images.

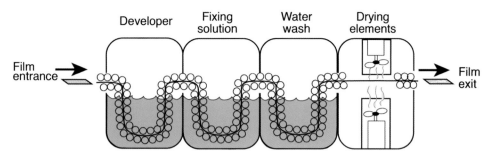

FIG. 3.2 ● **Processing of radiographic films.** Reprinted with permission from Wilkins EM. *Clinical Practice of the Dental Hygienist.* 12th ed. Philadelphia, PA: Wolters Kluwer; 2017.

Screen

An intensifying screen is primarily made of scintillator materials, which convert incident X-ray exposure into visible light photons, whose wavelengths fall into the sensitive range of the film.

In selecting the appropriate thickness of an intensifying screen, there is a trade-off between the spatial resolution of the image and the efficiency of X-ray absorption. When the screen thickness increases, more incident X-ray photons are absorbed by the screen, but the visible light photons have a broader spread before reaching the film, leading to a blurred image. When the screen thickness decreases, less blurring of the image is expected at the expense of a more grainy/noisy image.

Speed is a common term used to describe the efficiency of X-ray absorption by a radiographic image receptor. The higher the speed, the less radiation it takes for a certain level of signal output (the optical density of the film is the signal output for screen-film radiography).

Screen-Film Configuration

Radiographic applications often use screen-film cassettes with a double-emulsion and double-screen configuration, in which the film has two emulsion layers and is placed in between two screens for the maximum efficiency of X-ray absorption (Figure 3.3). The configuration becomes different for applications where high spatial resolution is desired, like mammography; only a single screen is used and placed behind the film along the X-ray path so that X-ray photons hit the film first. In this configuration, there are more X-ray photons absorbed by the screen at places near the film because of X-ray attenuation, and the resulting light spread is limited; if X-ray photons hit the screen first, there would be more photons absorbed by the screen at places far from the film and there would be more light spread.

Computed radiography

In computed radiography, the screen-film cassette is replaced by a photostimulable phosphor (PSP) plate. A PSP imaging plate is typically made of a mixture of BaFBr and BaFI, activated with a small quantity of Eu (europium). When X-ray energy is absorbed by the phosphor, electrons associated with the europium atoms are excited and become mobile, and then a fraction of them will get trapped locally in a higher energy state. The number of trapped excited electrons per unit area of the imaging plate is proportional to the intensity of X-rays incident at each location of the detector during the X-ray exposure. When a red laser beam scans the exposed imaging plate, the trapped electrons absorb energy from the light photons and become mobile again (Figure 3.4); when these electrons return to their ground state, they release energy in

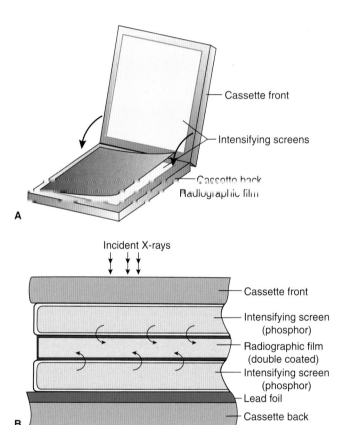

FIG. 3.3 ● A screen-film cassette whose configuration is featured by a double-emulsion sheet in between two phosphor screens (A). Compared to the use of single-emulsion film and/or single screen, this configuration has high sensitivity to incoming X-rays at the expense of compromised spatial resolution (cross-sectional view shown in B). Reprinted with permission from Smith WL. *Radiology 101.* 4th ed. Philadelphia, PA: Wolters Kluwer Health/Lippincott Williams & Wilkins; 2014.

the form of blue light photons. The photons will be captured by a light guide and measured for image formation.

The light released by the imaging plate has higher energy and shorter wavelength than the stimulating laser light. In fact, the stimulating laser light used by readers of PSP imaging plates is red in color (~600-700 nm wavelength), and the emitted photons coming out of the screen are blue (~400-450 nm wavelength). The separation in the wavelength profiles between the two groups of light photons allows efficient detection and accurate quantification of the light photons and the incident X-ray exposures.

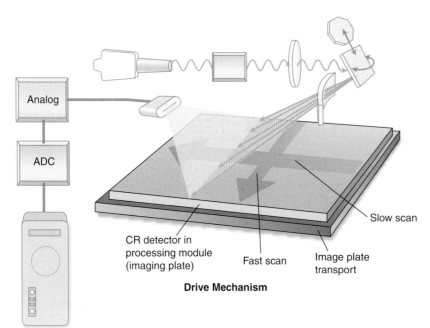

FIG. 3.4 ● **Image readout of a photostimulable phosphor plate inside a reader.** Reprinted with permission from Orth D. *Essentials of Radiologic Science.* 2nd ed. Philadelphia, PA: Wolters Kluwer; 2017.

Digital radiography

Flat panel detectors (FPDs), as a digital X-ray imaging technology, have the following advantages: (1) the images are instantaneously available after the exposure and (2) its area is sufficiently large to support most clinical applications without the need of optical coupling. X-ray detection by FPD is a two-step process: first, detected X-ray photons are converted into charges; then these charges are collected and read out by dedicated electronics. Although there are different designs for converting X-ray photons to charges, the handling of the charges in the second step is nearly the same for all FPDs.

An FPD is made on a flat piece of amorphous semiconductor material. It is divided into a large array of squared pixels arranged in a row by column matrix. Regardless of the design in converting X-ray photons to charges, each pixel has at least the following components: an electrode for charge collection, a storage capacitor to hold the charge, and a thin-film transistor to coordinate the readout of the charge. The entire array of pixels forms an active matrix structure, through which charges collected by each individual pixel can be read out in a coordinated fashion.

The conversion from X-ray photons to electrical charges may be either indirect or direct (Figure 3.5).

Indirect Conversion Detector

Indirect conversion FPD uses a scintillator mounted on the front surface of the detector. The scintillator functions in the same way as that in a screen-film cassette by converting incident X-ray photons to light photons. The light photons then reach the pixels, and each individual pixel, with its photodiode, converts the light photons to electrical charges before their readout. Light photons produced inside the scintillator layer diffuse in all directions while exiting the scintillator, eventually causing a blurring of the signal and a loss of resolution in the formed image. To reduce such resolution loss, most indirect conversion detectors use cesium iodide (CsI) as the scintillator material. CsI has a columnar crystal structure that acts like light pipes to reduce lateral spread of light.

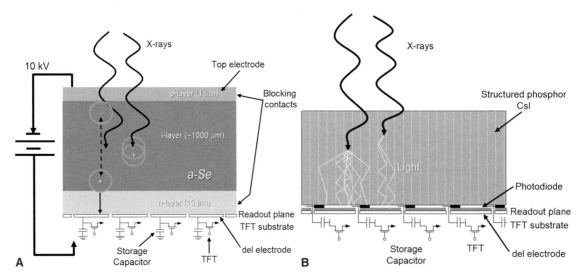

FIG. 3.5 ● A and B: Cross-sectional views of both indirect conversion and direct conversion detectors. Reprinted with permission from Kandarpa K, Machan L, Durham J. *Handbook of Interventional Radiologic Procedures.* 5th ed. Philadelphia, PA: Wolters Kluwer; 2016.

Direct Conversion Detector

Direct conversion FPDs eliminate the production of light photons and directly convert X-ray photons into charges. Amorphous selenium is the semiconductor material most commonly used for fabricating the layer at the entrance of the detector. The semiconductor layer produces electron-hole pairs in proportion to the incident X-ray intensity, and the ion pairs are instantly collected by the applied voltage across the layer and transferred to individual pixels for subsequent readout. This design minimizes the spread of signals and results in high spatial resolution in the acquired images.

Scatter management

X-ray imaging follows a straight-line assumption, that is, each X-ray remains on a straight-line trajectory while traveling through tissues, regardless of the interactions it may have with the tissues. Scattered X-rays often deviate from their original trajectory after interactions with tissues and cause displacement of information, overlapped with information from the nonscattered or primary X-rays on the image receptor. Effects of scattered radiation include reduction in image contrast and loss of spatial resolution.

The amount of scattered radiation in an image is characterized by the scatter to primary ratio (SPR), defined as the amount of energy from scattered X-rays, divided by that from primary X-rays. The SPR is a function of both tissue thickness and the field of view used for acquisition (Figure 3.6). In acquiring an abdominal X-ray image for a normal-sized adult patient (~25 cm tissue thickness), the SPR is about 4, meaning that, if uncorrected, 80% of the photons used for forming the image are scattered radiation.

Antiscatter grid

Antiscatter grids are widely used in X-ray imaging for scatter reduction (Figure 3.7). It is placed in between the patient and the image receptor and made of a large number of highly absorbing lead septa with interspace supporting materials in between. All the septa are aligned with the focal spot of the X-ray tube so that most primary photons reach the image receptor with minimal attenuation from interspace materials, whereas the scattered photons, deviating from their original paths, largely get absorbed by the septa. Lead is typically used for making the grid septa, whereas carbon fiber, giving little attenuation and providing necessary structural support, is a common interspace material.

Most antiscatter grids used in routine radiographic examinations are linear or one-dimensional, meaning the septa and interspace materials alternate along one dimension only. Two-dimensional grids have found uses in mammographic applications.

It is worth mentioning that antiscatter grids absorb both scattered and primary X-ray photons. Therefore, the reduction of

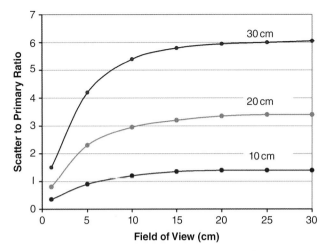

FIG. 3.6 ● **Scatter to primary ratio as a function of anatomy size and field size.** Reprinted with permission from Bushberg JT, Seibert JA, Leidholdt EM, Boone JM. *Essential Physics of Medical Imaging.* 3rd ed. Philadelphia, PA: Wolters Kluwer Health/Lippincott Williams & Wilkins; 2012.

scatter by the use of grids comes at a penalty of increased radiation to the tissues, because an increase in radiation is necessary to compensate for the loss of signal detected by the image receptor. This increase is described by the Bucky factor. Typical Bucky factors for grids used in abdominal X-ray imaging are between 3 and 8. The Bucky factor has more relevance in screen-film radiography than digital radiography. This is because screen-film cassettes have a fairly narrow dynamic range and the loss of signals by the use of grids would result in an underexposed film, whereas digital detectors have a wider dynamic range and allow for postprocessing that may compensate for at least part of the loss.

The septa of a grid cast shadows on the image receptor because of their absorption of primary photons, and the pattern of the septa may show up on the image if detector pixels have similar or smaller sizes with respect to the septa thickness. A solution to this issue is to move the grid with a reciprocating motion during the exposure. This type of grid is referred to as Bucky grid (not to be confused with Bucky factors).

Because of the alignment of septa and interspace materials with the X-ray source, each grid needs to be used with the intended range of source-to-detector distances and properly aligned, otherwise undesired artifacts may arise.

Air-gap geometry

The use of an air-gap geometry may also reduce scatter. In this geometry, a gap of air is purposely introduced between the patient and the detector so that scattered X-rays may fall out of the

FIG. 3.7 ● **Illustrations of linear grid, cellular grid, and air-gap geometry.** Reprinted with permission from Huda W. *Review of Radiologic Physics.* 4th ed. Philadelphia, PA: Wolters Kluwer; 2016.

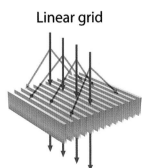

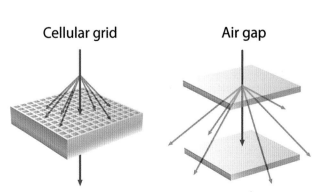

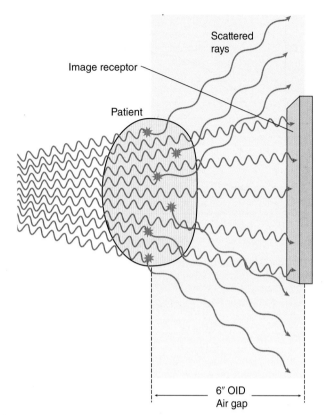

Scattered
rays

Image receptor

Patient

6″ OID
Air gap

FIG. 3.8 • Illustration of the air-gap geometry. Reprinted with permission from Fosbinder RA, Orth D. *Essentials of Radiologic Science.* Philadelphia, PA: Wolters Kluwer Health; 2012.

The adjustable set of parameters include the following:

- tube voltage (or kVp)—it affects image contrast because X-ray attenuation coefficients of materials vary by photon energy
- tube current (typically in mA)—it affects image noise because it affects the number of photons absorbed by the detector and therefore the level of signal fluctuation because of quantum effect
- exposure time (typically in milliseconds)—it also affects image noise by affecting the number of photons absorbed by the detector; it also affects temporal resolution as the longer the exposure time is, the more motion-caused image blur there may be
- product of tube current and exposure time (typically in the unit of mAs)—mAs includes the effects of both tube current and exposure time on image noise
- focal spot size—the use of different focal spot sizes affects spatial resolution. Smaller focal spot sizes result in higher spatial resolution than larger ones.
- filter material and thickness—filters at the exit of X-ray tubes alter the energy spectrum of the X-rays; they affect image contrast because of the changes they make in the number of photons at different energies; they also affect image noise because they absorb photons and result in loss of signals on detector and increase in image noise
- the use of antiscatter grid—because of the decrease in image contrast caused by scattered photons, the use of antiscatter grid improves image contrast and reduces undesired artifacts caused by scatter
- scan geometry—it includes the source-to-detector distance, the source-to-surface distance, and field size; scan geometry may affect image quality in numerous ways; examples include (1) the distances affect spatial resolution and (2) field size affects contrast resolution because of its effect on scatter

FLUOROSCOPY

Overview

Fluoroscopy produces a time series of X-ray images to allow real-time monitoring of events inside the human body. As a clinical imaging tool, it provides guidance for numerous diagnostic, surgical, and interventional procedures. Clinical settings in which fluoroscopy is used include gastrointestinal suites, urology suites, surgical rooms, interventional rooms, cardiac catheterization labs, and electrophysiology labs.

Fluoroscopy shares many physics principles with radiography, both as projectional X-ray imaging modalities. A major difference between the two is their radiation output rate, resulting from the different goals of their clinical applications. Radiography often aims at a single-view X-ray image with sufficient signal to noise ratio for diagnostic purposes; to minimize motion-caused blur, the exposure time is very short (typically tens of milliseconds or shorter) and the radiation output rate from the X-ray tube is usually high by the use of high mA. Fluoroscopy has much longer exposure time for monitoring the underlying event, and, in order to keep the total radiation output low, the radiation output rate from the X-ray tube is considerably lower (by 1-2 orders of magnitude), compared to radiography.

Fluoroscopic systems used today can be divided into two categories, image intensifier (II)- and FPD-based systems, mainly depending on the type of its image capturing device (Figure 3.9). II-based systems use II, an analog device to produce visible light signals for the exposed anatomy, and additional components to

detector (Figure 3.8). Drawbacks of this technique include: (1) the supported field of view becomes smaller for the same image receptor and (2) the spatial resolution of the images may become poorer because of more blurring by the focal spot when the detector is farther away from the source.

Automatic exposure control

Automatic exposure control on radiographic systems adjusts X-ray output from the X-ray tube based on the size of the anatomy to be imaged. Its goal is to reduce the probability of human error and produce uniform image quality across a wide range of anatomy size. It works by building a phototimer-controlled feedback mechanism between the image receptor and the X-ray tube. The phototimer measures the exposure incident upon the image receptor and, once the measured exposure exceeds a preset level, sends signals to the X-ray tube to terminate the exposure. The phototimer may be ion chambers placed right in front of or behind the image receptor, or just part of the image receptor, like a cluster of pixels, if it is digital.

Radiographic techniques: image quality versus technical parameters

It is a highly nontrivial task to select proper technical parameters for any diagnostic imaging task. The goal is the best achievable image quality with reasonable radiation dose to the exposed tissues. Image quality aspects of clinical relevance include contrast resolution (affected by both image contrast and image noise), spatial resolution, temporal resolution, presence of artifacts, and others.

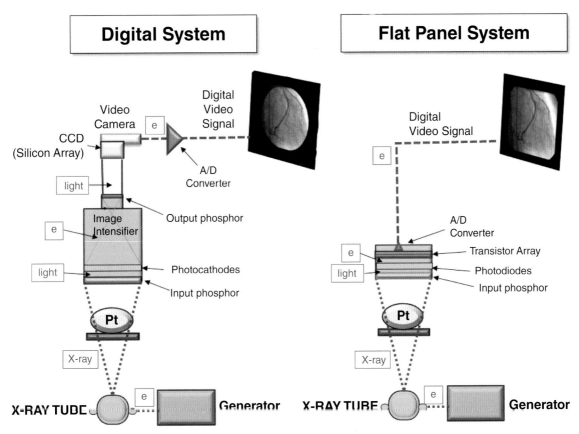

FIG. 3.9 ● **Comparison of image intensifier–based and flat panel detector–based fluoroscopic systems.** Reprinted with permission from Kern MJ. *SCAI Interventional Cardiology Board Review*. 2nd ed. Philadelphia, PA: Wolters Kluwer; 2014.

digitize and store these signals. FPD-based systems use integrated digital receptors to produce digital images directly.

II-based fluoroscopic systems

Image intensifier

An II is made of several major components enclosed by a vacuum housing; these components include the input screen, the electron focusing system, and the output port (Figure 3.10). Their structure and function are described as follows.

Input Screen

Following the direction of the incoming X-rays, the input screen can be divided into a few layers: (1) The first layer is the vacuum housing, typically made of aluminum. It separates the vacuum from outside and maintains the conditions critical for electron focusing. (2) The second layer is the vacuum. (3) The third layer is a support layer, made of thin aluminum, to both provide structural support and serve as part of the electron steering system. (4) The fourth layer is the input phosphor, which absorbs the incoming X-ray photons and converts them to fluorescent light photons. (5) The fifth layer is the photocathode, which converts fluorescent light photons to electrons.

Electron Focusing System

The electron focusing system consists of several pairs of electrodes. The electrons as well as the cathode and the anode are connected to different electrical potentials, and they together form electrical fields that drive the electrons originated from the cathode toward

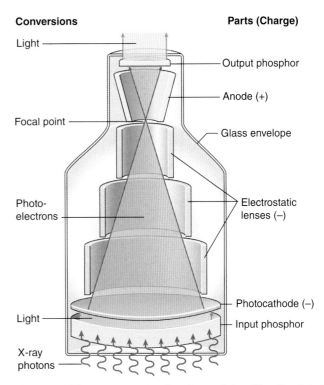

FIG. 3.10 ● **The components of an image intensifier.** Reprinted with permission from Fosbinder RA, Orth D. *Essentials of Radiologic Science*. Philadelphia, PA: Wolters Kluwer Health; 2012.

the anode at the output port. The electrons are also accelerated by the electrical fields and gain substantial amounts of kinetic energy before they strike on the anode. The amplification of the signal to achieve the desired brightness at the output is mainly accomplished by this component (Figure 3.11).

The curved shape of the input phosphor and the photocathode is purposely made to facilitate the focusing process. At the same time, it leads to geometric distortions. These distortions are nonexistent at the center of the field of view, but become more and more pronounced when moving away from the center. They are best demonstrated when a mesh grid is imaged; one would observe the most distortions of the squares at the boundaries of the field of view.

Output Port

The output port is made of three layers: the anode, the output phosphor, and the window. The anode attracts the electrons and also directs them away when they stop within the output phosphor. The output phosphor is where the electrons lose their kinetic energy through emission of visible light photons. The window is the final layer through which the produced light photons exit the II.

Optical coupling

The light output of the II needs to be coupled to the video camera using appropriate optics. The coupling may be implemented using either light guides made by optic fibers or lens-based systems (Figure 3.12).

Video camera

The video camera reads images from the output port of the II and sends them onto the viewing monitor. The video camera can be either an analog TV camera or a digital camera, depending on the type of the viewing monitor. Analog TV cameras work with analog monitors, like the cathode ray tube monitors, but they have been largely replaced by digital cameras, which work along with digital monitors, like a liquid crystal display.

FPD-based fluoroscopic systems

FPDs on fluoroscopic systems share the same principles as those used on radiographic systems. FPDs offer a number of benefits compared to IIs in fluoroscopic uses. They are more compact in size and thus give more room around the patient. They are also free of geometric distortions.

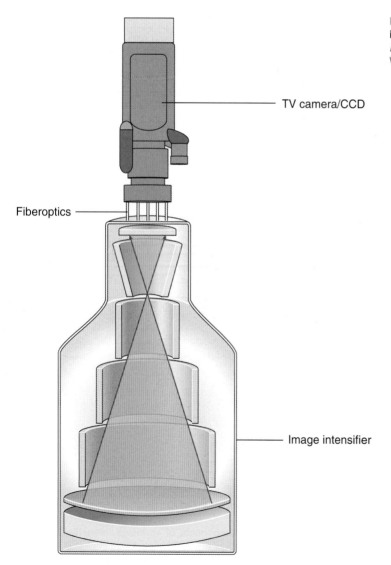

FIG. 3.11 ● **Illustration of image "intensification" by an image intensifier.** Reprinted with permission from Orth D. *Essentials of Radiologic Science.* 2nd ed. Philadelphia, PA: Wolters Kluwer; 2017.

TV camera/CCD

Fiberoptics

Image intensifier

FIG. 3.12 ● Optical coupling of the output of an image intensifier with video camera. Reprinted with permission from Orth D. *Essentials of Radiologic Science*. 2nd ed. Philadelphia, PA: Wolters Kluwer; 2017.

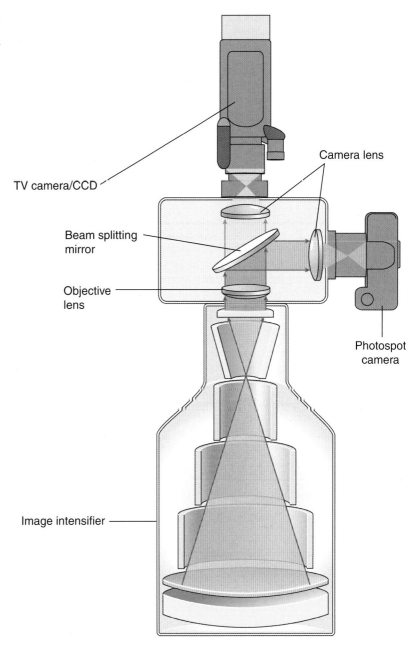

TV camera/CCD

Camera lens

Beam splitting mirror

Objective lens

Photospot camera

Image intensifier

Operating modes

Continuous fluoroscopy

Although continuous X-ray exposure is used in this mode (Figure 3.13), signals on the output screen of the II can be digitally sampled before they are displayed frame by frame on digital monitors. The duration of each frame, equal to the inverse of the sampling rate, determines the temporal resolution of the acquired frames; the shorter the duration, the less the motion blur and the higher the temporal resolution.

Pulsed fluoroscopy

X-ray exposures were made at constant pulse rates in this mode (Figure 3.13). The exposure duration, or the pulse width, is made shorter than the time between two successive exposures. The temporal resolution is determined by the pulse width instead of the pulse rate. Compared to continuous fluoroscopy, the temporal

resolution can become markedly higher without radiation penalty, as long as the product of exposure duration (for each frame) and mA remains constant. One may also use a lower frame rate as a means to reduce radiation dose when lower frame rates are deemed acceptable for characterizing the underlying motion.

Magnification mode

Magnification modes on a fluoroscopic system allow magnified view of small anatomic areas for improved spatial resolution. Its implementation on FPD-based systems is often by the use of different detector areas. On II-based systems, it works by changing the voltages of the electrodes in the electron focusing system so that only a small central area of the input screen has its generated electrons to be directed to cover the entire area of the output port (Figure 3.14). The X-ray field also adjusts its size accordingly so that only the area showing on the output port gets exposed.

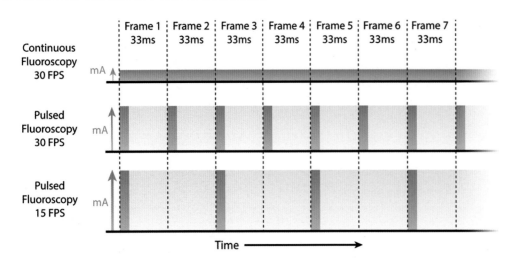

FIG. 3.13 ● **Continuous versus pulsed fluoroscopy of different frame rates.** Reprinted with permission from Huda W. *Review of Radiologic Physics.* 4th ed. Philadelphia, PA: Wolters Kluwer; 2016.

When switching from the normal mode to the magnification mode, the system typically increases its radiation output rate from the X-ray tube to maintain a constant brightness or signal level for its output image.

Frame averaging

Frame averaging reduces image noise by averaging over successive frames. Its drawback is motion blur and lower temporal resolution, because the frame duration becomes longer effectively. Frame averaging is used in applications where high temporal resolution is not crucially important and on systems with limited output.

Digital subtraction angiography

During angiographic procedures, the viewing of the vessels can be difficult when they are overlapped by the adjacent anatomy on the projectional views, even with the injection of iodinated contrast materials. Digital subtraction angiography removes the anatomic background through subtraction to leave enhanced vasculature alone on the frames, thereby boosting the image contrast (Figures 3.15 and 3.16). The subtraction can be done between two frames at different time points, one before and the other after the iodinated contrast materials arrive at the vasculature of interest. Alternatively, it can be done between two frames acquired with different X-ray beams, one filtered and the other unfiltered but at nearly identical time points.

Cone-beam computed tomography

The need to navigate complex anatomy in certain interventional procedures would be better served with three-dimensional imaging capabilities because projectional views at a few angles become rather limited in these applications. On C-arm fluoroscopic systems with FPD, cone-beam computed tomography (CT) acquisition is made available by rotating the assembly of X-ray tube and detector continuously around the anatomy of interest through an angular range of about 200° (varies by system design) and the hundreds of projectional views acquired during the rotation are reconstructed into a three-dimensional data set. Note that cone-beam CT on these systems is designed for image guidance instead of diagnosis; as a result, their image quality is generally inferior to that of diagnostic CT systems.

Automatic Brightness Control

Automatic brightness control (ABC) is a common feature on fluoroscopic systems that automatically adjust the radiation output rate to ensure a constant level of brightness on the image receptor. This term started on II-based systems and is straightforward there because the brightness at the II output primarily determines the operator's perception of image quality; as FPD-based systems became popular, it is often called automatic exposure rate control, but fundamentally they both involve adjustment of exposure rate to meet image quality requirements

The automatic adjustment of exposure rate on the detector surface is made through changes in kVp and mA as well as other parameters on certain systems. When the anatomy in the X-ray beam path becomes thicker, the decreased X-ray

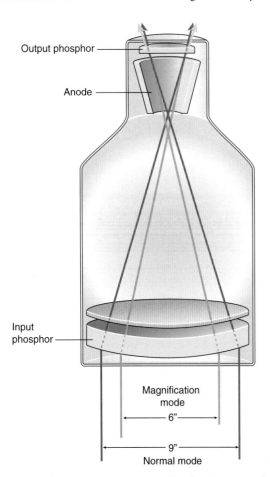

FIG. 3.14 ● **Illustration of how magnification works on image intensifiers.** Reprinted with permission from Fosbinder RA, Orth D. *Essentials of Radiologic Science.* Philadelphia, PA: Wolters Kluwer Health; 2012.

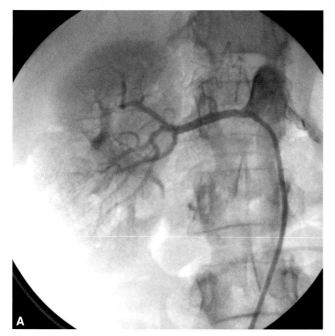

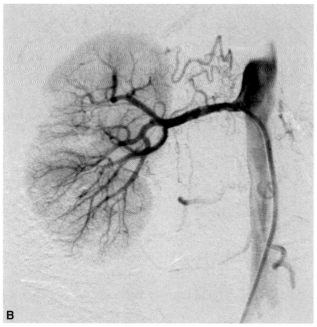

FIG. 3.15 ● Digital subtraction angiography of right renal arteries without (A) and with (B) the overlapping anatomy subtracted. Reprinted with permission from Casserly IP, Sachar R, Yadav JS. *Practical Peripheral Vascular Intervention*. 2nd ed. Philadelphia, PA: Wolters Kluwer Health/Lippincott Williams & Wilkins; 2011.

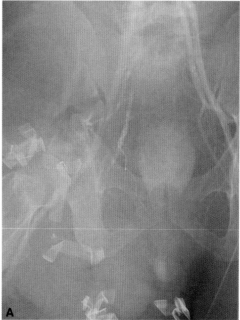

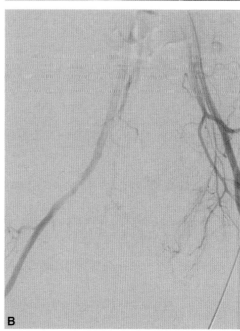

FIG. 3.16 ● Digital subtraction angiography of arteries near pelvis without (A) and with (B) the overlapping anatomy subtracted. Reprinted with permission from Kupinski AM. *The Vascular System*. 2nd ed. Philadelphia, PA: Wolters Kluwer; 2018.

exposure rate at the detector surface triggers the X-ray tube to use different kVp and/or mA to compensate for the decrease. Fluoroscopic systems have their specific kVp-mA curves that govern their adjustments of key technical parameters. The kVp-mA curves also differ in different modes (Figure 3.17). In the low-dose mode, kVp increase is primarily used when tissue thickness increases; higher kVp results in lower skin dose at the same detector signal level compared to lower kVp, but soft tissue contrast is compromised at the same time. In the high-contrast mode, mA increase is mainly employed for increasing detector signal when thicker tissues are imaged; soft tissue

contrast is preserved, but skin dose experiences a more rapid increase, proportional to mA.

DOSIMETRY FOR RADIOGRAPHY AND FLUOROSCOPY

In projectional X-ray imaging like radiography and fluoroscopy, it is typically the skin (or other tissues at shallow depth) at the X-ray beam entrance to body that receives the most radiation dose among all tissues, primarily because of the exponential decay of X-ray intensity as a function of tissue depth (Figure 3.18).

Automatic Brightness Control (ABC) Curves

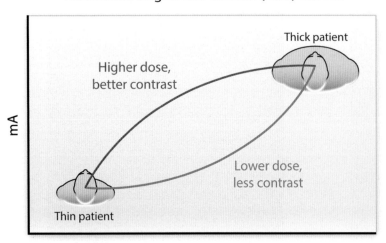

FIG. 3.17 ● Different kV-mA curves under different operating modes. Reprinted with permission from Huda W. *Review of Radiologic Physics.* 4th ed. Philadelphia, PA: Wolters Kluwer; 2016.

Air kerma is a commonly used radiation metric that is closely related to skin dose and can be readily measured. Air kerma is the in-air measurement of the photon energy released to air resulting in the production of ion pairs, in units of joule per kilogram or, equivalently, Gy. Air kerma at the skin entrance is used by radiographic and fluoroscopic systems to assist in the assessment of skin dose. Two other metrics related to air kerma, kerma-area-product (KAP) and air kerma rate (AKR), are also in common use. KAP incorporates the area of irradiated skin into an estimation of the total photon energy deposited in air at the skin entrance. AKR is only used in fluoroscopy as an indicator of the rate of X-ray energy deposition into air. Newer systems have live display of air kerma and/or AKR to allow real-time monitoring of radiation dose at the assumed skin entrance, as well as estimation of the incurred skin dose.

Regulation limits are often placed on the AKR of fluoroscopic systems to reduce the likelihood of excessive radiation to patient caused by typically long exposure times. Excessive radiation to skin is known to cause skin erythema, ulcer, and other severe reactions. In the United States, the AKR at the skin entrance cannot exceed 10 roentgens per minute (R/min) in the regular mode or 20 R/min in the high-level mode.

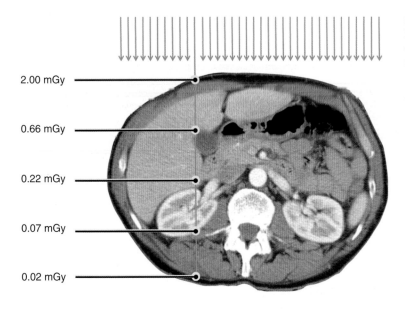

FIG. 3.18 ● Decay of tissue dose as a function of depth by a single-view X-ray exposure. In this example, tissue dose decays by about 100 times at the exit of body compared to at the entrance. Reprinted with permission from Bushberg JT, Seibert JA, Leidholdt EM, Boone JM. *Essential Physics of Medical Imaging.* 3rd ed. Philadelphia, PA. Wolters Kluwer Health/Lippincott Williams & Wilkins; 2012.

Suggested Readings

Bushberg JT, Seibert JA, Leidholdt EM, Boone JM. *The Essential Physics of Medical Imaging.* 3rd ed. Philadelphia, PA: Lippincott Williams & Wilkins; 2011.

Casserly IP, Sachar R, Yadav JS. *Practical Peripheral Vascular Intervention.* 2nd ed. Philadelphia, PA: Lippincott Williams & Wilkins; 2011.

Christman R. *Foot and Ankle Radiology.* 2nd ed. Philadelphia, PA: Lippincott Williams & Wilkins; 2014.

Fosbinder RA, Orth D. *Essentials of Radiologic Science.* Philadelphia, PA: Lippincott Williams & Wilkins; 2011.

Huda W. *Review of Radiologic Physics.* 4th ed. Philadelphia, PA: Lippincott Williams & Wilkins; 2016.

Kern MJ. *SCAI Interventional Cardiology Board Review.* 2nd ed. Philadelphia, PA: Lippincott Williams & Wilkins; 2013.

Moscucci M. *Grossman & Baim's Cardiac Catheterization, Angiography, and Intervention.* 8th ed. Philadelphia, PA: Lippincott Williams & Wilkins; 2013.

Orth D. *Essentials of Radiologic Science.* 2nd ed. Philadelphia, PA: Lippincott Williams & Wilkins; 2017.

Smith WL. *Radiology 101.* 4th ed. Philadelphia, PA: Lippincott Williams & Wilkins; 2013.

CHAPTER SELF-ASSESSMENT QUESTIONS

1. Which of the following is NOT true regarding an X-ray tube for medical imaging?

   A. It typically provides two or more focal spots.

   B. X-ray tubes with rotating anode are primarily used in radiography.

   C. Tungsten is commonly used as the target material.

   D. The majority of the input electrical energy is converted into X-ray photons.

2. Which of the following is true regarding the use of antiscatter grids in radiography?

   A. When available on the system, the grid should be used at all times to reduce scatter.

   B. The use of grid is an effective way of radiation dose reduction.

   C. The grid needs to be placed at its intended distance and well centered during its use.

   D. The use of grid is beneficial in imaging of hands and wrists.

3. Which of the following is NOT true regarding radiographic image quality?

   A. Short exposure time can be used to reduce motion-caused blur on image.

   B. Spatial resolution is the same everywhere on the image.

   C. Automatic exposure control keeps image noise constant regardless of object size.

   D. Changes in kVp (all other parameters unchanged) affect both image contrast and image noise.

4. Which of the following is NOT true regarding comparisons between II-based and FPD-based fluoroscopy?

   A. FPD-based systems support magnification modes, whereas II-based systems do not.

   B. FPD-based systems give more room around patient than II-based systems.

   C. FPD-based systems are less affected by geometric distortions as II-based systems.

   D. FPD- and II-based systems both have ABC or equivalent to ensure constant signal level on image receptor.

Answers to Chapter Self-Assessment Questions

1. D The majority of the input electrical energy is converted into heat.

2. C Since antiscatter grids remove both scattered and primary photons, the use of antiscatter grids involves trade-off between image quality improvement and dose penalty. Typically, an increase in radiation dose is necessary for the desired image quality (compared with when there is no scatter). Their use in imaging of small-sized anatomy is not well justified because the amount of scatter is relatively insignificant.

3. B Spatial resolution varies with the location in the field. The projected focal spot size, a major factor affecting spatial resolution, is not the same everywhere in the field (typically smaller near the anode).

4. A Magnification modes are supported on both FPD- and II-based systems.

X-ray Imaging: Mammography

4

Huimin Wu, PhD

LEARNING OBJECTIVES

1. Describe the main difference between the X-ray beams used for mammographic and radiographic imaging.
2. Name the commonly used materials for the anode target on a mammographic system.
3. Explain the role of the added beam filter in mammography.
4. Explain why molybdenum is never used as the filter when rhodium is the material for the anode target.
5. Name the main differences between screen-film cassettes used for mammography and those used for radiography.
6. Name the main reasons for breast compression in mammography.
7. List the methods commonly used for scatter reduction in mammography.
8. Explain how magnification mode works in mammography.
9. Explain the benefit of breast tomosynthesis in comparison with standard mammography.

OVERVIEW

Mammography is an X-ray imaging examination of breast tissues, primarily for detecting breast cancers. Breast cancers have both high morbidity and high mortality rates in the female population around the world. By estimate, one in eight women worldwide are affected by breast cancer. Early detection of breast cancer is considered crucial because treatment outcomes are typically better for breast cancers at earlier stages. Mammography plays a key role in the screening of breast cancer among asymptotic women, for the following reasons:

- Mammography excels at detecting certain early signs of breast cancer, including microcalcifications, speculated masses, and distorted tissues.
- Mammography demonstrates both high sensitivity and high specificity of cancer detection by clinical studies.
- Mammography poses minimal risk to the subject with very low radiation dose.
- Mammography is cost-effective and supports high throughput among a large population.

Mammography shares the same fundamental principles with radiography, but has its dedicated equipment and techniques to meet the unique challenges in breast imaging. For example, mammographic systems use X-ray beams of significantly lower energies than do standard X-ray equipment to increase the difference in attenuation between normal and cancerous tissues that would otherwise be too subtle for detection. Mammographic systems also use smaller focus spots and other measures to improve their spatial resolution for detecting microcalcifications. In addition, the level of radiation used by mammography is adjusted for each subject's breasts and kept low to pose minimal risk to the subject.

X-RAY BEAM

Mammography requires the use of X-ray beams of lower energies compared to those of radiography, as a result of the inherently small difference in X-ray attenuation between normal and cancerous tissues (Figure 4.1). At X-ray energies of 40 keV or higher (the mean energy level standard radiography uses), the difference between the two types of tissues becomes too subtle to detect; so low-energy X-rays are preferred. On the other hand, X-ray energy cannot be too low because nearly all X-ray photons would be absorbed without reaching the detector, leading to unnecessary radiation dose to breast tissues. X-ray beam with photon energies around 20 keV is considered optimal for breast imaging, and this principle is integrated into the design of mammographic X-ray tubes.

The difference between mammography and radiography in their X-ray beam quality can be seen in differences in their half-value layers (HVLs). HVLs of an X-ray beam, defined as the thickness of a reference material (aluminum is most often used) needed to attenuate the beam intensity by half, are commonly used to characterize its beam quality. The higher the HVL, the higher mean energy the X-ray beam has. As an example (Figure 4.2), the HVL of a mammographic X-ray beam (assuming the use of molybdenum as anode target) is about 0.3 mm at 27 kVp, an order of magnitude smaller than that of a typical radiographic X-ray beam at 80 kVp.

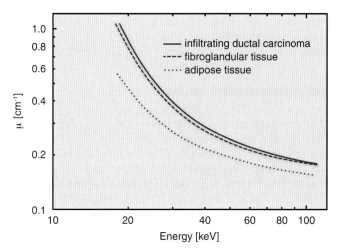

FIG. 4.1 ● **X-ray attenuation of breast tissues as a function of X-ray photon energy.** Reprinted with permission from Andolina VF, Lillé SL. Mammographic Imaging. 3rd ed. Philadelphia, PA: Wolters Kluwer Health/Lippincott Williams & Wilkins; 2011. From Johns PC, Yaffe MJ. X-ray characterization of normal and neo-plastic breast tissues. *Phys Med Biol.* 1987;32(6):675-695. Copyright © 1987 Institute of Physics and Engineering in Medicine. Reproduced by permission of IOP Publishing. All rights reserved.

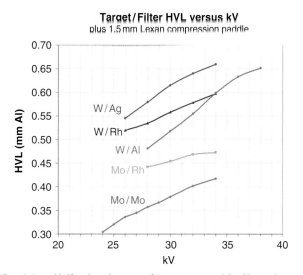

FIG. 4.2 ● **Half-value layers of mammographic X-ray beams.** Reprinted with permission from Bushberg JT, Seibert JA, Leidholdt EM, Boone JM. *Essential Physics of Medical Imaging.* 3rd ed. Philadelphia, PA: Wolters Kluwer Health/Lippincott Williams & Wilkins; 2012.

Tube voltage

Low kVp is used by mammographic X-ray tubes to ensure that the average energy of produced X-ray beams is near 20 keV. For normal-sized breasts, tube voltage of 25 to 28 kVp is often used.

Cathode

A mammographic X-ray tube often has two filaments installed to produce two focal spot sizes; 0.3 and 0.1 mm are typical nominal values for the large and small focal spot sizes, respectively. In comparison, the focal spots on a radiographic X-ray tube are typically a few times larger. Tube currents available on a mammographic tube are also substantially lower than those by a radiographic tube, because of the overheating issues associated with smaller focal areas on the target for the interactions between electrons and the target.

Anode target

Molybdenum (Mo) and rhodium (Rh) have long been used as anode target materials in screen-film and digital mammography. Characteristic X-rays, highly dependent on the electron-shell structure of the anode material, account for a large fraction of the X-ray photons produced by the X-ray tube; Mo and Rh both have an electron structure that results in abundant X-ray photons near 20 keV (17.5 and 19.6 keV for Mo, and 20.2 and 22.7 keV for Rh), the desired energy range for breast imaging.

Tungsten (W) is another anode target material mostly used in digital mammography. With digital detectors, despite an unfavorable choice regarding characteristic X-ray production, W shows the following advantages as the target material: W provides higher X-ray production efficiency, because of its higher atomic number, and much improved heat loading, because of its higher melting point, compared to Mo and Rh; in addition, wider dynamic range and postprocessing capabilities of digital detectors relax the requirement for X-ray beam energy, making characteristic radiation from Mo or Rh not as crucial as it is in screen-film mammography.

Table 4.1 shows a comparison of the three anode target materials in their physical properties related to mammography.

Beam filter

Both the tube port, as part of the inherent filtration, and the added beam filters play important roles in shaping the X-ray energy spectrum produced by a mammographic X-ray tube. Beryllium (Be) is typically used for the tube port where the beam exits the tube. Be has a low atomic number of 4 and is strong enough to be made thin. The thin tube port window made by Be absorbs low-energy X-ray photons that are unable to penetrate breasts and lets through those with higher energies.

Table 4.1 **MATERIAL PROPERTIES OF MOLYBDENUM, RHODIUM, AND TUNGSTEN, RELATED TO BEING ANODE TARGET OR BEAM FILTER FOR PRODUCING MAMMOGRAPHIC X-RAY BEAM.** Those physical properties highly favorable for mammographic imaging are highlighted in **bold**; these include the energies of the characteristic x-rays from Mo and Rh and the high melting point of W.

	Molybdenum (Mo)	Rhodium (Rh)	Tungsten (W)
Atomic no.	42	45	74
Physical density (g/cm³)	10.2	12.4	19.3
K_α X-ray energy (keV)	**17.5**	**20.2**	59.3
K_β X-ray energy (keV)	**19.6**	**22.7**	67.2
K-edge (keV)	20.0	23.2	69.5
Melting point (°C)	2620	1966	**3410**

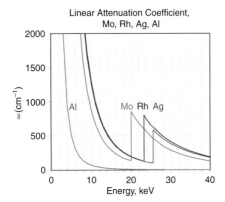

FIG. 4.3 ● **The attenuation characteristics of filter materials used on mammographic systems, including Mo, Rh, Ag, and Al. Mo, Rh, and Ag all have K-edges between 20 and 30 keV, useful for removing photons of high energy that could compromise tissue contrast otherwise.** Reprinted with permission from Bushberg JT, Seibert JA, Leidholdt EM, Boone JM. *Essential Physics of Medical Imaging.* 3rd ed. Philadelphia, PA: Wolters Kluwer Health/Lippincott Williams & Wilkins; 2012.

Added X-ray tube filtration further shapes the energy spectrum of the X-ray beam by selectively removing undesired X-ray photons with either too high or too low energies. It is often accomplished using materials that have K-edge energies that are slightly above the upper bound of the optimal energies for breast imaging. The K-edge of an element is the energy level at which X-ray photons have just enough energy to knock out atomic electrons on the K-orbit and a substantial increase in X-ray absorption results. Mo, Rh, and Ag are typical elements with suitable K-edge energies for providing added beam filtration for mammography (Figure 4.3). The added filter heavily absorbs both low-energy photons (<15 keV), due to high photoelectric absorption, and

high energy ones (above the K-edge), due to dramatically increased absorption beyond the K-edge. The result is selective transmission of X-rays in a narrow band of energies from about 15 keV up to the K-absorption edge of the filter.

Target-filter combination

The selection of the appropriate combination of target-filter materials is a nontrivial matter in mammographic tube design. When Mo or Rh is used as the target material, because of the abundant characteristic X-rays in the produced spectrum, the K-edge of the added filter needs to be slightly above the energies of those characteristic X-rays so as not to absorb these useful photons (Figure 4.4). If Mo is used as the target material, both Mo and Rh can be used as the filter materials. If Rh is used as the target material, then Rh itself is an acceptable filter material, but Mo would not be a good candidate because its K-edge is lower than the energies of characteristic X-rays produced by an Rh target.

When W is used as the target material, practical choices of filter materials include Rh, Ag, and Al. Because of its large atomic number, W produces a smaller fraction of characteristic X-rays than do Mo and Rh as a target, and these photons are at higher energies than the K-absorption edges of the filter materials listed. Rh is routinely used for imaging of normal-sized or smaller breasts. The energy band of transmitted X-rays for Ag is shifted toward the higher end compared to that for Rh, so Ag is often the choice when imaging larger than normal breasts. Figure 4.5 shows X-ray spectra of the target-filter combinations of W/Rh and W/Ag. Al is mostly used for tomosynthesis acquisition, a mode of multiview acquisition for producing a 3D-like image set. Al does not have a sufficiently high K-edge to reject higher energy photons, so it primarily serves to remove low-energy ones for dose savings. The rejection of higher energy photons is not a strong need in tomosynthesis for image contrast considerations, because of the improvement in image contrast that comes with the reconstruction process in tomosynthesis.

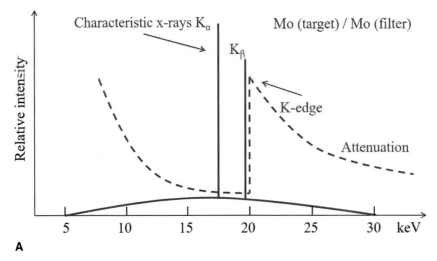

A

FIG. 4.4 ● A-D: Choice of appropriate target-filter combinations when Mo and Rh are used as target and filter. Mo/Mo, Mo/Rh, and Rh/Rh all provide X-ray spectra suitable for mammography with mean energies around 20 keV; the combinations with Rh as filter have higher average energy because the spectra are cut off at higher energy by the K-edge of Rh. Rh/Mo would not work well for mammography because Rh-produced characteristic X-rays are removed by the K-edge absorption by the Mo filter.

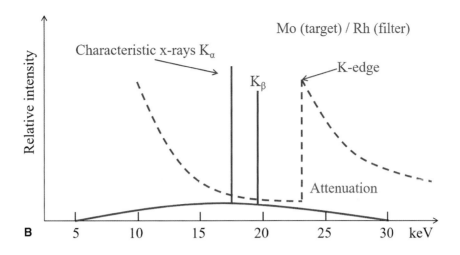

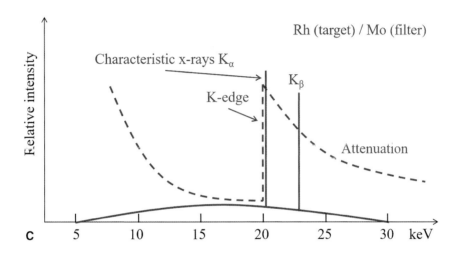

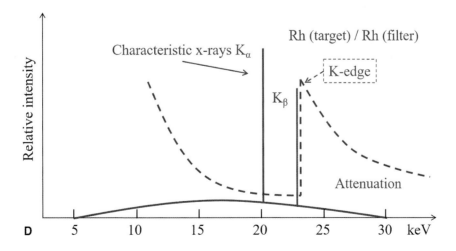

FIG. 4.4 ● (*continued*)

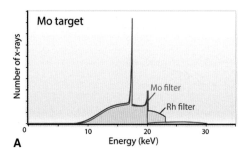
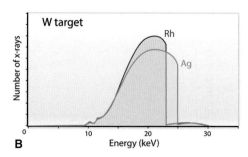

FIG. 4.5 ● A, B: Target-filter combinations of Mo/Mo, Mo/Rh, W/Rh, and W/Ag, and their produced X-ray spectra. Reprinted with permission from Huda W. *Review of Radiologic Physics*. 4th ed. Philadelphia, PA: Wolters Kluwer; 2016.

Tube tilting and orientation

The X-ray tube is particularly oriented such that the cathode is close to the patient and the anode is away, to account for the heel effect (Figure 4.6). As discussed in radiography, the heel effect

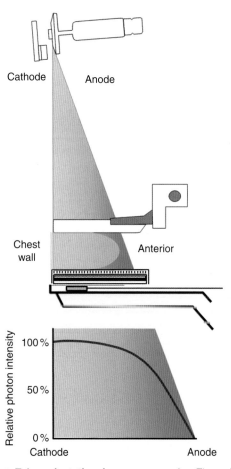

FIG. 4.6 ● **Tube orientation in mammography.** The axis of the cathode-anode is perpendicular to the chest wall and the cathode is closer to the chest wall. The orientation is largely based on heel effect. The heel effect refers to the decrease in X-ray intensity from the cathode side to the anode side, due to interactions between X-ray and the target surface. The thickness of the breast also sees a decrease moving away from the chest wall toward the nipple. Therefore, the specific tube orientation allows thicker tissues to be exposed by X-rays of higher intensities for more uniform image quality. Reprinted with permission from Bushberg JT, Seibert JA, Leidholdt EM, Boone JM. *Essential Physics of Medical Imaging*. 3rd ed. Philadelphia, PA: Wolters Kluwer Health/Lippincott Williams & Wilkins; 2012.

refers to the fact that the intensity of the X-rays emitted from the focal spot varies, with the greatest intensity on the cathode side of the projected field and the lowest intensity on the anode side. In a clinical examination, the positioning of the X-ray tube, as described earlier, allows higher X-ray intensity to match with thicker breast tissues near the chest wall and lower intensity with thinner tissues around the nipple.

The X-ray tube is also mounted with its cathode-anode axis at an angle with respect to the horizontal level (Figure 4.7). This angled configuration is necessary because of the following considerations: (1) the bounding plane of the X-ray field proximal to the standing patient is parallel to the chest wall so that minimal radiation is given to the chest wall and tissues behind; and (2) the X-ray field is sufficiently large to cover the examined breast without the use of larger anode angle, which would compromise the system's performance in spatial resolution.

IMAGE RECEPTOR

Screen-film cassettes have been used as image receptors in mammography for decades before the recent trend in digital mammography. Clinical studies have found that the statistical difference between the clinical performances of the two types of image receptors is not significant for the entire women population, although digital detectors do demonstrate advantages for certain subgroups, including women younger than 50 years, women with dense breasts, and premenopausal or perimenopausal women. Given here is a brief discussion of the two major types of image receptors for mammography.

Screen-film cassette

Mammographic screen-film cassettes are largely similar to radiographic ones in their design. Special considerations specific to mammography are reflected in their design, including (but not limited to):

- The encasing cassette is made of low-attenuation carbon fiber to allow transmission of lower energy X-ray photons.
- Its typical configuration is featured by a single emulsion film and a single phosphor screen, with the screen mounted on the beam-exit side of the cassette. With this configuration, X-rays go through the film first before interactions with the screen. Owing to the exponential decay of X-rays, a larger fraction of X-ray photons interacts near the surface of the screen than at the depths; much more visible light photons are therefore produced closer to the film than farther away, resulting in a narrower light diffusion and therefore higher spatial resolution compared to the configuration in which the screen is on the beam-entranced side of the cassette.

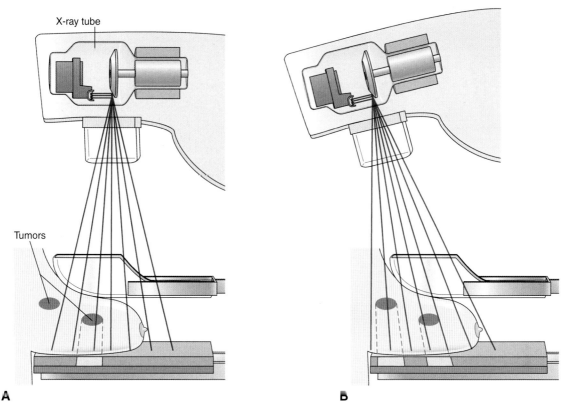

FIG. 4.7 ● A, B: Tube tilting in mammography. Tilting allows more effective coverage of the entire breast with minimal X-ray exposure to the chest wall. It also allows an increase in X-ray field size without the need for a larger anode angle, which would compromise spatial resolution of images if used. Reprinted with permission from Fosbinder RA, Orth D. *Essentials of Radiologic Science.* Philadelphia, PA: Wolters Kluwer Health; 2012.

- Mammographic cassettes typically have lower speed ratings than do the conventional radiographic ones. Speed in the discussions of X-ray image receptors is linked to the level of X-ray exposure clinically required to reach the desired signal level; the higher the speed, the less exposure it takes to produce the desired optical density on film. The use of a single emulsion film, for spatial resolution considerations discussed earlier, accounts for the higher exposure necessary to expose the film to the desired optical density.

Mammographic films also have different requirements in viewing conditions compared to the conventional radiographic films. View boxes for the reading of mammographic films must provide sufficiently high luminance (a measure of brightness level of a light source) so that small differences in optical densities on the film may be perceived by eye. The luminance of a mammography view box should exceed a minimum of 3000 cd/m^2 and are commonly at levels higher than 6000 cd/m^2. In comparison, the luminance of a view box for general radiology is about 1500 cd/m^2.

Digital detector

A major advantage of digital detectors over screen-film cassettes is their much wider exposure latitude. The latitude is the ratio of the maximum exposure to the minimum exposure of the range within which the image receptor exhibits a linear response

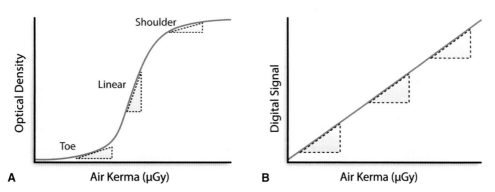

FIG. 4.8 ● A, B: Comparison between screen-film and digital receptors in their response to radiation. The linear range over which the response remains linear is much wider for digital receptors compared with screen-film receptors. Reprinted with permission from Huda W. *Review of Radiologic Physics.* 4th ed. Philadelphia, PA: Wolters Kluwer; 2016.

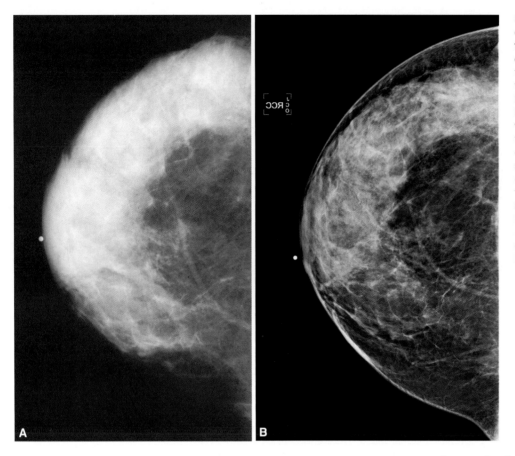

FIG. 4.9 ● A clinical case demonstrating the benefits of digital mammography in imaging dense breast. Using screen-film technique (A), this patient's breast tissue appears dense and shows little intrinsic contrast, possibly allowing for obscuration of a cancer, which may be of similar attenuation to normal tissue. However, the digital technique, used 1 year subsequently (B), provides improved dynamic range, resulting in greater tissue contrast. Reprinted with permission from Harris JR, Lippman ME, Osborne CK, Morrow M. *Diseases of the Breast.* 4th ed. Philadelphia, PA: Wolters Kluwer Health/Lippincott Williams & Wilkins; 2009.

(Figure 4.8). The variations in the thicknesses, for example, skin lines versus the middle section, and compositions, fatty versus glandular tissues, within the breasts may result in exposures varying by more than a few hundred times across the detector. Screen-film cassettes, whose exposure latitude is approximately 25:1, have limited capabilities in displaying the entire breast appropriately; highly glandular tissues could get underexposed, while fatty tissues could get overexposed. Digital detectors have a wider latitude to match with the variations in tissue thickness and composition across the breast and ensure high image contrast for all regions within the breast. The use of digital detectors is therefore beneficial for imaging dense and thick breasts (Figure 4.9).

BREAST COMPRESSION

Firm compression of the breast during exposure is necessary for high image quality (Figure 4.10). The benefits of breast compression include (1) tissue contrast is improved because of reduced overlapping and fewer scattered X-rays, (2) the likelihood of tissue motion and the associated blurring becomes less, (3) a narrower range of exposures across the detector leads to more potential for improved contrast, (4) radiation dose to the breast tissues may be lower, and (5) more breast tissues can be pressed away from the chest wall and included within the field of view.

Foot-pedal-controlled, motor-driven compression paddles are typically used for breast compression with additional manual controls for fine adjustment. A full-field compression paddle typically applies a mechanical force of 25 to 45 lb to achieve a uniform breast thickness. A spot paddle may be used for a small region of interest for local enhancement.

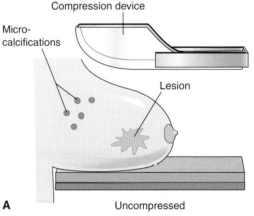

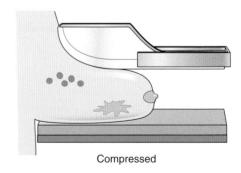

FIG. 4.10 ● Breast compression in mammography. When breast is compressed (B) and tissue penetration depth by x-ray is reduced, lesions may become more conspicuous and the micro-calcifications better resolved, compared with when there is no compression (A). Reprinted with permission from Fosbinder RA, Orth D. *Essentials of Radiologic Science.* Philadelphia, PA: Wolters Kluwer Health; 2012.

MAGNIFICATION MODE

In the magnification mode, the breast is placed on top of a support platform, aka the magnification stand, accompanied by the use of a small focal spot (~0.1 mm) and the retraction of the antiscatter grid (Figure 4.11). The major benefit of the magnification mode is improved spatial resolution, because of the magnified view and the resulting smaller effective pixel size; at the same time, the blurring effect by moving the object closer to the X-ray source is compensated for by the use of a smaller focal spot. The air gap introduced by the support platform also provides an effective way of scatter reduction in the absence of an antiscatter grid.

SCATTER MANAGEMENT

The intensity of scattered X-rays relative to that of primary ones, characterized by the scatter-to-primary ratio (SPR), is a function of breast thickness and the X-ray field size. Breast compression is an effective measure for reducing scattered X-ray photons (Figure 4.12). By compressing a breast from a 6- to 8-cm thickness in its uncompressed state to a nearly uniform 4-cm thickness, SPR reduces by approximately 50%.

Antiscatter grids are commonly used for scatter mitigation in mammography. In addition to 1D grids, cellular grids, made of copper septa in crossed patterns, have been used for

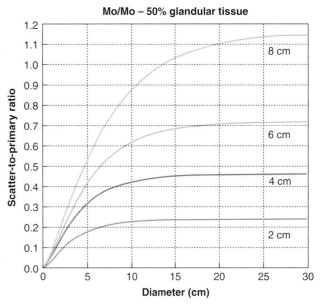

Mo/Mo – 50% glandular tissue

FIG. 4.12 ● **Plot of scatter-to-primary ratio as a function of the size (cross-field) and thickness of the breast.** Reprinted with permission from Bushberg JT, Seibert JA, Leidholdt EM, Boone JM. *Essential Physics of Medical Imaging.* 3rd ed. Philadelphia, PA: Wolters Kluwer Health/Lippincott Williams & Wilkins; 2012.

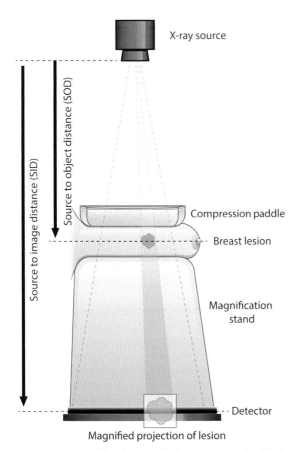

FIG. 4.11 ● **The magnification mode of mammography.** The breast is moved closer to the X-ray tube, but most of the time, only part of the breast is irradiated. The lesions appear larger compared with contact mammography, and overall image quality typically improves. Reprinted with permission from Huda W. *Review of Radiologic Physics.* 4th ed. Philadelphia, PA: Wolters Kluwer; 2016.

scatter rejection in two dimensions. The air-gap technique, used in the magnification mode (described previously), provides an alternative means of scatter reduction to antiscatter grids. Figure 4.13 illustrates two types of antiscatter grids and the air-gap technique.

STEREOTACTIC BREAST BIOPSY

Stereotactic breast biopsy systems use mammographic images to determine, with high accuracy and precision, the 3D locations of breast lesions and to guide the sampling of lesion tissues.

A stand-alone stereotactic breast biopsy system is typically designed in a pendulant geometry. During the procedure, the patient lies prone on the table, with one of the breasts dropping through a hole and being imaged and accessed from below (Figure 4.14). The X-ray tube, the detector, and the biopsy needle guide are mounted on a platform beneath the table. X-ray images are used to determine the exact spatial location, in particular the depth, and guide the needle to extract the tissue with high precision. The imaging part of the procedure is as follows. After an initial scout image taken at 0° (when the central ray connecting the source and the center of the detector is perpendicular to the compressed breast by paddle), two other images are taken at typically +15° and −15°. Assume the horizontal and vertical axes within the detector plane are the x- and y-axes, respectively, and the axis perpendicular to the detector plane is the z-axis. The x- and y-coordinates of the lesions are determined from the 0° image. The z-coordinate, or the depth of the lesion within the compressed breast, is determined from the separation between the lesion's positions on the +15° and −15° images, utilizing trigonometry relationships (Figure 4.15). Digital detectors of the charge coupled device type are used on these systems, because the required field of view for such application is small, that is, approximately 5 × 5 cm².

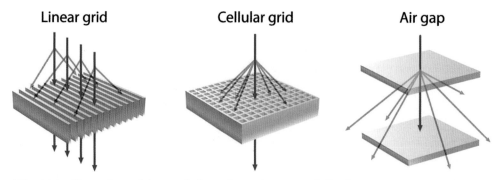

Linear grid   Cellular grid   Air gap

FIG. 4.13 ● **Illustrations of three techniques for scatter removal.** The first two use antiscatter grids, either 1D (left) or 2D (middle). Air-gap technique (right) introduces the gap between the breast and image receptor for scatter removal. Reprinted with permission from Huda W. *Review of Radiologic Physics.* 4th ed. Philadelphia, PA: Wolters Kluwer; 2016.

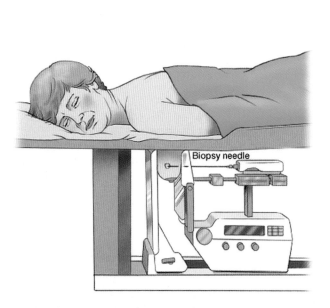

FIG. 4.14 ● **Illustration of the setup of stereotactic breast biopsy.** The patient is placed in the prone position on a table and the breast to be biopsied is compressed firmly between two plates. Reprinted with permission from Lippincott Nursing Advisor, 2014. © Wolters Kluwer.

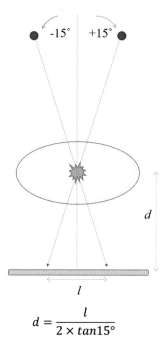

$$d = \frac{l}{2 \times tan15°}$$

FIG. 4.15 ● **Illustration of how the depth of the target lesion is determined in stereotactic breast biopsy.** The depth of the target lesion can be derived from the distance between the locations of the target lesion on the images acquired at −15° and +15° (X-ray source rotates but detector remains stationary).

TOMOSYNTHESIS

Mammography has a fundamental limitation in lesion detection because of its 2D nature, that is, tissue overlapping lowers image contrast and obscures lesion detection. Breast tomosynthesis is a novel acquisition method that addresses the limitation by acquiring multiple projection views over a limited angular range (Figure 4.16). After an image reconstruction process, a stack of images become available, each of which represents a plane through the breast volume and displays all the in-plane structures "in focus" while any out-of-the-plane structure gets "blurred out" effectively.

Breast tomosynthesis is made possible by digital detector technologies, that is, rapid acquisition of multiple images using flat panel detectors. One of the commercially available systems

acquires 15 projection views of the compressed breast over an angular range of 15° (−7.5° to +7.5°) in approximately 4 seconds. The anode uses a tungsten target together with an aluminum filter to produce the X-ray beam. In clinical settings, tomosynthesis acquisition may be either accompanied by a conventional mammography acquisition in a so-called combo mode, with the former accounting for slightly less than 50% of total radiation, or stand-alone with software capabilities to synthesize virtual mammographic images to reduce radiation dose.

RADIATION DOSE

Radiation dose to the breast by mammography is of concern because of its impact on a large population through screening. Regulations as per the Mammography Quality Standards Act

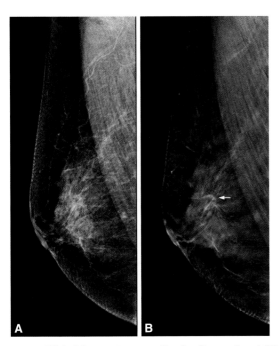

FIG. 4.16 ● **Digital breast tomosynthesis.** Conventional 2D mediolateral oblique digital mammogram (A) and single image from a 3D digital breast tomosynthesis (DBT) scan (B) depicting a small irregular/spiculated mass (arrow) just above the nipple in the middle one-third of the breast. Note that the conspicuity of the mass is significantly improved on the DBT Image. Reprinted with permission from Smith WL. *Radiology 101*. 4th ed. Philadelphia, PA: Wolters Kluwer Health/Lippincott Williams & Wilkins; 2014.

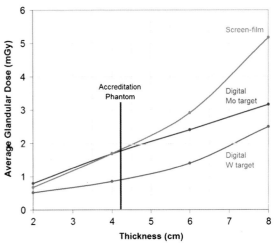

FIG. 4.17 ● **Average glandular doses of several mammographic systems made with different technologies and designs, including screen-film detector with Mo target and Mo/Rh filtration (green), a digital system using a-Se direct conversion detector with Mo target and Mo/Rh filtration (purple), and a digital system using a-Se direct conversion detector with W target and Rh/Ag filtration (blue).** The accreditation phantom (4.5-cm thickness) is indicated with the vertical black bar for comparison of average glandular dose noted in Mammography Quality Standards Act reports. Reprinted with permission from Bushberg JT, Seibert JA, Leidholdt EM, Boone JM. *Essential Physics of Medical Imaging*. 3rd ed. Philadelphia, PA: Wolters Kluwer Health/Lippincott Williams & Wilkins; 2012.

require that the average glandular dose for a compressed breast thickness of 4.2 cm and a composition of 50% glandular and 50% adipose tissue not exceed 3 mGy per view (view may be either cranial-caudal or medial-lateral oblique).

The average glandular dose is not easily measured even on phantoms, because of the heterogeneity of radiation dose within the breast. The intensity of X-ray decreases exponentially as it goes through tissues, and radiation dose follows approximately the same trend. With typically a pair of views acquired for each breast, skin tissues at beam entrance receive much higher radiation dose than those at depth. A practical method to determine average glandular dose is to derive it from the entrance exposure using a lookup table; the lookup table is determined with extensive experiment and careful measurement under a variety of conditions and considers factors like kVp, X-ray beam quality, and so on.

Radiation dose to the breast of a mammographic system is affected by its technologies and designs. Figure 4.17 shows average glandular doses measured on several mammographic systems with different technologies and designs; the trend shows the benefits of the tungsten target in general and the digital detector in imaging thicker breasts.

Suggested Readings

Bushberg JT, Seibert JA, Leidholdt EM, Boone JM. *The Essential Physics of Medical Imaging*. 3rd ed. Philadelphia, PA: Lippincott Williams & Wilkins; 2011.

Fosbinder RA, Orth D. *Essentials of Radiologic Science*. Philadelphia, PA: Lippincott Williams & Wilkins; 2011.

Huda W. *Review of Radiologic Physics*. 4th ed. Philadelphia, PA: Lippincott Williams & Wilkins; 2016.

Smith WL. *Radiology 101*. 4th ed. Philadelphia, PA: Lippincott Williams & Wilkins; 2013.

CHAPTER SELF-ASSESSMENT QUESTIONS

1. Which of the following is NOT true regarding mammographic X-ray tubes using tungsten as anode target material?

   A. Tungsten targets are often used on digital mammography systems.

   B. Tungsten targets produce X-ray spectra with higher mean energies than do molybdenum or rhodium targets.

   C. Tungsten targets allow the tubes to operate at higher power than do molybdenum or rhodium targets.

   D. Tungsten targets are less affected by heel effects than are molybdenum or rhodium targets.

2. Which of the following is NOT true regarding the magnification mode in mammography?

   A. Magnification mode has a smaller field of view than the normal mode.

   B. Magnification mode has poor image contrast because antiscatter grid is not used.

   C. Magnification mode has improved spatial resolution compared to normal mode.

   D. Magnification mode uses the small focal spot.

3. Which one of the following is NOT true regarding breast compression in mammography?

   A. It brings more tissues near the chest wall into the field of view.

   B. It reduces overlapping of breast tissues and improves image contrast.

   C. It leads to substantial increases in radiation dose compared to no compression.

   D. It reduces the chances of motion caused by image blur.

Answers to Chapter Self-Assessment Questions

1. D Tungsten targets are less affected by heel effects than are molybdenum or rhodium targets.

2. B Magnification mode has poor image contrast because antiscatter grid is not used.

3. C It leads to substantial increases in radiation dose compared to no compression.

X-ray Imaging: Computed Tomography

5

Zhihua Qi, PhD

LEARNING OBJECTIVES

1. Define computed tomography (CT) number and name two materials whose CT numbers stay constant regardless of the X-ray beam energy spectrum.
2. Explain the role of bow-tie filters on a CT scanner.
3. Explain the importance of the slip ring on diagnostic CT scanners.
4. Compare analytic reconstruction with iterative reconstruction and state their differences.
5. Explain the benefits of helical scan compared to axial scan and define helical pitch.
6. Explain how tube current modulation (TCM) works and why it is desired on diagnostic CT scanners.
7. Explain how various technical parameters affect CT image quality.
8. Recognize common artifacts on CT images and understand their causes.
9. Explain the concepts of Computed Tomography Dose Index (CTDI), dose length product (DLP), and effective dose.
10. Name approaches one may take in pediatric CT to minimize unnecessary radiation.

INTRODUCTION

CT produces cross-sectional images of the object of interest through acquisition of multiple views, typically with X-ray radiation (although its principles have been widely used in applications outside of X-rays). The exploration of clinical use of CT began in the 1960s; G.T. Hounsfield and McCormack made independent investigations at that time, and were later awarded the Nobel Prize in Physiology and Medicine for their pioneering work. Since then, CT has gone through tremendous development and growth to become a highly valuable imaging tool in routine clinical use.

A number of different configurations have been used by CT; the most commonly used configuration in today's CT scanners is referred to as the third generation (Figure 5.1). This design is also referred to as a "rotate-rotate" geometry. It is typically featured by the use of one or two assemblies of X-ray tube and detector which are fixed relative to each other and rotate around the patient for data acquisition. The X-ray beam emanating from the X-ray tube is divergent in all dimensions; usually, its divergence is discussed separately in the plane of rotation (the transverse plane or the *x-y* plane) and in the axial direction (or the *z*-direction) (Figures 5.2 and 5.3). The angle of the X-ray beam in the plane of rotation is referred to as the fan angle, usually about 60° to cover the body cross-section of a normal-sized patient. The angle of the X-ray beam in the axial direction, referred to as the cone angle, is much smaller than the fan angle. If the cone angle is so small that the X-ray beam divergence in the axial direction can be neglected without significant impact on image quality, it is often called fan beam; otherwise it is often called cone beam.

Compared to projectional X-ray imaging, CT eliminates tissue overlapping and allows an object to be characterized at each individual point, resulting in substantially improved contrast. In a reconstructed CT image, the value associated with each individual point is essentially its attenuation coefficient at the effective

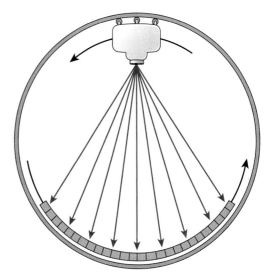

Rotating detector system

FIG. 5.1 ● The illustration of the third-generation computed tomography. Reprinted with permission from Orth D. *Essentials of Radiologic Science.* 2nd ed. Philadelphia, PA: Wolters Kluwer; 2017.

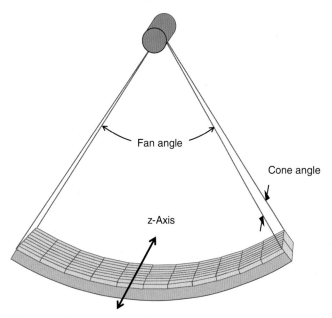

FIG. 5.2 ● **The concepts of fan angle and cone angle.** Reprinted with permission from Bushberg JT, Seibert JA, Leidholdt EM, Boone JM. *Essential Physics of Medical Imaging.* 3rd ed. Philadelphia, PA: Wolters Kluwer Health/Lippincott Williams & Wilkins; 2012.

X-ray beam energy used for acquisition. CT number is a quantity defined for the convenience of clinical use on the basis of X-ray attenuation coefficient. Its definition is

$$CT\# = \frac{\mu - \mu_{water}}{\mu_{water}} \times 1000,$$

where μ and μ_{water} are the X-ray attenuation coefficients of the image point and water, respectively, at the effective X-ray beam energy used for acquisition. By definition, CT numbers for water and air are constant regardless of X-ray beam energy. For water, its CT number is always zero, whereas for air, its CT number is always -1000. Other than these two materials, CT number for a certain material generally varies by X-ray beam energy. Typical CT numbers of human tissues are shown in Figure 5.4.

CT SYSTEM

The components of a modern CT system include the X-ray tube, the detector, the gantry, the data acquisition system (DAS), the patient table, the control console, the reconstruction engine, and others. The inside of a CT scanner when the cover is off is shown in Figures 5.5 and 5.6. Several of these components are discussed in more detail later.

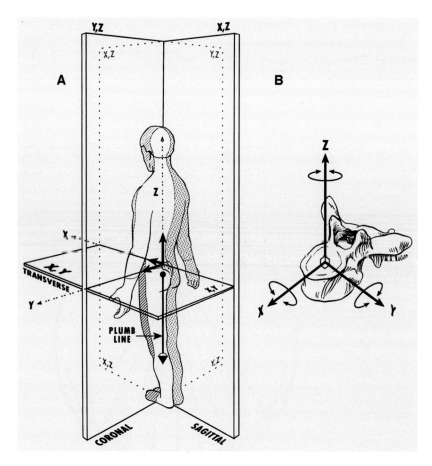

FIG. 5.3 ● **The patient coordinate system.** Reprinted with permission from Bridwell KH, DeWald RL. *Textbook of Spinal Surgery.* 3rd ed. Philadelphia, PA: Wolters Kluwer Health/Lippincott Williams & Wilkins; 2011.

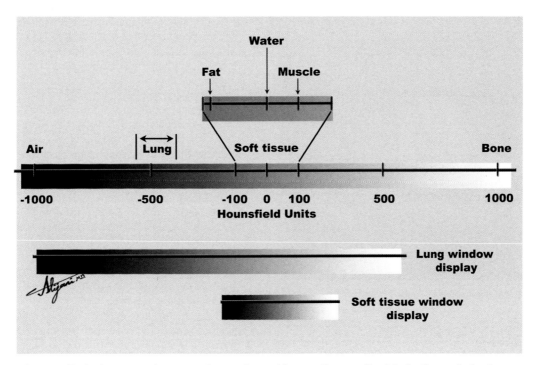

FIG. 5.4 ● Typical computed tomography numbers of human tissues. Reprinted with permission from Huda W. *Review of Radiologic Physics.* 3rd ed. Philadelphia, PA: Wolters Kluwer Health/Lippincott Williams & Wilkins; 2010.

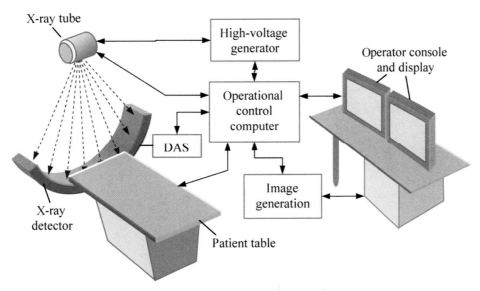

FIG. 5.5 ● The block diagram of a computed tomography system. DAS, data acquisition system. From Hsieh J. *Computed Tomography Principles, Design, Artifacts, and Recent Advances.* 2nd ed. Hoboken, NJ: John Wiley & Sons, Inc; 2009. Copyright © 2009 The Society of Photo-Optical Instrumentation Engineers. Reprinted by permission of John Wiley & Sons, Inc.

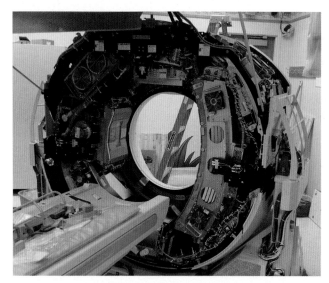

FIG. 5.6 ● A clinical CT scanner when the cover is off.

X-ray tube

As the X-ray-producing component of the system, the X-ray tube produces sufficient flux of X-ray photons at desired energy levels within a typically short scan time. It is important for the X-ray tube to be both powerful and robust to meet the clinical needs in a radiology department. The performance of the X-ray tube affects both image quality of the scans and radiation dose received by patients. Discussions of several important aspects regarding the tube are provided as follows:

• Heat management—the majority of the input electrical energy is converted into heat in the process of X-ray production.

An X-ray tube of high performance should be able to withstand high temperature and dissipate heat rapidly and efficiently. The use of liquid metal bearings is one example of X-ray tube designs that promote heat management. Liquid metal bearings support the anode and facilitate its rotation during an exposure, as conventional ball bearings do, but offer much improved efficiency in the conduction of the produced heat.

• X-ray beam energy—the energy spectrum of X-ray photons produced by an X-ray tube is mostly continuous within its range, with several discrete peaks characteristic of the anode material (Figure 5.7). The tube voltage, applied between the anode and the cathode, defines the maximum energy of the spectrum. The mean energy of the X-ray beam, in the unit of keV, is approximately between 1/3 and 1/2 of the kVp value. Most often, 120 kVp is used for head and body examinations of typical adult patients, but other kVps are available for the consideration of various patient sizes and different clinical tasks. On clinical scanners, 80 to 140 kVps in the increment of 20 kVp are typical offerings, but 70 and 150 kVp have become available on some newer models for advanced needs.

• Focal spots—two filaments are usually available in the X-ray tube to provide dual focal spots for imaging. The small focal spot is used for applications that require high spatial resolution, like imaging of extremities and small bony structures, whereas the large one is used for those that require high flux of X-ray photons, like body imaging. During the flight of high-speed electrons from the cathode to the anode, the electron beam may have broader lateral spread by the time it reaches the anode because of the repulsive force between electrons. Both kVp and mA affect the lateral spread, so the focal spot varies for different combinations of kVp and mA settings. Newer technologies have been introduced to allow active control of the lateral spread and therefore more constant focal spot size regardless of the choices of kVp and mA.

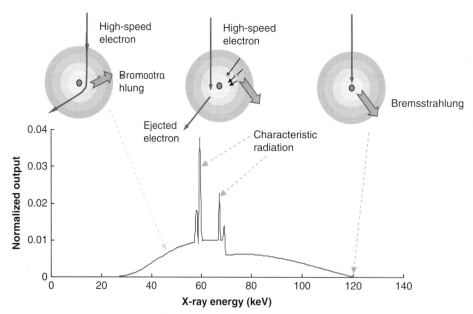

FIG. 5.7 ● **The typical X-ray spectrum for a computed tomography scanner when 120 kVp is used and the involved interactions of high-speed electrons.** Reprinted with permission from Bammer R. *MR and CT Perfusion and Pharmacokinetic Imaging: Clinical Applications and Theoretical Principles.* Philadelphia, PA: Wolters Kluwer; 2016.

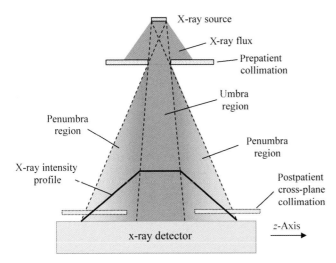

FIG. 5.8 • **Pre- and postpatient X-ray beam collimators used on computed tomography scanners.** From Hsieh J. *Computed Tomography Principles, Design, Artifacts, and Recent Advances.* 2nd ed. Hoboken, NJ: John Wiley & Sons, Inc; 2009. Copyright © 2009 The Society of Photo-Optical Instrumentation Engineers. Reprinted by permission of John Wiley & Sons, Inc.

X-ray beam collimator

Collimators are important components of a CT system. A CT scanner has both a prepatient collimator and a postpatient collimator, which work together to limit radiation to only the area of clinical interest (Figure 5.8). The use of a postpatient collimator is necessitated because the focal spot usually has a finite size and produces nonnegligible penumbra beyond the boundaries defined by the prepatient collimator.

X-ray collimation is also served by the antiscatter grid, mounted on the surface of the detector. The purpose of an antiscatter grid is to keep scattered photons from reaching the detector for image quality improvement. 1D grids are common, although some high-end models have employed 2D grids for improved reduction in scatter.

X-ray beam filter

Filters are devices mounted at the beam exit port of an X-ray tube to further modify the intensity and energy characteristics of the X-ray beam before it interacts with patients.

Two types of filters are typically used. The first is a thin flat filter made of metal and applied to "harden" the X-ray beam by preferentially removing low-energy photons in the beam. The second is often called a bow-tie filter, whose profile is to account for the oval shape of the human body. When a homogeneous X-ray field is incident upon the human body, the center of the detector receives the lowest signal because of the longest X-ray attenuation path, whereas peripheral areas of the detector corresponding to body boundaries receive the highest signal because of little attenuation along the path. This is undesired because the range of signals received by the detector may be too wide to handle and the body periphery receives much higher radiation than is necessary. The bow-tie filter provides an effective solution to this problem by equalizing the X-ray flux across the detector within the axial plane (Figure 5.9). A CT scanner typically has several bow-tie filters optimized for different body sizes.

Detector

Solid-state detectors are the most common type of detectors used on diagnostic scanners today. These detectors can use either an indirect conversion or direct conversion process for X-ray detection (Figure 5.10).

Indirect conversion detector

Indirect conversion detectors are used in nearly all clinical CT scanners today. With this technology, a detector is made of a block of scintillating material coupled to a photodiode array. An incident X-ray photon undergoes a photoelectric interaction with the scintillator, and, as a result, produces a freely moving photoelectron, which goes on to excite electrons in other atoms. When these excited electrons return to their ground state, characteristic photons are emitted in the visible or ultraviolet light spectrum. Those light photons traveling toward the photodiode array will

FIG. 5.9 • **The role of bow-tie filter in signal equalization.** Reprinted with permission from Bushberg JT, Seibert JA, Leidholdt EM, Boone JM. *Essential Physics of Medical Imaging.* 3rd ed. Philadelphia, PA: Wolters Kluwer Health/Lippincott Williams & Wilkins; 2012.

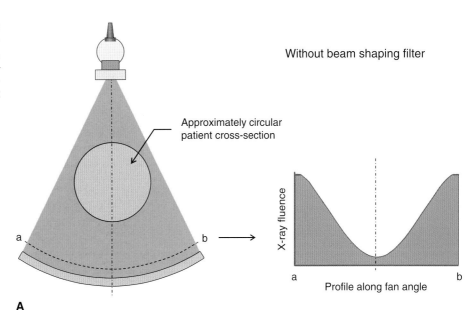

FIG. 5.9 ● (*continued*)

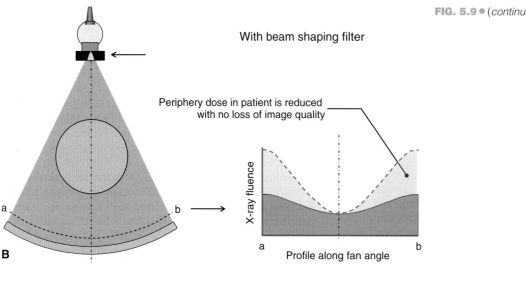

With beam shaping filter

Periphery dose in patient is reduced
with no loss of image quality

X-ray fluence

a

b

Profile along fan angle

B

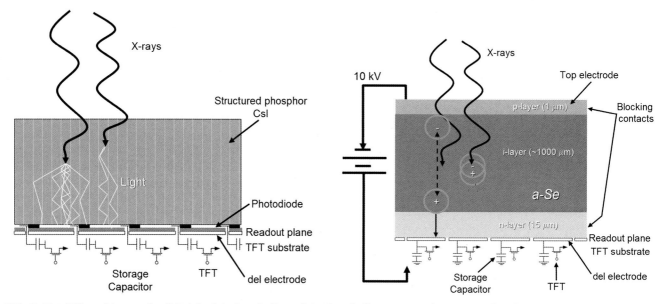

FIG. 5.10 ● **Different types of solid-state detectors in X-ray detection: indirect conversion versus direction conversion.** TFT, thin-film transistor. Reprinted with permission from Kandarpa K, Machan L, Durham J. *Handbook of Interventional Radiologic Procedures.* 5th ed. Philadelphia, PA: Wolters Kluwer, 2010.

convert their energies to electrical signals, which are subsequently processed, digitized, and stored by the electronics of the DAS.

The light photons produced by the scintillation process travel in all directions. To direct more light photons toward the photodiode array, the scintillator block is often divided into an array of columns and reflective coatings are applied at the boundaries of individual columns. When light photons travel in directions other than the forward, they will be reflected toward the photodiode array for higher detection efficiency.

Geometric configuration

A CT detector is a 2D array of individual detector elements or pixels. It can be viewed as multiple identical rows stacking up along the longitudinal axis (*z*-axis). Scanners nowadays typically have 16, 32, 64, 128, or more row of detectors, and within each row, there are thousands of detector pixels distributed along an arc (~60°) concentric to the X-ray source (if the source is at the

same plane defined by the arc). The detector pixel, the smallest unit of X-ray detection, has comparable sizes in both dimensions; when projected to the isocenter, the pixel sizes are typically within the range of 0.5 to 0.625 mm.

The configuration of detector rows in the longitudinal direction varies by both hardware design and clinical use. This is illustrated in Figure 5.11.

Detector performance

The performance of the detector closely impacts image quality of CT. Some clinically relevant aspects of its performance are discussed as follows:

- Primary speed—during the acquisition of each projection view, the scintillation process takes time to complete before the scintillator can return to its ground state and be ready for the acquisition of the next view. In general, the faster the primary speed of a detector is, the less contamination from previous views

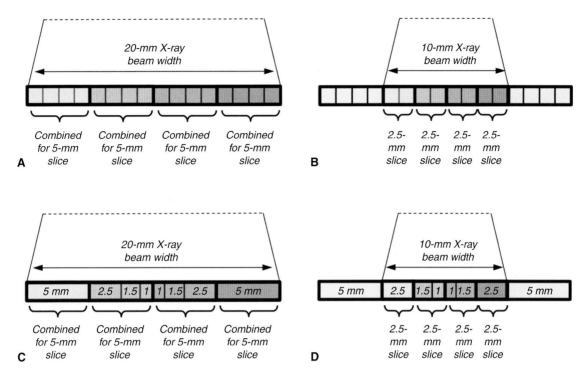

FIG. 5.11 ● The configuration of detector rows in the longitudinal direction. Some detectors use uniform detector row thicknesses (A, B), whereas others use variable thicknesses with thinner ones near the center (C, D). The rows may also be combined to provide choices of different slice thicknesses needed by clinical applications. Reprinted with permission from Bammer R. *MR and CT Perfusion and Pharmacokinetic Imaging: Clinical Applications and Theoretical Principles.* Philadelphia, PA: Wolters Kluwer; 2016.

there is in the data for each view. For those studies that require the fastest rotation speed and/or the highest view sampling rate a scanner can afford, detector primary speed needs to be fast enough to reduce or eliminate blurring caused by signal contamination between neighboring views.

- Radiation history—the gain of a detector changes after its scintillator is exposed to X-ray flux. Although such changes may be subtle within a short period, they can result in substantial differences across the detector array and therefore in artifacts on CT images. This issue can be addressed by (1) avoiding unnecessary exposures to detector channels by choosing the appropriate scan field of view and (2) routine calibrations or corrections. New materials insensitive to radiation damage are also of interest to minimize radiation history–related artifacts.

- Uniformity—the pixels of a detector are typically grouped into channels along the angular direction. Channel-to-channel uniformity is crucial in producing artifact-free CT images. If the response of a channel to radiation deviates substantially from that of the others, artifacts arise on images, typically in the form of arcs or rings on the images.

- Cross-talk—ideally, the signal of a detector pixel should be separate and independent from that of its neighboring pixels, but, in practice, there are often leakage signals for each pixel from its neighbors. Cross-talk causes loss of spatial resolution and degradation of image quality.

Direct conversion detector

In recent years, direct conversion detectors have been extensively investigated for their use in CT. This type of detector is made of a layer of photoconductor, like selenium and cadmium zinc telluride, with a bias voltage applied across the detector structure. The X-ray photons generate electron-hole pairs in the photoconductor layer and each pair, once generated, is swiftly swept to the electrodes by the electric field to produce its electrical signal. When built with ultrafast readout electronics, the direct conversion detector may allow each individual photon to be measured for its energy, which opens up opportunities for applications like multienergy imaging, low-dose CT, and so on. One of the major challenges faced by this excitingly new technology includes the robustness of the detector and its capability of handling high X-ray photon flux.

Gantry

The gantry of a modern CT scanner needs to support high-speed transfer of power, data, and signals. At any time during a CT scan, between the moving parts, rotating at high speed, and the stationary gantry, large amounts of electrical energy, data, and control signals need to be transferred within a very short time. Slip ring is an enabling technology for high-speed continuous rotation on a CT scanner (Figure 5.12). Slip ring includes essentially high-performance electrical brushes that maintain close contact between the moving and nonmoving parts and ensure timely transmission between them.

The gantry also requires high mechanical standards to fulfill the requirements of clinical CT scans. The rotating components of a CT scanner can easily weigh over 1000 lb, and, while such a large load is rotating at high speed, high degrees of mechanical accuracy and precision are also desired. A simple fact in the mechanical design is that the centrifugal force a gantry needs to withstand increases with the square of the rotation speed. Therefore, for a scanner to improve its rotation time from 0.35 to 0.25 seconds, that is, an improvement by 40%, the centrifugal force the gantry has to withstand nearly doubles.

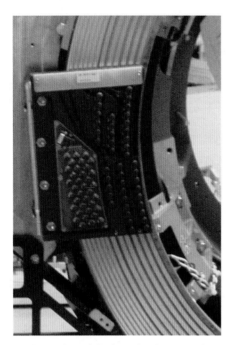

FIG. 5.12 ● **A close view of the junction between the rotating and nonrotating components of a slip ring system.** Reprinted with permission from Bammer R. *MR and CT Perfusion and Pharmacokinetic Imaging: Clinical Applications and Theoretical Principles.* Philadelphia, PA: Wolters Kluwer; 2016.

Original Object   Sinogram

Backprojection   Filtered Backprojection

FIG. 5.13 ● **The comparison of back projection (BP) and filtered back projection (FBP) in the reconstruction a digital phantom.** BP reconstructs only a blurred version of the true image, whereas FPB, in comparison, reconstructs an accurate image (aliasing artifacts are due to insufficient sampling rate in simulation). Reprinted with permission from Sadock BJ, Saddock VA, Ruiz P. *Kaplan and Sadock's Comprehensive Textbook of Psychiatry.* 10th ed. Philadelphia, PA: Wolters Kluwer; 2017.

CT RECONSTRUCTION

There are largely two types of reconstruction algorithms for CT, analytic and iterative reconstruction algorithms. Filtered back projection (FBP) is the basis of most analytic algorithms and has been used as primary for a long time on clinical scanners. Iterative algorithms did not gain popularity in early days of CT, but have moved rapidly into clinical practice in recent years, mainly due to advances in computation speed and demands in imaging with lower radiation dose.

Analytic reconstruction

Back projection

Back projection (BP) is not practically used, but, as an intuition-based concept, is helpful to the understanding of the later introduced FBP. With this algorithm, the reconstructed image starts as a matrix of zeroes at all locations. Then, at each view angle and for each detector element, the image pixels encompassed by the X-ray beam illuminating the detector element are identified, and the value of the detector element is added to each of these identified pixels. By projecting the signal back along its path, the process is intuitively a reversal of the signal production. One may easily notice that BP reconstructs a blurred version of the original image (Figure 5.13). Such a blur comes as no surprise in that, along each ray path, each image pixel contributes differently to the value of the detector pixel, and such nonuniformity is lost while the same value is back projected to each image pixel in the reconstruction. A deblurring step is necessary to ensure the exactness of reconstruction.

Filtered back projection

FBP is the basis of the vast majority of analytic algorithms used on CT scanners. An FBP algorithm consists of two steps: first, in the "filtering" step, projection data of each view, are filtered by a specially designed function, often called "filter" or "kernel," and then, in the "back projection" step, each detector element, with its data filtered, back projects and adds its contribution to the pixels along the ray path that produces its signal. With the added filtering step, FBP is able to give a theoretically exact reconstruction of the image (Figure 5.13).

The concept of k-space, the concept used extensively by magnetic resonance imaging, is helpful in understanding how FBP works. It is a domain in which any object is viewed as a summation of spatially oscillating patterns of various frequencies and characterized by its intensity distribution over these different frequencies. Assuming a CT scan in which a parallel x-ray beam (a beam of x-rays parallel to each other) rotates around the patient, the projection data acquired at each view is essentially a line in the k-space which goes through the origin and is angled specifically to the view angle; with projection data from all different views, the k-space counterpart of the desired image can be assembled and the image recovered through a well-defined mathematical transform, aka the Fourier transform. This is called central slice theorem, as is illustrated in Figure 5.14. In short, the problem of reconstructing an image turns into solving its k-space counterpart followed by a well-defined transform back into the spatial domain. In practice, one could only acquire a finite number of view angles, and, at each of them, acquire data at only a finite number of points. With the view angles and data points on each view typically evenly spaced,

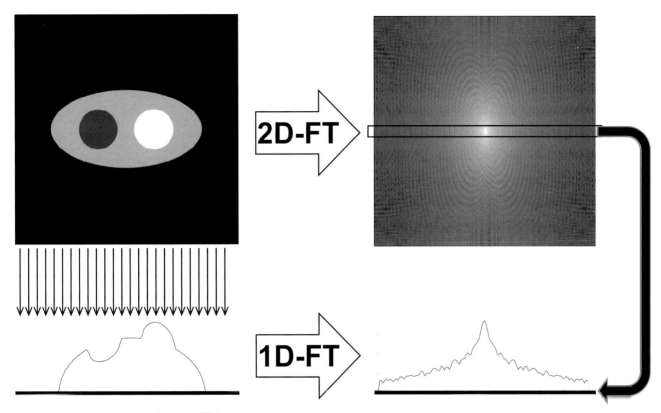

FIG. 5.14 ● The central slice theorem. FT, Fourier transform. Reprinted with permission from von Schulthess GK. *Molecular Anatomic Imaging.* 3rd ed. Philadelphia, PA: Wolters Kluwer; 2016.

k-space regions near the origin (low-frequency regions) are covered at a density higher than those far away (high-frequency regions). To compensate for this nonuniformity in sampling density, it becomes necessary to give higher weighting to high-frequency data points than to low-frequency ones at each view angle. This explains why filtering is a necessary step of the reconstruction and why the applied filter is in a "ramp" shape, namely, it increases linearly, from zero at the origin toward higher frequency.

Although the filter is, in theory, a ramp function to ensure the exactness of the reconstruction, it is often modified to enhance certain aspects of image quality depending on the clinical application. A "body" filter is designed to suppress noise and give the resulting images a smoother look to resolve subtle signal differences between lesions and normal tissues in body examinations. This filter is nearly the same as the ramp filter in the low-frequency range, but as the frequency gets higher, it starts to roll off instead of continuing to increase for the desired suppression of noise in the high-frequency range. A "bone" filter, on the other hand, is designed to enhance features of tiny sizes to detect bone fractures, calcified specks, and others alike. Therefore, one should expect higher values in the high-frequency range of the filter compared to those of the ramp filter.

FBP algorithms gain popularity in their clinical use because of simplicity and speed. At the same time, their simplicity, mostly due to assumptions of rather ideal systems, has led to limitations in addressing issues affecting practical systems.

Iterative reconstruction

In an iterative algorithm, models accounting for practical aspects of a CT scan are incorporated into the reconstruction process. As an analytic solution in one step becomes unattainable, an iterative algorithm utilizes a numerical approach to solve for the desired image; this approach starts with an estimated image, and iteratively updates it following a model-driven guidance until the level of consistency between the image and the projection measurements becomes acceptable. Figure 5.15 illustrates a typical workflow of iterative reconstruction.

Compared to the standard FBP algorithms, iterative reconstruction algorithms are able to make improvements in image quality through lowering image noise, suppression of artifacts, and others. Their capability of lowering image noise can be translated to reduction in radiation dose to patients. Despite the potential clinical benefits of iterative reconstruction algorithms, special attention should be paid to their uses in clinical applications, with considerations such as (1) they may introduce substantial change in the texture of image noise, which may produce undesired artifacts and interfere with visual detection of subtle features on images; (2) they may introduce changes in the quantitative aspects of CT images and make necessary changes in the existing standards on the basis of traditional algorithms. The capability of radiation dose reduction by an iterative reconstruction algorithm needs to be carefully evaluated for each diagnostic task with considerations of their impact on diagnostic performance.

CT TECHNIQUES

Axial scan

In an axial scan (Figure 5.16), the tube-detector assembly rotates around the patient while the patient couch stays still. To cover

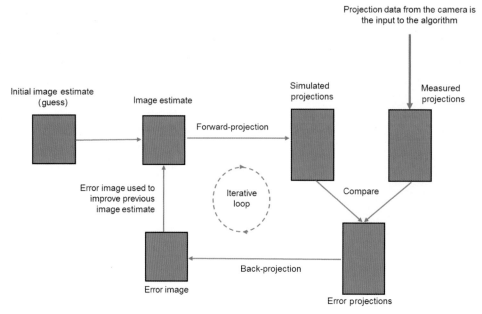

FIG. 5.15 ● **A typical workflow of iterative reconstruction.** Reprinted with permission from Chandra R, Rahmim A. *Nuclear Medicine Physics: The Basics.* 8th ed. Philadelphia, PA: Wolters Kluwer; 2018.

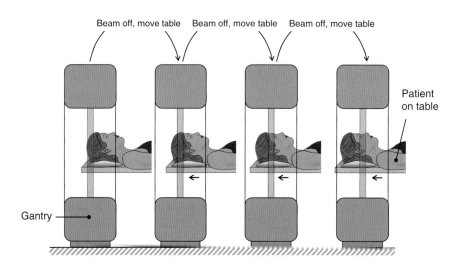

FIG. 5.16 ● **Illustration of axial computed tomography scan, aka step-and-shoot scan.** Reprinted with permission from Bushberg JT, Seibert JA, Leidholdt EM, Boone JM. *Essential Physics of Medical Imaging.* 3rd ed. Philadelphia, PA: Wolters Kluwer Health/Lippincott Williams & Wilkins; 2012.

anatomy longer than the longitude coverage of a single axial scan, a step-and-shoot mode may be employed, in which the couch steps through a series of locations with an axial scan performed at each step but with no radiation between steps.

Helical scan

In a helical scan (Figure 5.17), the tube-detector assembly rotates around the patient while the patient is continuously translated through the center of rotation. It allows a fast scan through an anatomic volume.

Helical pitch is a common concept used in the characterization of how fast the patient table moves relative to the width of the detector coverage. It is defined as the table feed per 360° gantry rotation divided by the width of the detector coverage at the isocenter.

Cine scan

A cine scan (Figure 5.18) refers to a series of axial scans at the same couch location for the characterization of temporal changes in the anatomy of interest.

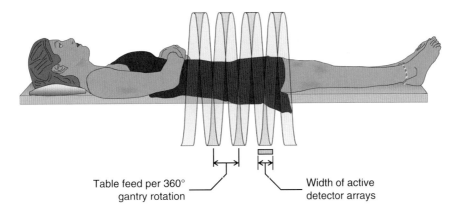

Table feed per 360°
gantry rotation

Width of active
detector arrays

Helical or spiral CT acquisition

FIG. 5.17 ● Illustration of a helical computed tomography scan. Reprinted with permission from Bushberg JT, Seibert JA, Leidholdt EM, Boone JM. *Essential Physics of Medical Imaging.* 3rd ed. Philadelphia, PA: Wolters Kluwer Health/Lippincott Williams & Wilkins; 2012.

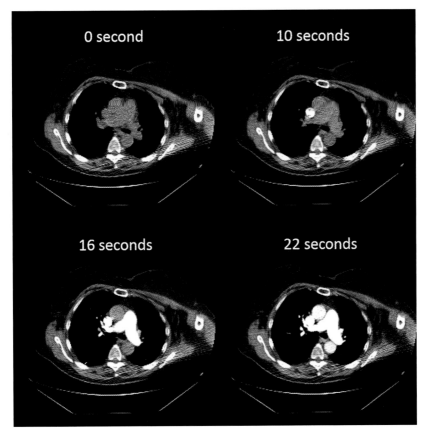

FIG. 5.18 ● An example of cine computed tomography (CT), in which a series of CT scans are performed at a fixed chest location to monitor the arrival of contrast in the aorta so that a subsequent computed tomography angiography may be triggered at the right time point.

Gated scan

With a gated scan, exposure to the patient is made only when the patient is at a desired physiologic state. A gated scan is often desired in imaging organs subject to breathing and/or cardiac motion. The differences in the images when the cardiac structures are scanned with and without gating are shown in Figure 5.19.

Although a gated scan may intuitively mean a scan in which the beam is only on at certain time points, it may refer to two different scan modes. The first is the prospectively gated scan, as the intuitive

meaning of a gated scan. The other is the retrospectively gated scan, in which the beam is always on (may vary in its X-ray flux), but images for a certain physiologic state may be retrospectively reconstructed using only the data acquired at the intended state. Illustrations of the two different modes are shown in Figure 5.20.

Tube current modulation

Tube current may be modulated for optimizing image quality and/or minimizing radiation to certain radiation-sensitive

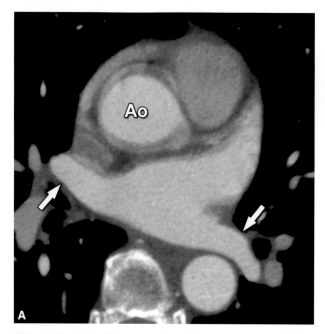
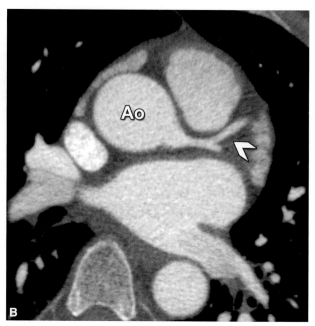

FIG. 5.19 ● A, B, The comparison of gated versus nongated scans of cardiac structures. Ao, aorta. Reprinted with permission from Higgins CB, de Roos A. *MRI and CT of the Cardiovascular System.* 3rd ed. Philadelphia, PA: Wolters Kluwer Health/Lippincott Williams & Wilkins; 2013.

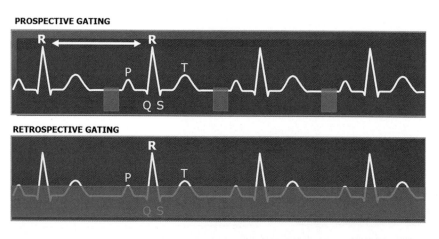

FIG. 5.20 ● **Illustrations of prospectively versus retrospectively gated computed tomography scans.** Reprinted with permission from Webb WR, Higgins CB. *Thoracic Imaging.* 3rd ed. Philadelphia, PA: Wolters Kluwer; 2017.

organs. Tube current modulation (TCM) may be applied in a variety of scenarios, including, but not limited to, the following: (1) When a body part, like the shoulder or pelvis, varies in its thickness (X-ray penetrating path length) at different tube angles, tube current may increase when X-ray beams go through longer path lengths and decrease when they go through shorter ones, to minimize streak artifacts along the long axis of the scanned body part. See Figure 5.21 for an illustration. (2) When the attenuation of different body parts varies substantially along the long axis, tube current may vary as the scanner scans through different body parts to maintain a relatively constant image noise at all locations. See Figures 5.22 and 5.23 for illustrations. (3) During a cardiac CT scan where images at all phases are desired, one may increase tube current within a certain phase window for high quality and decrease tube current outside the window to meet typically lower image quality requirements there. See Figure 5.24 for an illustration. (4) To minimize radiation to certain radiation-sensitive organs (like

the breasts for scanning young female patients), tube current may reduce when the tube is closer to them. This is often called organ-based modulation or selective organ shielding.

Dual-source CT

Dual-source CT acquires data using two sets of X-ray tube and detector installed on the same scanner gantry (Figure 5.25). Dual-source CT proves valuable in the following clinical applications:

• The temporal resolution of dual-source CT is superior to that of single-source CT with the same rotation time. For any point near the isocenter, single-source CT needs at least 180° rotation to acquire sufficient data for its reconstruction. For dual-source CT on which the two sets of X-ray tube and detector are 90° relative to each other, the data needed can be acquired with only 90° rotation because the two of them together will cover 180°. Hence, the effective temporal window for any point near the isocenter on a dual-source CT is only half of that on a single-source CT.

FIG. 5.21 ● A, B, Angular modulation of tube current in computed tomography. Reprinted with permission from Bushberg JT, Seibert JA, Leidholdt EM, Boone JM. *Essential Physics of Medical Imaging*. 3rd ed. Philadelphia, PA: Wolters Kluwer Health/Lippincott Williams & Wilkins; 2012.

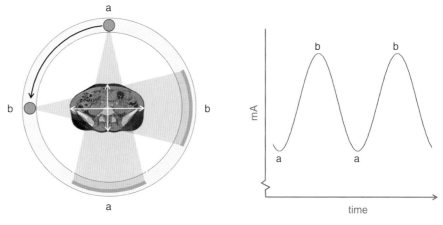

A. Tube rotation around oval patient   **B.** mA modulation

FIG. 5.22 ● **Longitudinal modulation of tube current in computed tomography.** Reprinted with permission from Bushberg JT, Seibert JA, Leidholdt EM, Boone JM. *Essential Physics of Medical Imaging*. 3rd ed. Philadelphia, PA: Wolters Kluwer Health/Lippincott Williams & Wilkins; 2012.

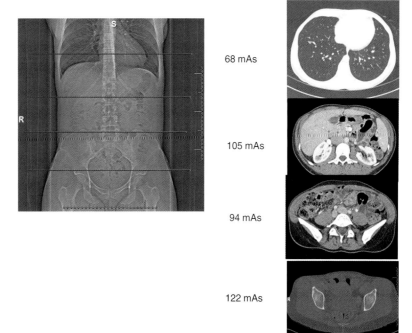

68 mAs

105 mAs

94 mAs

122 mAs

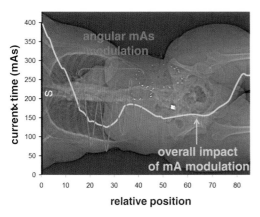

FIG. 5.23 ● **Simultaneous angular and longitudinal modulation of tube current in computed tomography.** Reprinted with permission from Bushberg JT, Seibert JA, Leidholdt EM, Boone JM. *Essential Physics of Medical Imaging*. 3rd ed. Philadelphia, PA: Wolters Kluwer Health/Lippincott Williams & Wilkins; 2012.

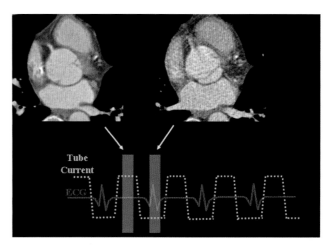

FIG. 5.24 ● **Electrocardiography (ECG)-based tube current modulation in computed tomography.** Reprinted with permission from Garcia MJ. *NonInvasive Cardiovascular Imaging: A Multimodality Approach*. Philadelphia, PA: Wolters Kluwer Health/Lippincott Williams & Wilkins; 2010.

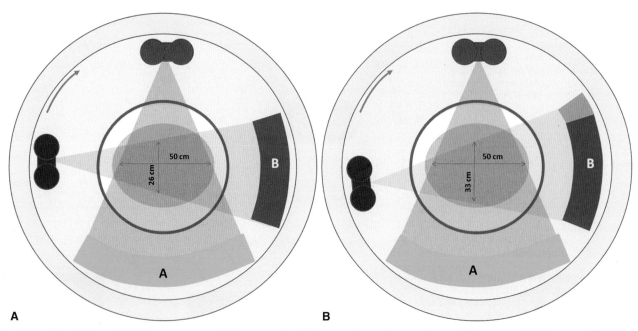

FIG. 5.25 ● **Illustrations of dual-source computed tomography (CT) geometry on two versions of CT scanners by Siemens.** While the two X-ray tubes are identical, the two detectors differ in size. On the earlier version (A), the larger detector supports a 50-cm field of view and the smaller a 26-cm field of view. On the later version (B), the smaller detector increases its coverage to support a 33-cm field of view. Reprinted with permission from Saremi F. *Perfusion Imaging in Clinical Practice.* Philadelphia, PA: Wolters Kluwer; 2015.

This is particularly valuable in cardiac CT, where temporal resolution is crucial for minimizing motion artifacts.

- The speed of volumetric coverage nearly doubles with the use of two sets of X-ray tubes and detectors. Single-source CT supports helical pitches up to 1.6, whereas dual-source CT allows for helical pitches as high as 3.4. Assuming a rotation time of 270 ms and detectors of 6 cm in longitudinal coverage (at the isocenter), the travel speed of the patient table, the volumetric coverage speed can also reach 71 cm/s. The scan of the whole heart (assuming 16 cm in length) can be completed under 250 ms, with each local point in the heart effectively acquired under 65 ms. Other clinical benefits of faster volumetric coverage include savings on iodinated contrast and less use of sedation for patients; the former is beneficial to patients with impaired renal function when contrast-enhanced studies are necessary, whereas the latter is of importance in pediatric applications.

- Dual-source CT offers a unique implementation of dual-energy CT. When the two X-ray tubes are operating at different kVps, two scans using different X-ray energy spectra are acquired nearly at the same time; the two sets of acquired images can be processed to provide more information than single-source CT for improved material differentiation, quantitative imaging, artifact reduction, and other benefits.

Dual-energy CT

Dual-energy CT makes two sets of acquisitions of the subject using different energy spectra with the goal of providing clinically valuable information that would be impossible with CT numbers for a single-energy spectrum. Its applications include material differentiation, iodine quantification, and others.

The underlying principles of dual-energy CT can be explained as follows. The CT number of any tissue reflects the probability of interactions between X-ray photons and the tissue. In the energy range of diagnostic X-ray, the interactions primarily involve two types: photoelectric effect and Compton scatter. The probability of interaction as a function of the photon energy differs between the two. With acquisitions using two different X-ray energy spectra, one can mathematically solve for individual contributions from the two types of interactions, which would be impossible with a single acquisition. Knowing individual contributions from the two interactions not only provides new perspectives for differentiation and separation of tissues and materials but also allows quantitative determination of parameters of potential clinical values, including electron density, atomic number, iodine concentration, and others (Figure 5.26).

A number of technical designs for dual-energy CT have been implemented on clinical scanners in recent years. These designs include the following:

- Dual-source CT—Two sets of X-ray tube and detector are installed on a CT gantry, about 90° apart from each other (Figure 5.25).
- Fast kVp switching—The X-ray tube switches its kVp, back and forth between two preset values, for every two neighboring views in its acquisition (Figure 5.27).
- Dual-layer detector—The front layer of the detector attenuates mostly low-energy X-ray photons and collects their signal, while the back layers collect signal from photons that go through the front layer undetected (Figure 5.27).
- Dual-scan CT—Two scans with different kVps are performed sequentially. To reduce motion effect on the two datasets, this is by far only available on scanners with wide coverage for applications in which a single rotation is sufficient to cover the anatomy of diagnostic interest (Figure 5.27).
- Split filter—A metal filter is inserted into the beam path and splits the X-ray field into two halves along the longitudinal direction. Therefore, half of the X-ray field is filtered for higher effective energy and the other half has no interaction with the filter for relatively lower effective energy.

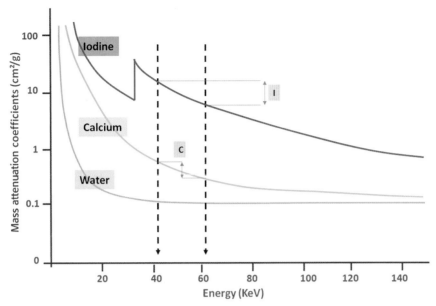

FIG. 5.26 ● **The principle of material differentiation by dual-energy computed tomography (CT).** By having CT numbers at two different X-ray energy levels, one may differentiate between two different materials, fundamentally as a result of the two interactions contributing to their attenuation of X-rays (photoelectric effect and Compton scatter). Reprinted with permission from Saremi F. *Perfusion Imaging in Clinical Practice.* Philadelphia, PA: Wolters Kluwer; 2015.

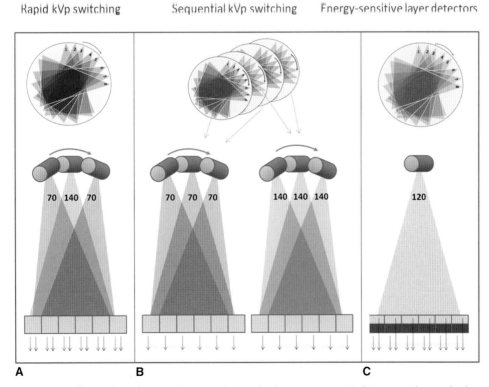

FIG. 5.27 ● **Illustration of several approaches to dual-energy computed tomography on single-source scanners.** Reprinted with permission from Saremi F. *Perfusion Imaging in Clinical Practice.* Philadelphia, PA: Wolters Kluwer; 2015.

Dual-energy CT has found values in a series of diagnostic applications (Figures 5.28-5.33). Selected examples of these applications include the following:

● Renal stone characterization—The management of patients with renal stones is highly dependent on the type of the stones. Dual-energy CT offers an excellent noninvasive diagnostic tool

for stone characterization; with the additional information provided by dual-energy CT, excellent clinical results have been achieved (Figure 5.28).

● Imaging of gout—The diagnosis of gout relies on the identification of monosodium urate crystals in synovial fluid or tissue aspirates. The unique capability of material differentiation by

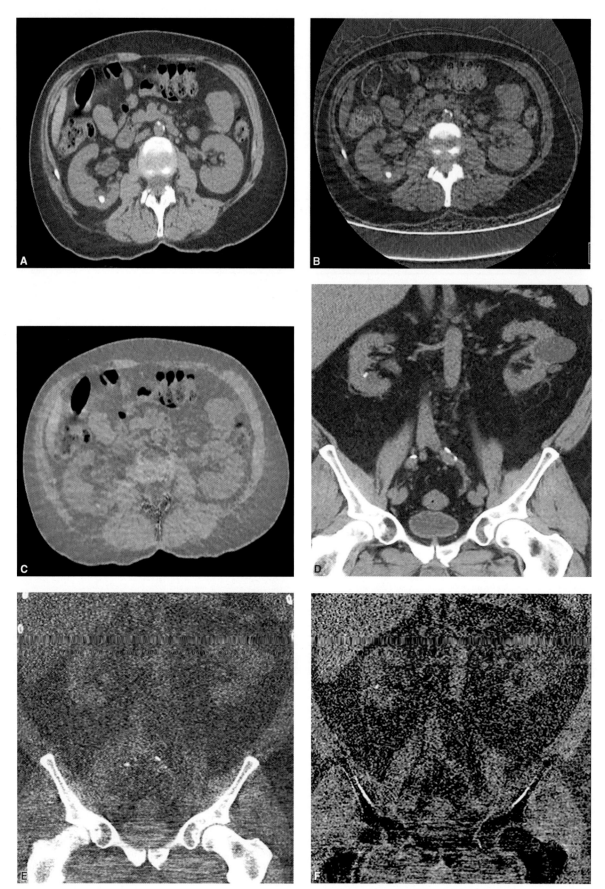

FIG. 5.28 ● A-F, The use of dual-energy computed tomography in the characterization of renal stones. Reprinted with permission from Dunnick NR, Newhouse JH, Cohan RH, Maturen KE. *Genitourinary Radiology*. 6th ed. Philadelphia, PA: Wolters Kluwer; 2018.

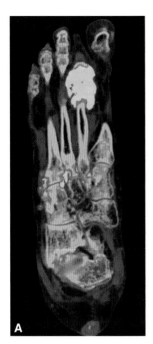
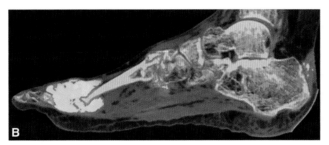
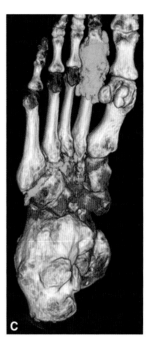

FIG. 5.29 ● A-C, The use of dual-energy computed tomography in the diagnosis of gout. Reprinted with permission from Greenspan A, Gershwin ME. *Imaging in Rheumatology.* Philadelphia, PA: Wolters Kluwer, 2018.

dual-energy CT has proved to be valuable for this clinical task (Figure 5.29).

● Tumor characterization through iodine quantification— Hounsfield unit (HU) enhancement by iodine on contrast-enhanced CT images often provides information for the diagnosis of cancer. The additional capability of quantifying the iodine concentration by dual-energy CT allows characterization of the tumor and improves understanding of the pathology (Figure 5.30).

● Metal artifact reduction—The pronounced beam hardening effect when metal is included in the imaging field of view is a

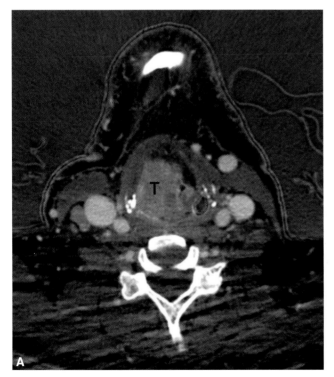
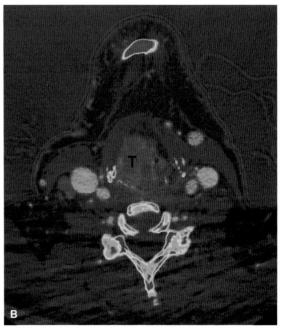

FIG. 5.30 ● A, B, Iodine quantification and overlay by dual-energy computed tomography. Reprinted with permission from Myers J, Hanna E. *Cancer of the Head and Neck.* 5th ed. Philadelphia, PA: Wolters Kluwer; 2017.

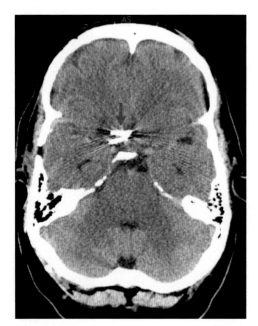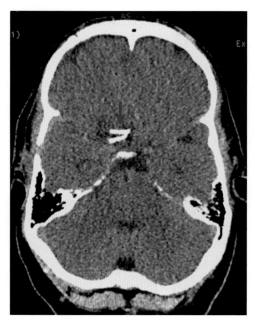

FIG. 5.31 ● **The use of dual-energy computed tomography in the reduction of metal artifacts.** Reprinted with permission from Gean AD. *Brain Injury: Application from War and Terrorism.* Philadelphia, PA: Wolters Kluwer Health/Lippincott Williams & Wilkins; 2014.

major source of metal artifacts. The use of a monochromatic X-ray beam (with the same energy for all photons) of high energy level would be ideal for minimizing metal artifacts but is unrealistic on clinical systems; dual-energy CT allows creation of images that are virtually the same as those acquired with such an X-ray beam to minimize metal artifacts (Figure 5.31).

● Image optimization with virtual monochromatic images. With dual-energy CT, because of the additional information made available, one may simulate a virtual monochromatic scan at any selected photon energy level (within a range) and choose the one that gives the highest contrast resolution and the fewest artifacts (Figure 5.32).

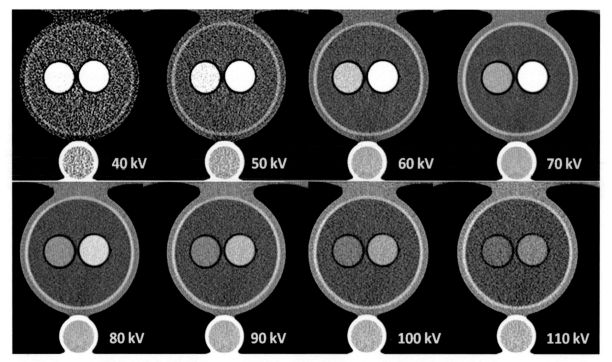

FIG. 5.32 ● **Examples of monochromatic images from dual-energy computed tomography.** An example of monochromatic images from 40 to 110 keV created from a dual-energy scan. Display window level and width are 40 and 400 HU, respectively. From Yu L, Christner JA, Leng S, Wang J, Fletcher JG, McCollough CH. Virtual monochromatic imaging in dual-source dual-energy CT: radiation dose and image quality. *Med Phys.* 2011;38(12):6371–6379. Copyright © 2011 American Association of Physicists in Medicine. Reprinted by permission of John Wiley & Sons, Inc.

CT IMAGE QUALITY

Three aspects of CT image quality are discussed here, including contrast resolution, spatial resolution, and temporal resolution.

Contrast resolution

Contrast resolution refers to the capability of resolving different types of tissue. Contrast resolution depends primarily on two components: the contrast (the signal difference between tissues of interest), and the noise (the fluctuation of signal within the same tissue).

Image contrast

The contrast is a function of both inherent differences in different materials' attenuation characteristics and the X-ray energy spectrum. Both may be utilized clinically to boost the contrast on CT images. For the former, an example application is the use of iodine- or barium-based contrast medium to enhance certain clinical features in CT examinations. For the latter, lower kVp is preferred for contrast-enhanced CT examinations because of improvements in image contrast.

Image noise

The amplitude of image noise is often characterized by the standard deviation of pixel values within a user-defined homogeneous region. It is affected by a variety of scan parameters. The relationships between CT image noise and these parameters are as follows:

- kVp—The higher the kVp, the lower the image noise. This is because, at higher energies, a larger fraction of X-ray photons from the tube can penetrate through the patient and get detected by the detector.
- Effective mA—Effective mA is defined as the product of tube current (with mA as the unit) and rotation time (with a second as the unit), divided by the pitch of the scan. The higher the effective mAs, the lower the image noise.

- Slice thickness—The thicker the slice is, the lower the image noise because of the more photons used in reconstructing a thicker slice.
- Reconstruction—When the reconstruction algorithm belongs to the traditional analytic type, a reconstruction using a sharp kernel will result in higher image noise than the one using a standard kernel, and, similarly, a reconstruction using a smooth kernel will result in lower image noise than the one using a standard kernel. When the reconstruction algorithm is iterative, the strength setting of the algorithm affects CT image noise; typically, a higher strength setting of the iterative reconstruction algorithm results in lower image noise.

Contrast-to-noise ratio

Contrast resolution has been traditionally characterized by the ratio of the contrast to the noise amplitude, also called contrast-to-noise ratio (CNR). CNR has been often used for comparing contrast resolution across different techniques and protocols. The effects of scan parameters on CNR can be derived from how they affect image contrast and image noise separately. A summary is provided as follows:

- kVp—The effect of kVp on CNR is not straightforward. Image contrast increases when kVp decreases, and decreases when kVp increases (Figure 5.34). The same trend applies to the relationship between image noise and kVp. Therefore, CNR, as a ratio between image contrast and image noise, does not have a clear trend to follow. Given a fixed amount of radiation output from the X-ray tube, the CNR of the imaged object peaks at a certain kVp point and drops when kVp is away from the point, and the peak point of kVp is a function of the object size. This explains why different kVps should be used for patients of different sizes for body examinations with iodinated contrast: for normal-sized adults, 100 and 120 kVp are most commonly used, but for pediatric patients, 80 kVp or lower is typically considered, and for obese patients, 140 kVp gives the best results.

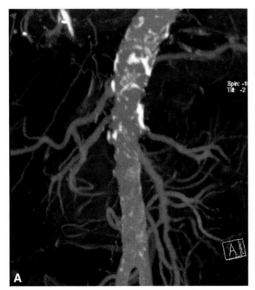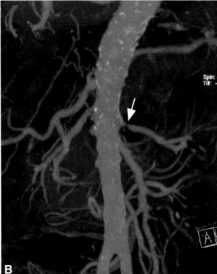

FIG. 5.33 ● **The use of dual-energy computed tomography in the removal of plaques to aid the visualization of vessel lumens.** Reprinted with permission from Geschwind J, Dake M. *Abrams' Angiography.* 3rd ed. Philadelphia, PA: Wolters Kluwer Health/Lippincott Williams & Wilkins; 2014.

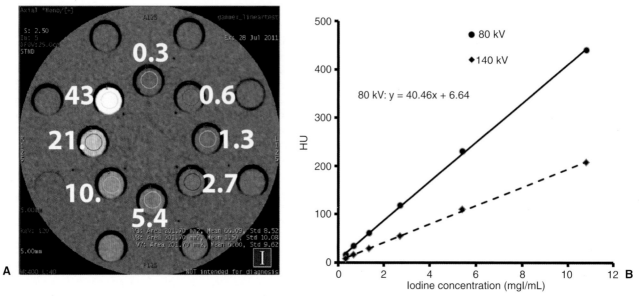

FIG. 5.34 ● **The effect of kVp on image contrast of iodine solutions.** The left is an axial computed tomography (CT) slice of a phantom containing eight vials of iodine solutions of different concentrations (as indicated by numbers next to the vials). The right shows plots of Hounsfield units (HU) for these vials at both 80 and 140 kVp. For the entire range of iodine concentrations, the HUs at 80 kVp nearly double those at 140 kVp. Because soft tissues typically have HUs near 0, it shows the contrast of iodine (at any concentration) with respect to soft-tissue increases as kVp decreases. Reprinted with permission from Bammer R. *MR and CT Perfusion and Pharmacokinetic Imaging: Clinical Applications and Theoretical Principles.* Philadelphia, PA: Wolters Kluwer; 2016.

- Effective mA—Effective mA affects only image noise, not image contrast. As a result, CNR increases as effective mA increases, and decreases as it decreases (Figure 5.35).
- Slice thickness—Slice thickness typically has little to no effect on image contrast. CNR increases as slices become thicker, and decreases as they become thinner.
- Reconstruction—Reconstruction does not alter image contrast; so its effect on CNR is straightforward. For analytic reconstructions, a smooth kernel results in higher CNR, whereas a sharp kernel lowers CNR in general (Figure 5.36).

A major limitation of CNR is its inability to characterize noise texture, which appears to be another important factor in affecting readers' ability to make confident and accurate diagnosis. Noise amplitude, which is frequently approximated as the standard deviation of CT numbers over a homogeneous region, does not account for any spatial correlation of signals in an image. Noise texture, on the other hand, depicts spatial relations of noise with an image.

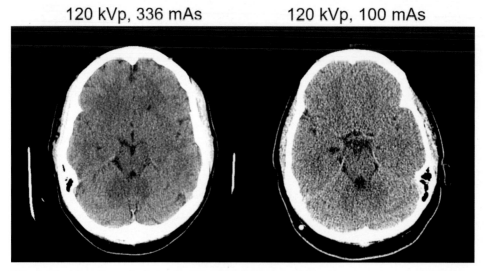

FIG. 5.35 ● **The effect of mAs on image noise.** The two axial head computed tomography images were acquired with the same parameters except for different mAs. Higher mAs results in less image noise than lower mAs. Image contrast is not affected by mAs.

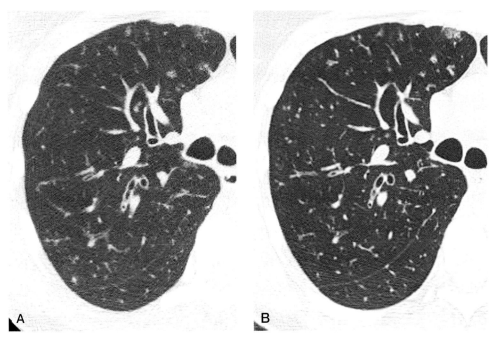

FIG. 5.36 ● A, B, The effect of filter kernel on image noise. Reprinted with permission from Webb WR, Muller NL, Naidich DP. *High-Resolution CT of the Lung.* 5th ed. Philadelphia, PA: Wolters Kluwer; 2015.

Spatial resolution

Spatial resolution refers to the capability of resolving small-sized features in the anatomy of interest. Spatial resolution of a CT study can be further classified into two categories: in-plane resolution (x-y plane) and longitudinal resolution (z-axis).

The in-plane resolution of a CT image is affected by the following:

- Detector pixel size—a smaller detector pixel size in the x-y plane results in improved in-plane resolution.
- Angular sampling rate—when the scanner increases its angular sampling rate, that is, acquires more views per rotation, the in-plane resolution of the CT images improves.
- Reconstruction algorithm—when the algorithm is of analytic type, it is the kernel used in the filtering step that affects the in-plane resolution of the reconstructed images; when the algorithm is of iterative type, the in-plane resolution is typically affected by how the algorithm keeps balances between image noise and edge sharpness.

The longitudinal resolution of a CT image is affected by the following:

- Detector pixel size—a smaller detector pixel size in the longitudinal direction, often called detector thickness, leads to improved longitudinal resolution.
- Helical pitch—for a helical scan, a smaller pitch means more overlapping of data in the longitudinal direction and often higher spatial resolution.
- Longitudinal sampling rate—one way of increasing longitudinal sampling rate is to use the technology of z-flying focal spot, in which the focal spot is moved between two different z-positions on the anode by electromagnetic deflection of the electron beam generated by the cathode; longitudinal sampling rate doubles effectively, leading to improved longitudinal resolution.

- Reconstruction algorithm—it is, in particular, true for helical scans in which the reconstruction of any slice needs some data from adjacent slices and how such data are located and used affects the longitudinal resolution of the images.

Temporal resolution

Temporal resolution refers to the capability of resolving temporally varying features or events in the anatomy of interest. Temporal resolution has the most relevance in cardiac imaging; in addition, it is also important in the imaging of other moving structures or dynamic processes. Intuitively, temporal resolution of any image point depends on the time span used to acquire the data used for reconstructing the point. Therefore, rotation time and reconstruction technique are two major factors affecting the temporal resolution of a CT study. Understandably, cardiac CT always prefers the shortest rotation time and specialized reconstruction algorithms to minimize motion artifacts.

Summary of CT image quality

A summary of how CT image quality is affected by various acquisition parameters is included in Table 5.1.

CT ARTIFACTS

Beam hardening

Beam hardening refers to the fact that the X-ray beam, as it traverses the anatomy being scanned, has its energy spectrum shifted toward higher energy, that is, the X-ray beam becomes hardened. Beam hardening artifacts are often seen in head CT studies. The shift is caused by the fact that more photons at lower energies than those at higher energies are absorbed by tissues and removed from the beam as it traverses the anatomy. The shift contributes to a decrease in the reconstructed CT number for image pixels along any X-ray path through the anatomy. See Figure 5.37 for

Table 5.1 **THE SUMMARY OF THE EFFECTS OF ACQUISITION PARAMETERS ON CT IMAGE QUALITY**

	Image Contrast	Image Noise	Image Contrast-to-Noise Ratio (CNR)	Spatial Resolution	Temporal Resolution
kVp	−	−	Depends	No impact	No impact
mA	No impact	−	+	No impact	No impact
Rotation time	No impact	−	+	No impact	+
Helical pitch	No impact	+	−	+ (z only)	No impact
Detector pixel size (x-y plane)	No impact	−	+	+ (x-y only)	No impact
Detector row thickness (z-direction)	No impact	−	+	+ (z only)	No impact
Reconstruction algorithm	No impact	Depends	Depends	Depends	Depends

"+" indicates that the image quality aspect increases/decreases as the acquisition parameter increases/decreases, in the same trend; "−" indicates that the image quality aspect decreases/increases as the acquisition parameter increases/decreases, in the opposite trend.

an illustration of the spectrum-shifting effect in beam hardening. Such effects are the most pronounced in two scenarios. First, for a round or an elliptical object, image pixels located near the center experience the most beam hardening effect because of the long X-ray path for each X-ray through them, and, as image pixels get away from the center, the effect becomes less and less. The artifacts on the image are called cupping artifacts because the image visually appears dark in the center and progressively brighter toward the periphery (Figure 5.38). Second, pixels located in between highly attenuating objects are affected by beam hardening more than others, and therefore a dark band is observed over them. Brain tissues near the posterior fossa in the skull are a great example of this scenario (Figure 5.39).

Photon starvation

Photon starvation occurs when the signal on the detector becomes so low that it is near the electronic noise level. Streak artifacts are observed along the X-ray paths along which photon attenuation is the most. These artifacts may be found on images for the shoulder, pelvis, and large body habitus (Figure 5.40).

Photon starvation can be addressed in several ways. One way is to adapt tube current to body thicknesses at different view angles and locations so the detector signal always stays within an expected range. This is often called tube current modulation (TCM). It works by first modeling the patient's attenuation profile through one or more projectional views acquired immediately before the CT scan and then applying the appropriate tube current at each view angle and scan location. Another way to address the problem is through the reconstruction process. The contribution of the signals where detected photons are too few may be suppressed in the reconstruction algorithm for fewer streaks on the image.

Aliasing

Aliasing arises when the signals are being sampled at a frequency lower than is desired. Insufficient sampling of projection views within each rotation is a typical example of undersampling and a source of view aliasing artifacts (Figure 5.41). Aliasing-caused artifacts typically present themselves as streaks at all angles through the affected object. Objects with sharp boundaries are more likely to become a source of aliasing artifacts,

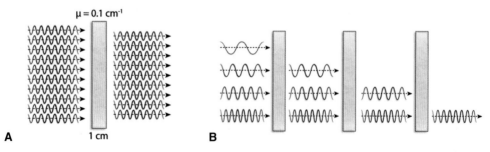

FIG. 5.37 ● Illustration of beam spectrum shift due to beam hardening. The lower energy X-rays (lower wave frequency) are preferentially attenuated when traveling through materials because of higher attenuation coefficients. After traveling through a certain distance, the higher energy X-rays become dominant in the spectrum. Reprinted with permission from Huda W. *Review of Radiologic Physics*. 4th ed. Philadelphia, PA: Wolters Kluwer; 2016.

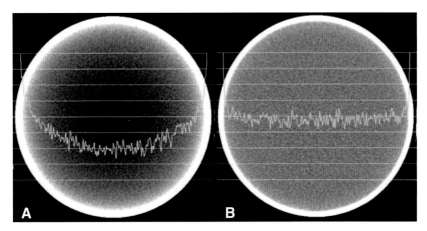

FIG. 5.38 ● Cupping artifacts in computed tomography images of a homogeneous water phantom before (A) and after (B) beam hardening correction. Reprinted with permission from Bammer R. *MR and CT Perfusion and Pharmacokinetic Imaging: Clinical Applications and Theoretical Principles.* Philadelphia, PA: Wolters Kluwer; 2016.

FIG. 5.39 ● **Shading artifacts in computed tomography head images before and after beam hardening correction.** Reprinted with permission from Bammer R. *MR and CT Perfusion and Pharmacokinetic Imaging: Clinical Applications and Theoretical Principles.* Philadelphia, PA: Wolters Kluwer; 2016.

Cupping   **Water precorrected**

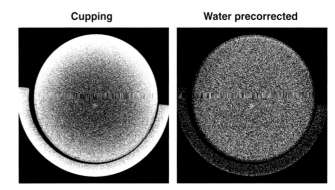

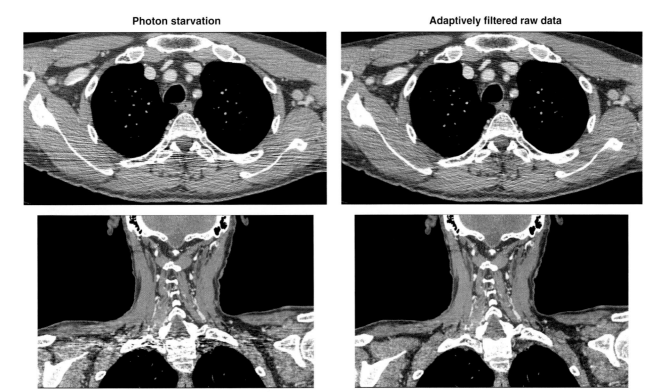

FIG. 5.40 ● **An example of photon starvation near the shoulder region on computed tomography images.** Reprinted with permission from Bammer R. *MR and CT Perfusion and Pharmacokinetic Imaging: Clinical Applications and Theoretical Principles.* Philadelphia, PA: Wolters Kluwer; 2016.

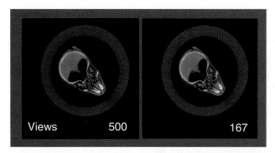

A. Image of mouse with different numbers of views

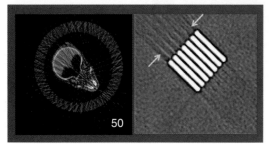

B. Streaks near the resolution bar pattern
(made by metal) in an image quality phantom

FIG. 5.41 ● A, B, View aliasing artifacts in computed tomography. Reprinted with permission from Bushberg JT, Seibert JA, Leidholdt EM, Boone JM. *Essential Physics of Medical Imaging*. 3rd ed. Philadelphia, PA: Wolters Kluwer Health/Lippincott Williams & Wilkins; 2012.

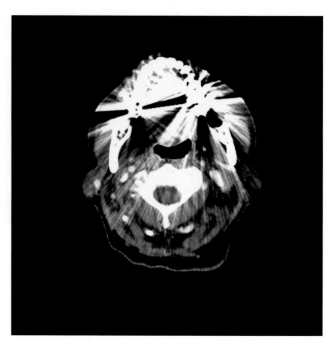

FIG. 5.42 ● An axial computed tomography image showing metal artifacts as a result of dental fillings.

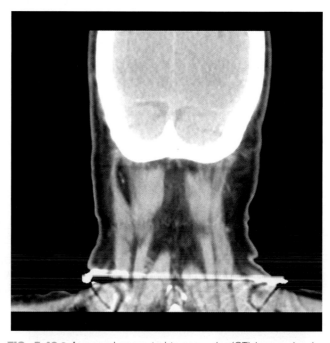

FIG. 5.43 ● A coronal computed tomography (CT) image showing metal artifacts because of a necklace worn during CT scan.

because the high-frequency signals inherent in the transition at sharp boundaries often exceed the sampling frequency of the scanner.

Metal

Highly attenuating metal objects present near or inside the patient create a number of issues that result in artifacts. Both beam hardening and photon starvation effects become much more pronounced because of the metal's high attenuation of X-ray photons. Typical metal artifacts on clinical images are shown in Figures 5.42 to 5.44.

Metal artifacts can be reduced in a number of ways, including the use of higher kVps during acquisition and the use of specialized correction algorithm during reconstruction.

Truncation

Truncation artifacts occur when any body part extends outside the scan field of view. Areas near where the boundary of the field of view intersects with the patient's body will appear brightened markedly (Figure 5.45). Best efforts should be made at the time of scanning to keep the area of clinical interest centered within the scan field of view and to minimize any unnecessary truncation.

Motion

Motion causes inconsistencies in acquired projection data in CT, leading to artifactual appearances on reconstructed images. Examples of motion artifacts include (1) gross movement of body parts (Figure 5.46), (2) breathing motion (Figures 5.47 and 5.48), (3) cardiac motion (Figure 5.49), and so on.

There are numerous ways of mitigating motion artifacts. For gross movement by the patient, one may shorten the scan time using shorter rotation time or higher pitch. For body parts affected by periodic motion, one may monitor surrogate signals of the motion and gate the scan to be performed at specific motion phases to improve consistency within data. Advanced processing and reconstruction algorithms represent another category of methods to address motion artifacts.

Detector nonuniformity

A detector is composed of a large array of pixels, which ideally should have a uniform response to X-ray exposure. In practice,

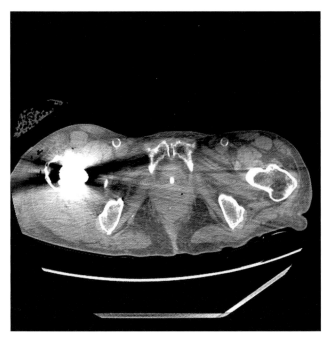

FIG. 5.44 ● An axial computed tomography (CT) image showing metal artifacts on pelvic CT images.

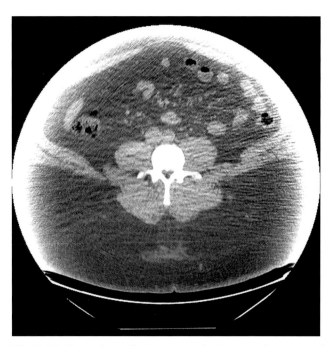

FIG. 5.45 ● Truncation artifacts on computed tomography images of patients with large body habitus.

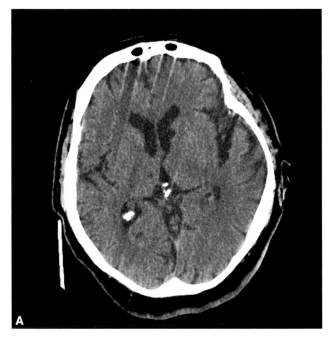

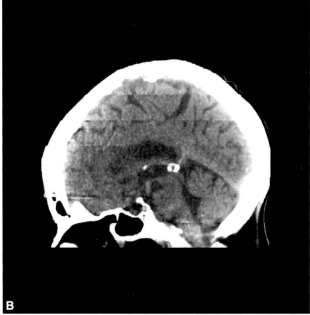

FIG. 5.46 ● Axial (A) and sagittal (B) computed tomography images showing artifacts caused by head movement during the scan.

each pixel has more or less a different response from one another, and, it is through a calibration process that these pixels produce the same digital signal in response to a uniform X-ray field. If a pixel has its response out of its expected range, the image points whose reconstructed values primarily rely on signals from the affected pixel will be darker or brighter than are expected and therefore form artifacts; because such image points lie on a circle whose radius is dependent on the faulty pixel's location, the artifacts have the appearance of a ring or arc and are often called ring artifacts. Dead pixels are the extreme case of detector nonuniformity, in

which recalibration is unable to address the issue. Typical ring artifacts on clinical images are shown in Figures 5.50 to 5.53.

RADIATION DOSE IN CT

Radiation dose to patients from CT examinations has attracted a lot of attention in recent years. It is partly based on the fact that CT is a diagnostic imaging tool of very common use in clinical settings. A recent survey showed that CT accounts for about a quarter of radiation exposures to the entire US population

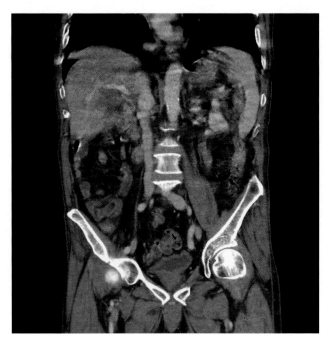

FIG. 5.47 ● A coronal computed tomography image showing breathing motion artifacts near the dome of the liver.

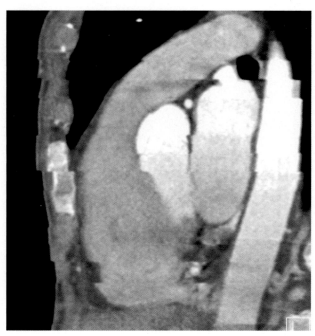

FIG. 5.48 ● **Motion artifacts on cardiac computed tomography images due to breathing.** Reprinted with permission from Garcia MJ. *NonInvasive Cardiovascular Imaging: A Multimodality Approach.* Philadelphia, PA: Wolters Kluwer Health/Lippincott Williams & Wilkins; 2010.

FIG. 5.49 ● A, B. Motion artifacts on cardiac computed tomography images. Reprinted with permission from Saremi F. *Perfusion Imaging in Clinical Practice.* Philadelphia, PA: Wolters Kluwer; 2015.

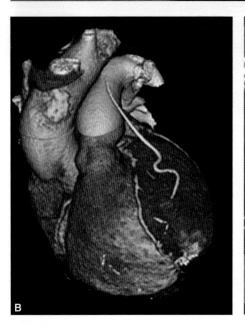

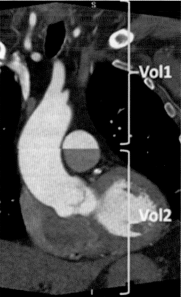

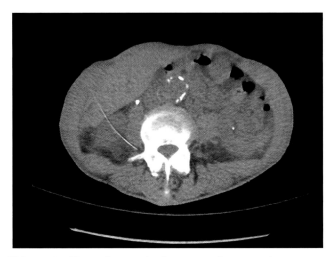

FIG. 5.50 ● Ring artifacts on body computed tomography.

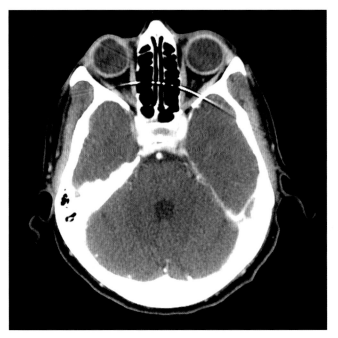

FIG. 5.51 ● Ring artifacts on head computed tomography.

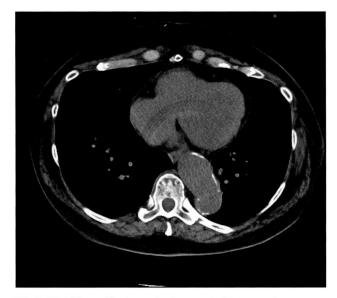

FIG. 5.52 ● Ring artifacts on chest computed tomography.

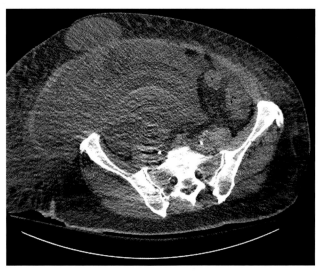

FIG. 5.53 ● Ring artifacts on body computed tomography for a patient with large body habitus.

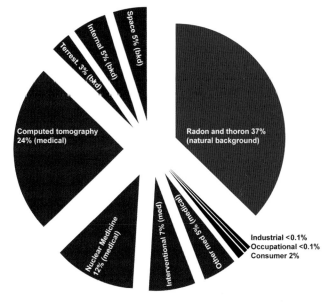

FIG. 5.54 ● **The contributors of radiation exposures to US population in 2006.** Reprinted with permission from Moscucci M. *Grossman & Baim's Cardiac Catheterization, Angiography, and Intervention.* 8th ed. Philadelphia, PA: Wolters Kluwer Health/Lippincott Williams & Wilkins; 2014.

(Figure 5.54). Although extensive discussions about CT radiation dose go beyond the scope of this chapter, a brief discussion of commonly used dose metrics is provided as follows.

Computed Tomography Dose Index (CTDI)

CTDI is a radiation metric used to quantify the radiation output by scanner for a CT protocol. For most CT examinations today, volumetric coverage is achieved by performing either a helical scan or a step-and-shoot axial scan. For either scan mode, the final radiation dose distribution can be viewed or approximated as the summation of dose distributions of many individual single axial scans at various locations.

Despite its widespread use, one should not interpret CTDI as patient dose. It is measured using an acrylic phantom with a diameter of 16 or 32 cm, depending on the size of the body part to be scanned. Therefore, it is very limited in depicting radiation dose to patients of any arbitrary size. However, it is very effective in making comparison of radiation usage by CT protocols across different scanners on similar patients.

Dose Length Product (DLP)

DLP is the product of CTDIvol and the scan length. It is an indicator of the total amount of X-ray energy delivered to the patient, because CTDIvol describes X-ray energy delivered to the patient per unit volume and the scan length is related to the volume of tissue being scanned.

Size-specific Dose Estimate

Size-specific dose estimate (SSDE) is a recently introduced metric that attempts to address CTDI's limitations in quantifying patient dose. In its methodology, SSDE is the product of CTDIvol and a conversion factor dependent on the attenuation characteristic of the body part of interest. For the body part of interest, its water-equivalent size can be determined and used to look up a table for an appropriate size-dependent factor for the calculation of SSDE (Figure 5.55).

Effective dose

Effective dose is used for quantifying the cancer risk caused by the radiation the patient receives. It includes in its consideration many factors affecting an exposure individual's risk of cancer, including age, gender, type of radiation, radiation sensitivity of different organs, and others.

A common practice in effective dose estimation for CT is based on DLP and risk-conversion factors, or k-factors. It is found that, for a specific body section, like the head, abdomen, or chest, the effective dose can be approximated by the product of the DLP and a k-factor, which is specific to the exposed body section and the subject's age. For a CT scan encompassing multiple body sections, the total effective dose is the summation of all effective doses to individual body sections.

CT FOR PEDIATRIC PATIENTS

There are millions of pediatric CT studies performed every year in United States. Like pharmaceuticals used in managing diseases, radiation, too, needs to be appropriately administered for diagnostic purposes. CT has received scrutiny because of concerns over the impact of its radiation on pediatric patients; these concerns typically include the following:

- Children are more sensitive to radiation than are adults.
- Children have a longer life expectancy than do adults, resulting in higher likelihood for expressing radiation damage, mostly in the form of cancers.
- Children, when having their imaging studies performed at adult facilities (not uncommon), may receive a higher radiation dose than necessary if CT protocols are not adapted for children.

Safe use of radiation in pediatric CT can be achieved by following proper guidelines. Here is a discussion of some of these guidelines:

- Consider lower kVp for examinations with iodinated contrast— kVp affects both the brightness of iodine signals and the image noise in competing ways: lower kVp increases the brightness of iodine signals, but, at the same time, results in higher image noise if all other parameters remain unchanged. So, for a certain body size, there is an optimal range of kVp for the highest CNR; 120 kVp seems to be the choice for adult patients, whereas the optimal kVp gets lower for pediatric patients. For young pediatric patients, 100 kVp or even 80 kVp should be considered for CT examinations with iodinated contrast being used. Note

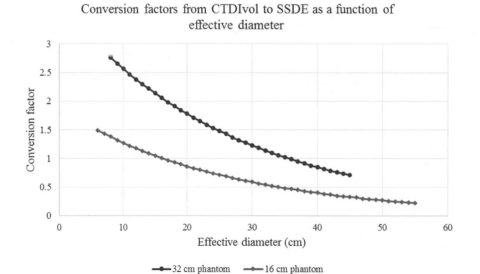

FIG. 5.55 ● The conversion factor from CTDIvol to size-specific dose estimate (SSDE) as a function of size.

that, when using lower kVp, the mAs of the CT protocol often need to increase to compensate for noise increase for a balanced image quality.

- Use SSDE in protocol setup and radiation monitoring—For the same type of CT examination, the amount of X-ray radiation needed for a child patient varies, because of the large variation in the body sizes of pediatric patients. Therefore, a wide range of CTDIvol values result, even when the protocol properly adapts its radiation usage to patient size. It is beneficial to use SSDE in evaluating the radiation levels used by a CT protocol for various patient sizes, because SSDE, compared to CTDIvol, stays within a narrower range.
- Patient cooperation—In a pediatric CT examination, it is crucial for a young patient to stay still and stress-free and cooperate with instructions when applicable. The operator should employ all measures to achieve the goal. Effective measures include having parents stay inside the room, appropriate distraction to divert the patient's focus, and others.
- Minimize exposure time—Pediatric patients tend to have difficulties in following instructions and remain still as well, as is ideally expected for CT examinations. Reducing exposure time helps minimize the chances of motion artifacts. It helps cut down the usage of sedation and iodinated contrast and their related side effects on children when they need to be used.
- Modulate tube current to its advantage—TCM provides a useful tool in addressing large variation in body size in the pediatric population. It should be used in most body examinations whenever applicable.

Selective organ shielding is available on some CT scanners so that certain radiation-sensitive organs may get less radiation without negatively impacting image quality. Breast shielding is one such application in young female patients for concerns over radiation to breast tissues. With selective organ shielding, the current of the X-ray tube decreases when it rotates to the front of the patient (also closest to the breasts), and increases when it rotates to the back of the patient. In this way, the total photons contributing to image formation remain unchanged, while fewer of them are absorbed by the breasts.

- Patient centering and field of view selection—Because of the relative small sizes of pediatric patients, centering them and the choice of field of view become important in managing CT dose. Patient centering affects the effectiveness of TCM, which is commonly used in body examinations. TCM on most CT scanners estimates patient size depending on one or two X-ray views of the patient before the scan for correctly setting up the tube current and how it varies by time. When a patient is off-centered with respect to the isocenter, the estimated size may be incorrect and result in unintended tube current and often unnecessary radiation dose.

CONE BEAM CT

Traditionally, CT uses X-ray beam whose cone angle is substantially smaller than its fan angle, by approximately an order of magnitude or more. In the past two decades, more and more cone beam CT systems have come into clinical use, whose cone angle starts to become comparable to its fan angle, for both diagnostic and nondiagnostic applications. A substantially large cone angle brings both benefits and challenges to cone beam CT in its clinical use.

The uses of cone beam CT in diagnostic and nondiagnostic applications have been driven by different considerations and followed different pathways:

- For diagnostic CT, the introduction of cone beam CT is part of a so-called slice war, during which more and more rows of detectors are built into a CT scanner. More rows of detectors enable wider scan coverage along the longitudinal body axis and allow CT examinations to be completed in shorter time periods, which translate into fewer motion artifacts, less iodinated contrast usage, and other clinical benefits. Cone beam CT is, in particular, appealing in cardiac applications. If a heart can fit into the coverage of cone beam CT within one rotation, a single heartbeat cardiac CT becomes possible, which eliminates artifacts caused by heartbeat-to-heartbeat inconsistencies and gives a significant boost of image quality.
- For nondiagnostic CT used in interventions and radiation therapy applications, cone beam CT begins as an extension of the use of flat panel detectors. With the benefits of large area coverage, isotropic spatial resolution, and instantaneously available digital X-ray images, flat panel detectors have found widespread use for image guidance in nondiagnostic applications, and its extension to cone beam CT becomes natural for those applications where 3D definitions of body anatomy are desired.

Cone beam CT also faces a number of challenges in clinical use. On diagnostic scanners, challenges for cone beam CT include the following:

- Scatter
  Scattered X-ray photons detected by the detector increase substantially when the cone angle of the X-ray beam increases from $\leq 4°$ to $\geq 15°$. Increased scatter introduces shading and cupping artifacts, and lowers image contrast resolution (Figure 5.56). The amplitude of the scattered X-ray photons on the detector is strongly dependent on the size of the body parts inside the field of view: the larger the size, the more scattered X-ray photons detected. Effective ways to mitigate scatter in cone beam CT have been studied extensively. 2D antiscatter grids are preferred on cone beam CT systems for more effective removal of scatter signals.
- Cone beam artifacts
  For a single axial cone beam CT scan, the circular trajectory of the X-ray source defines a plane commonly referred to as the central plane. For any point on the central plane, all X-rays going through the point and contributing to signal measurements by detector are within the same plane. These measurements are sufficient for a theoretically exact reconstruction of any of these points. For all points out of the central plane, however, it is not the case; all X-rays passing through any of those points are oblique relative to the central plane. As a consequence, these measurements do not provide a complete data set for an exact reconstruction for these points and artifacts.

The cone beam artifacts can be demonstrated using a Defrise phantom, which is a stack of circular disks with interspace materials in between (Figure 5.57). In a coronal or sagittal view of the reconstructed image volume, the disks should ideally appear identical regardless of their locations. That is, however, not the case. With a standard analytic reconstruction algorithm, the disk at the central plane shows no artifacts, although the off-center disks show artifacts increasingly more pronounced as they move away from the central plane.

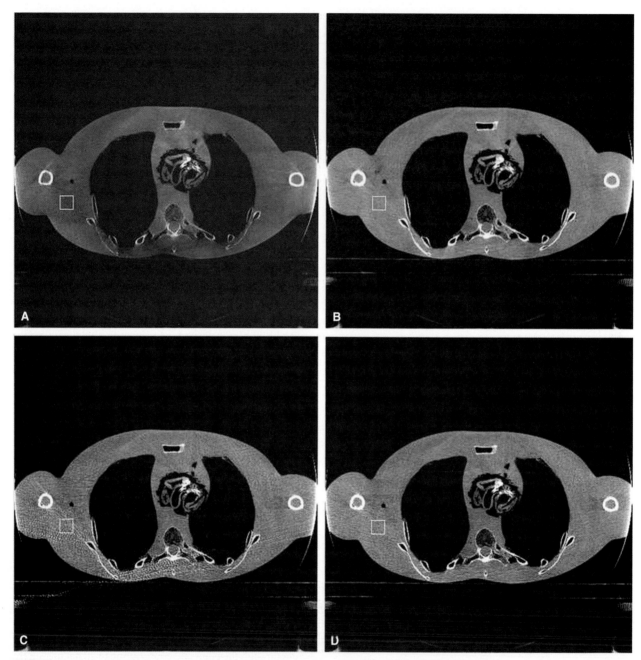

FIG. 5.56 ● **The effect of scatter on cone beam computed tomography (CT) image quality.** (A) shows the image of an anthropomorphic phantom by cone beam CT without any scatter correction, whereas (B-D) show images after corrections with different considerations for noise suppression. From Zhu L, Wang J, Xing L. Noise suppression in scatter correction for cone-beam CT. *Med Phys.* 2009;36:741–752. Copyright © 2009 American Association of Physicists in Medicine. Reprinted by permission of John Wiley & Sons, Inc.

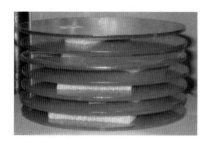

A. Defrise phantom

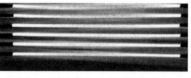

B. Some cone beam artifacts

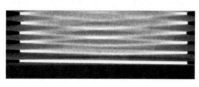

C. Pronounced cone beam artifacts

FIG. 5.57 ● A-C, The demonstration of cone beam artifacts using a Defrise phantom. Reprinted with permission from Bushberg JT, Seibert JA, Leidholdt EM, Boone JM. *Essential Physics of Medical Imaging.* 3rd ed. Philadelphia, PA: Wolters Kluwer Health/ Lippincott Williams & Wilkins; 2012.

Suggested Readings

Bammer R. *MR and CT Perfusion and Pharmacokinetic Imaging: Clinical Applications and Theoretical Principles*. Philadelphia, PA: Lippincott Williams & Wilkins; 2016.

Bridwell KH, Dewald RL. *Textbook of Spinal Surgery*. 3rd ed. Philadelphia, PA: Lippincott Williams & Wilkins; 2011.

Bushberg JT, Seibert JA, Leidholdt EM, Boone JM. *The Essential Physics of Medical Imaging*. 3rd ed. Philadelphia, PA: Lippincott Williams & Wilkins; 2011.

Chandra R, Rahmim A. *Nuclear Medicine Physics: The Basics*. 8th ed. Philadelphia, PA: Lippincott Williams & Wilkins; 2017.

Dunnick R, Sandler C, Newhouse J. *Textbook of Uroradiology*. 5th ed. Philadelphia, PA: Lippincott Williams & Wilkins; 2012.

Fosbinder RA, Orth D. *Essentials of Radiologic Science*. Philadelphia, PA: Lippincott Williams & Wilkins; 2011.

Garcia MJ. *Non-Invasive Cardiovascular Imaging: A Multimodality Approach*. Philadelphia, PA: Lippincott Williams & Wilkins; 2011.

Geschwind J, Dake M. *Abrams' Angiography*. 3rd ed. Philadelphia, PA: Lippincott Williams & Wilkins; 2013.

Greenspan A, Borys D. *Radiology and Pathology Correlation of Bone Tumors*. Philadelphia, PA: Lippincott Williams & Wilkins; 2015.

Higgins CB, de Roos A. *MRI and CT of the Cardiovascular System*. 3rd ed. Philadelphia, PA: Lippincott Williams & Wilkins; 2013.

Hsieh J. *Computed Tomography: Principles, Designs, Artifacts, and Recent Advances*. 2nd ed. Bellingham, WA: SPIE and New York, NY: John Wiley & Sons; 2009.

Huda W. *Review of Radiologic Physics*. 4th ed. Philadelphia, PA: Lippincott Williams & Wilkins; 2016.

Kandarpa K, Machan L, Durham J. *Handbook of Interventional Radiologic Procedures*. 5th ed. Philadelphia, PA: Lippincott Williams & Wilkins; 2016.

Moscucci M. *Grossman & Baim's Cardiac Catherization, Angiography, and Intervention*. 8th ed. Philadelphia, PA: Lippincott Williams & Wilkins; 2013.

Myers J, Hanna E. *Cancer of the Head and Neck*. 5th ed. Philadelphia, PA: Lippincott Williams & Wilkins; 2016.

Orth D. *Essentials of Radiologic Science*. 2nd ed. Philadelphia, PA: Lippincott Williams & Wilkins; 2017.

Sadock BJ, Sadock VA, Ruiz P. *Kaplan and Sadock's Synopsis of Psychiatry: Behavioral Sciences/Clinical Psychiatry*. 11th ed. Philadelphia, PA: Lippincott Williams & Wilkins; 2014.

Saremi F. *Perfusion Imaging in Clinical Practice*. Philadelphia, PA: Lippincott Williams & Wilkins; 2015.

Von Schulthess GK. *Molecular Anatomic Imaging*. 3rd ed. Philadelphia, PA: Lippincott Williams & Wilkins; 2015.

Webb WR, Muller, NL, Naidich DP. *High-Resolution CT of the Lung*. 5th ed. Philadelphia, PA: Lippincott Williams & Wilkins; 2014.

CHAPTER SELF-ASSESSMENT QUESTIONS

1. Which of the following scenarios would *not* benefit from the use of kVp lower than 120?

   A. Abdomen CT of a 3-year-old child

   B. Abdomen-pelvis CT of an obese patient

   C. Brain perfusion CT

   D. Abdominal CT angiography of an undersized patient for whom iodine contrast volume needs to be reduced because of impaired kidney function

2. Which of the following is *not* true regarding bow-tie filters in CT?

   A. It is made in the shape of a "bow-tie," that is, thin in the middle and thicker at the ends, to account for the oval shape of body in general.

   B. It narrows the range of signal levels detected by the detector and thus improves image contrast.

   C. It cuts down unnecessary radiation dose to tissues at the periphery of the body.

   D. It eliminates scattered photons from signals on the detector.

3. Which of the following is *not* true regarding dual-energy CT?

   A. It allows quantification of iodine quantification by separating signal contributions from water and iodine.

   B. It allows synthesis of CT images acquired with monochromatic X-ray beams, which may be used to reduce beam hardening artifacts.

   C. It allows characterization of kidney stones of different types by material differentiation.

   D. It allows for substantial reduction in radiation dose.

4. Which of the follow is *not* true regarding radiation dose in CT?

   A. Increase in mA alone leads to increases in both CTDIvol and DLP.

   B. Increase in longitudinal scan coverage alone leads to increases in DLP.

   C. Increase in helical pitch leads to increases in both CTDIvol and DLP.

   D. With the same CTDIvol, scans of an undersized patient have higher SSDE than do scans of oversized patients.

Answers to Chapter Self-Assessment Questions

1. B   Abdomen-pelvis CT of an obese patient.

2. D   Bow-tie filters help to mitigate scatter caused by artifacts; they, however, do not eliminate scatter.

3. D   The benefits of dual-energy CT do not include substantial reduction in radiation dose. Its clinical use today is typically with equivalent radiation dose to that used by traditional CT.

4. C   CTDIvol and DLP are inversely proportional to helical pitch.

Magnetic Resonance Imaging

6

Huimin Wu, PhD

LEARNING OBJECTIVES

1. Name the three main types of coils used in a magnetic resonance (MR) scanner.
2. Define the Larmor frequency and its relationship with the static magnetic field.
3. Describe the basic principles of the three main types of MR pulse sequences: spin echo (SE), gradient echo (GE), and inversion recovery (IR).
4. Explain the rationale of parameter selection for an SE pulse sequence to produce T1-, T2-, or proton-weighted images.
5. Identify different types of artifacts on MR images and explain their possible causes.
6. Define specific absorption rate (SAR).
7. Describe the four different MR safety zones.
8. Magnetic resonance imaging (MRI) is a commonly used and highly valued clinical imaging modality, primarily attributed to its offered exquisite soft-tissue contrast through a multitude of mechanisms and its use of nonionizing radiation. The phenomenon of MR is the underlying mechanism of MRI.

BASIC CONCEPTS

Magnetism

Magnetism results from the organized motion of electric charge. Magnetic fields exist as dipoles and are commonly depicted by lines that originate from the North Pole and return to the South Pole with the density of these lines, that is, the number of lines per unit area, proportional to the local field strength (Figure 6.1). Magnetic field strength produced by a dipole, B, decreases approximately as the inverse square of the distance from the dipole. Two commonly used units for B are Tesla (T) and Gauss (G), and 1 T = 10 000 G. The earth's magnetic field strength is about 0.5 G, whereas that of today's clinical MR scanners is typically on the order of a few Teslas.

Magnets

All MRI scanners need a main magnet that produces a strong, stable, and homogeneous magnetic field. MRI magnets can be classified into three types by the way the field is generated:

- Permanent magnets—They are made of materials magnetized to keep the magnetic field permanently. Permanent magnets use permanently magnetized iron (or other alloys). They require no power consumption, need no cooling, and are of low cost.
- Resistive electromagnets—They produce a magnetic field by running electric currents through wirings that are typically iron cored or air cored. These magnets require a large constant flow of current and significant cooling during operation due to electrical resistance of the magnet coils.

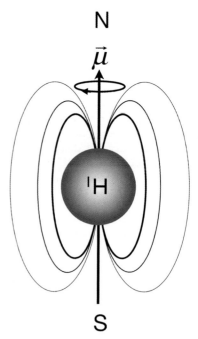

FIG. 6.1 ● A small magnetic dipole resulting from the spinning of a hydrogen nucleus (proton). It behaves like a bar magnet and can be depicted by field lines going from the north pole to the south pole. Reprinted with permission from Atlas SW. *Magnetic Resonance Imaging of the Brain and Spine.* 5th ed. Philadelphia, PA: Wolters Kluwer; 2017.

• Superconducting electromagnets—Superconductivity is a unique characteristic exhibited by certain types of metals with zero resistance to electric currents when their temperature drops below a critical point close to the absolute zero. A superconducting magnet is built by immersing metal wires made by special alloys like niobium-titanium in liquid helium whose temperature is below 4 K; in this way, electric currents large enough to produce a clinically desired field strength ($\geq$1 T) may run through the wires without overheating issues. Care should be taken to ensure the proper state and temperature of liquid helium because, once its temperature rises above the critical point, resistance heating from the electric current running through the wires will boil the helium and eventually lead to a quench of the system.

Superconducting magnets are predominantly used in diagnostic MR scanners, typically requiring a high field strength ($>$0.5 T) for sufficient signal-to-noise ratio (SNR). On the other hand, both permanent magnets and resistive electromagnets are mostly seen in low-field systems. Permanent magnets are limited by their bulk and weight, and resistive electromagnets by the maximum currents allowed without generating excessive heat by resistance.

Coils

An MR scanner consists of multiple coils of wire stacked or nested, each serving a different purpose (Figure 6.2).

Main coils

As previously mentioned, the main coils establish the main magnetic field to induce nonzero bulk magnetization as a foundation for signal production. Large currents run through the static coils to produce the desired field strength, typically at 1.5 or 3 T. The static coils are immersed in cryogen, whose temperature is near the absolute zero degree (Figure 6.3).

Shim coils

Shim coils are used to introduce small adjustments to the main magnetic field to increase its homogeneity within the imaging field of view (FOV).

Radiofrequency coils

RF coils transmit and receive signals. The RF transmit coil produces a rotating magnetic field to flip the magnetization. The

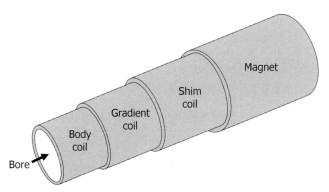

FIG. 6.2 ● **A simplified illustration of the relative positions of the coils on a cylindrical magnetic resonance scanner, including the main coils (aka the magnet), the shim coils, the gradient coils, and the radiofrequency (RF) coils (denoted as body coil as that is often the built-in RF coil of a system).** Reprinted with permission from Garcia MJ. *Noninvasive Cardiovascular Imaging: A Multimodality Approach.* Philadelphia, PA: Wolters Kluwer Health/Lippincott Williams & Wilkins; 2010.

MRI magnet bathed in cryogens

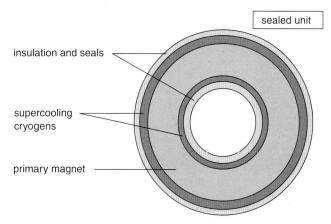

FIG. 6.3 ● **A cross-sectional view of the surroundings of the main coils on a scanner.** Reprinted with permission from Andolina VF, Lillé SL. *Mammographic Imaging.* 3rd ed. Philadelphia, PA: Wolters Kluwer Health/Lippincott Williams & Wilkins; 2011.

RF receive coil detects the induced electric current of precessing magnetization via electromagnetic induction. There are volume coils (eg, body coil in Figure 6.2), array coils, and surface coils.

Gradient coils

The gradient coils generate linearly varying magnetic fields in multiple dimensions; these gradient fields encode spatial information into the detected signal so that images can be correctly reconstructed. Three sets of gradient coils are typically mounted on an MR scanner, responsible for the gradient fields in the *x*-, *y*-, and *z*-directions separately (Figure 6.4).

Nuclei capable of MR signal production

Atomic and subatomic particles possess a property called spin angular momentum (also known as spin). Nuclear spin is traditionally denoted by the letter I. Protons, neutrons, and electrons all have spin = ½. Nuclei containing even numbers of both protons and neutrons have I = 0. Nuclei with odd numbers of both protons and neutrons have spin quantum numbers that are positive integers. The remaining nuclei (odd/even and even/odd) all have spins that are half integers. Only nuclei with nonzero spins (I $\neq$ 0) can absorb and emit electromagnetic radiation and undergo "resonance" when placed in a magnetic field. Only a small number of nuclei have the potential for MR signal production, and their values in clinical use are dependent on the strength of the nuclear magnetic moment, the physiologic concentration, and the isotopic abundance.

The nucleus of hydrogen (^{1}H), or the proton equivalently, becomes the major focus for MR signal production, because of its strong nuclear magnetic moment, its great abundance, and its wide availability in water (~70% of body weight in an adult) and fat molecules.

Some other nuclei, like ^{23}Na and ^{31}P, have also been used in clinical applications, but their use has been limited primarily due to their low abundance in human body.

While the notion of spin is fundamentally a quantum mechanical concept, one can use classical physics to understand most of the principles of MRI. Consider Figure 6.1, the spin of proton can be seen as a rotation of the nucleus about some axis, giving the proton a magnetic dipole moment (u) similar to a small bar magnet.

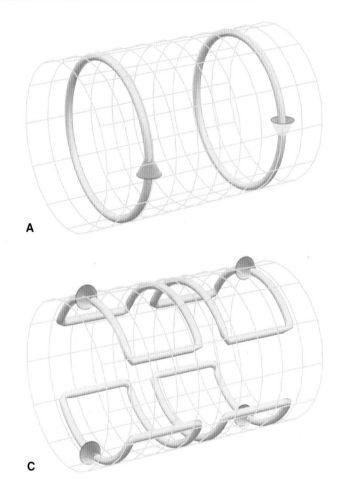

A

B

C

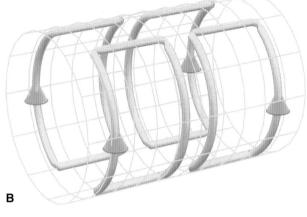

FIG. 6.4 ● The three sets of gradient coils on a magnetic resonance system, including the z-axis gradient coil (A), the x-axis gradient coil (B), and the y-axis gradient coil (C). The conical arrows indicate the flow of the current in the coils. Note that the x- and y-axis coils are equivalent but rotated by 90°. Reprinted with permission from Bammer R. *MR and CT Perfusion and Pharmacokinetic Imaging: Clinical Applications and Theoretical Principles.* Philadelphia, PA: Wolters Kluwer; 2016.

Behaviors of spins inside a static magnetic field

Precession

A spin placed inside a static magnetic field, $\vec{B}_0$, experience a torque that is perpendicular to both the magnetic field and angular momentum (Figure 6.5). The torque causes the spin to precess around the direction of the magnetic field similarly as a spinning top precesses around a gravitational field (Figure 6.6). The precessing frequency of the proton, proportional to the applied magnetic field strength, can be characterized by the Larmor equation:

$$f = \frac{\gamma}{2\pi} B_0,$$

where f is the precession frequency, B_0 is the magnitude of the static magnetic field, and $\frac{\gamma}{2\pi}$ is a constant called the

gyromagnetic ratio that depends on the type of the nucleus. The gyromagnetic ratio for the hydrogen nucleus, or the proton, is 42.58 MHz/T, so the Larmor frequency of the proton on 1.5 and 3 T systems are $42.58 \times 1.5 = 63.87$ MHz and $42.58 \times 3 = 127.68$ MHz, respectively.

The precessing directions of the spins, defined using the right-hand rule, are not the same for all spins. Some spins precess in the direction parallel to that of B_0, whereas others do so in the direction antiparallel. The two different directions, parallel and antiparallel, also correspond to two discrete different energy levels, with the former being the ground state and the latter at a higher level. The energy difference between the two states is proportional to B_0; the higher the field strength, the more energy separation between parallel and antiparallel spins.

FIG. 6.5 ● **Paramagnetic and diamagnetic materials in magnetic fields.** Paramagnetic materials increase the local magnetic field, whereas diamagnetic ones decrease the local field. They introduce inhomogeneity into the main magnetic field. Reprinted with permission from Bushberg JT, Seibert JA, Leidholdt EM, Boone JM. *Essential Physics of Medical Imaging.* 3rd ed. Philadelphia, PA: Wolters Kluwer Health/Lippincott Williams & Wilkins; 2012.

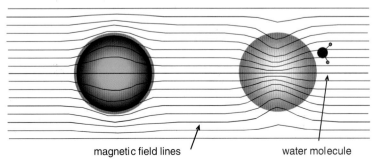

Diamagnetic: Paired electron spins

Paramagnetic: Unpaired electron spins

magnetic field lines

water molecule

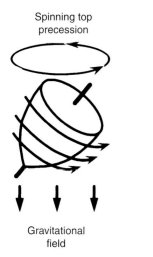
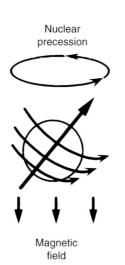

Spinning top precession

Nuclear precession

Gravitational field

Magnetic field

FIG. 6.6 ● The precession of an individual proton in the presence of an external magnetic field (in analogy to a spin top in the presence of a gravitational field). Reprinted with permission from Berquist TH. *MRI of the Musculoskeletal System.* 6th ed. Philadelphia, PA: Wolters Kluwer Health/Lippincott Williams & Wilkins; 2013; Adapted from Fullerton GD. Basic concepts for nuclear magnetic resonance imaging. *Magn Reson Imaging.* 1982;1:39–55. Copyright © 1982 Elsevier. With permission.

Net magnetization

At equilibrium, a slight majority exists in the parallel direction with lower energy. Owing to the excess of protons that precess in the parallel direction, a nonzero net magnetization vector forms as a combination of all individual spins, in the direction parallel to that of the static magnetic field (Figure 6.7). The net magnetization vector is referred to as $\vec{M}_0$, and varies linearly with $\vec{B}_0$. It serves as the source of the MR signal to be detected for imaging purposes.

Frame of reference

Two frames of reference have been used in understanding the behavior of the spins under the influence of static and RF magnetic fields. They are described as follows (Figure 6.8):

- The laboratory frame is a stationary reference frame from the observer's point of view. The sample magnetic moment vector precesses about the z-axis in a circular geometry.
- The rotating frame is a spinning axis system, whereby the x' to y' axes rotate at an angular frequency equal to the Larmor frequency. In this frame, the sample magnetic moment vector appears to be stationary when precessing at the resonance frequency.

FIG. 6.7 ● The formation of net magnetization. Each proton spin has its magnetic moment (left) inherent to the spin. When there is no external magnetic field, each individual moment has its random orientation, and, as a group together, they show zero net magnetization (middle). When there is an external magnetic field, proton spins align themselves with the field into two groups, one parallel to the external field, and the other antiparallel. There is always, however, a slightly larger number of parallel spins than antiparallel spins at equilibrium (because the parallel spins are at a more stable, lower energy state) and that results in a nonzero net magnetic moment, or magnetization vector, in the direction parallel to the applied external field (right).

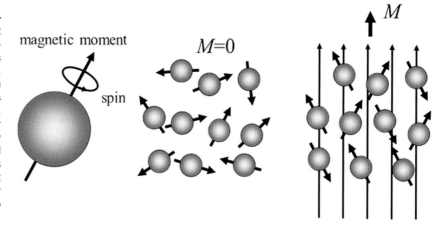

FIG. 6.8 ● The laboratory versus the rotating frames of reference in the depiction of proton spin's behaviors. A, The laboratory frame of reference is simply the stationary 3D Cartesian coordinate system, in which the precessing motion of proton spins in a magnetic field are observed. B, The rotating frame of reference is a 3D Cartesian coordinate system that is spinning at the Larmor frequency about the z-axis; the proton spins look stationary to the observer in this frame of reference. The rotating frame of reference is convenient in the understanding of proton spin's behaviors when the precessing motion is "removed." Reprinted with permission from Bushberg JT, Seibert JA, Leidholdt EM, Boone JM. *Essential Physics of Medical Imaging.* 3rd ed. Philadelphia, PA: Wolters Kluwer Health/Lippincott Williams & Wilkins; 2012.

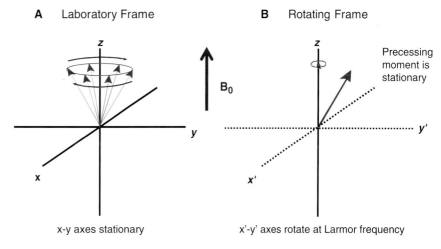

The RF excitation of the magnetization can be more clearly described using the rotating frame of reference, whereas the observed returning signal and its frequency content are explained using the laboratory (stationary) frame of reference.

As a convention, the direction of the applied magnetic field is considered the longitudinal direction, or the z-direction; in cylindrical scanners, this direction aligns with cranial-caudal axis, and is also referred to as the longitudinal axis. The plane perpendicular to the z-direction is the transverse plane in which the x-direction is typically aligned with the left-right direction of human body and the y-direction the anterior-posterior direction.

IMAGE FORMATION

Once nonzero net magnetic vectors are is in place within tissues, the process of image formation ensues by manipulation of these vectors. This process is divided into the following steps: signal production, signal detection, and signal localization.

Signal production

Excitation

Protons precess inside a static magnetic field at a frequency proportional to its strength, B_0; when an additional time-varying magnetic field, often denoted as $\vec{B_1}$, is applied whose oscillation frequency is equal to the precessional frequency of protons, MR occurs involving energy absorption and motion synchronization. The process of the resonance leads to changes in both the z- and the transverse (x-y) components of the net magnetization vector (Figure 6.9), described as follows:

- As $\vec{B_1}$ is applied, $\vec{M_z}$, the z-component of the net magnetization vector, initially equal to $\vec{M_0}$, first decreases until zero and then increases in the opposite direction until it reaches $-\vec{M_0}$. It can be explained as follows. The applied RF magnetic field, $\vec{B_1}$, can be considered as a train of energy packets; when the frequency of $\vec{B_1}$ matches that of the proton precession, the energy of each packet is equal to the difference between the energy levels of parallel and antiparallel spins, and as a result, the low-energy parallel spins will absorb the RF energy and become high-energy antiparallel spins. $\vec{M_z}$ becomes zero when the parallel and antiparallel spins are equal in number.
- In the meantime, $\vec{M_{xy}}$, the transverse component of the magnetization vector, increases from zero until it reaches the maximum at $\vec{M_0}$. This is due to the synchronization effect $\vec{B_1}$ has on the precessional phases of individual proton spins. Before $\vec{B_1}$ is applied, all proton spins are at random phases, and

their transverse components cancel out one another. After $\vec{B_1}$ is applied, its synchronization effect results in coherence in the precessional motion of the spins and a nonzero transverse component.

In rotating frame, the net magnetization M can be viewed as being progressively tipped away by continuous application of B_1. The flip angle is a quantity that describes the angle between $\vec{B_0}$ and the net magnetization vector at the end of the application of $\vec{B_1}$. The flip angle, depending on the needs of different pulse sequences, varies from 0° to 180°. A desired flip angle of $\vec{M_z}$ is achieved by varying the strength or the duration of $\vec{B_1}$ (Figure 6.10). Following Faraday's Law of Induction, wherein a changing magnetic field induces a voltage in a nearby conductor, the precessing magnetization induces an electrical current in the receive coil that's oriented perpendicular to the direction of the main magnetic field. This signal is then amplified, digitized, filtered, and stored as MR signal that will later be used for image reconstruction.

Once the RF field is turned off, the net magnetization vector will return to its equilibrium through a relaxation process. This relaxation process includes two separate subprocesses for $\vec{M_z}$ and $\vec{M_{xy}}$, in the longitudinal and transverse dimensions, respectively (Figure 6.11).

Longitudinal relaxation

For $\vec{M_z}$, once the RF field becomes zero, it will recover toward the net magnetization vector at equilibrium, $\vec{M_0}$. The underlying process is the turnover of individual proton spins, from higher energy antiparallel to lower energy parallel by releasing energy into the surrounding environment (often called the lattice). This recovery process, aka the spin-lattice relaxation, involves energy exchange between protons and the surrounding environment following an exponential behavior. The time constant of the relaxation process, defined as the time it takes for $\vec{M_z}$ to change from 0% to 63% of $\vec{M_0}$, is T1.

Energy emission from spins to the surrounding environment must be stimulated through encounter of the nucleus with another magnetic field fluctuating near the Larmor frequency. The trend of variation can be explained as follows (Figure 6.12 and Table 6.1):

- For tissues of solid type, all the molecules are tightly bound to each other; they form a lattice that vibrates at a narrow range of low frequencies, usually distinctly different from the Larmor frequency, and absorbs only a small fraction of the energy released during the longitudinal relaxation. As a result, such tissues have long T1.

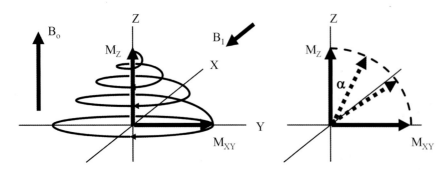

FIG. 6.9 ● **A net magnetization vector in a static magnetic field flips away from its initial vertical direction after a second radiofrequency pulse at the Larmor frequency is applied.** The trajectory followed by the vector differs because it is observed in the laboratory frame of reference (left) versus the rotating frame of reference (right). The rotating frame of reference is preferred due to the simplified view of the vector's behaviors. Reprinted with permission from Garcia MJ. *Noninvasive Cardiovascular Imaging: A Multimodality Approach.* Philadelphia, PA: Wolters Kluwer Health/Lippincott Williams & Wilkins; 2010.

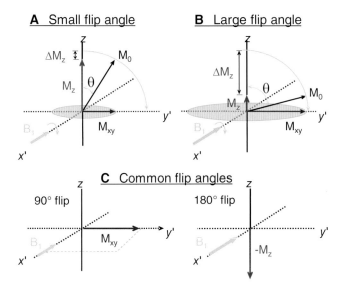

FIG. 6.10 ● **The flip angle of the net magnetization vector.** The flip angle is the angular displacement of the net magnetization vector from its initial or equilibrium position, viewed in the rotating frame. It is determined by both the amplitude and the duration of the applied B_1 field (at the Larmor frequency). The illustrations here include small (A; <45°), large (B; 75°-90°), and common (C; 90° and 180°) angles. Reprinted with permission from Bushberg JT, Seibert JA, Leidholdt EM, Boone JM. *Essential Physics of Medical Imaging.* 3rd ed. Philadelphia, PA. Wolters Kluwer Health/Lippincott Williams & Wilkins; 2012.

• For tissues of liquid type, like cerebral spinal fluid, or water itself, all the molecules are nearly free and form a highly loose lattice. Such a lattice allows a wide range of frequencies in their molecular vibration; only a small fraction of these frequencies may be close enough to the Larmor frequency to allow absorption of energy released during the longitudinal relaxation. These tissues too have long T1.

• For tissues that exhibit both solid and liquid behaviors, their molecular vibrations have a range of frequencies that are near the Larmor frequency, which leads to the absorption of a substantial amount of energy released during the longitudinal relaxation and therefore a shorter relaxation process back to the equilibrium. These tissues have a short T1 as a result.

T1 is not a constant for the same tissue; it varies by the strength of the static magnetic field, B_0. In general, T1 becomes longer as B_0 increases; longer T1 is expected for the same tissue at 3 T than at 1.5 T.

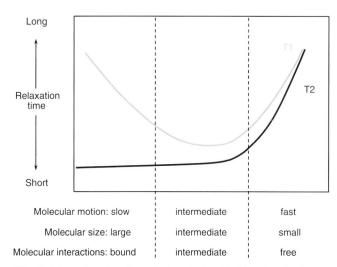

FIG. 6.12 ● **Relaxation times (T1 and T2) exhibit trends with tissue types.** They are fundamentally affected by tissue characteristics like molecular motion, molecular size, and interactions among molecules. Typically, solid tissues, fluid tissues, and tissues of certain viscosity fall on the left side, the right side, and the middle of the graph, respectively. Reprinted with permission from Bushberg JT, Seibert JA, Leidholdt EM, Boone JM. *Essential Physics of Medical Imaging.* 3rd ed. Philadelphia, PA: Wolters Kluwer Health/Lippincott Williams & Wilkins; 2012.

Table 6.1 **T1 AND T2 VALUES FOR COMMON TYPES OF TISSUES**

Tissue	T1 at 0.5 T (ms)	T1 at 1.5 T (ms)	T2 (ms)
Fat	210	260	80
Liver	350	500	40
Muscle	550	870	45
White matter	500	780	90
Gray matter	650	920	100
Cerebrospinal fluid	1800	2400	160

FIG. 6.11 ● **T1 and T2 relaxations as observed in a rotating frame of reference.** (A) shows changes in spin magnetization in the rotating frame, and (B) relaxation and decay curves. Reprinted with permission from Bammer R. *MR and CT Perfusion and Pharmacokinetic Imaging: Clinical Applications and Theoretical Principles.* Philadelphia, PA: Wolters Kluwer; 2016.

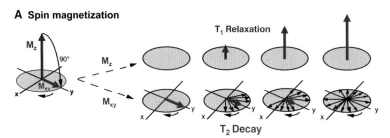

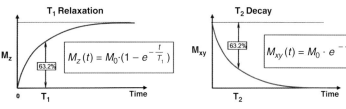

$$M_z(t) = M_0 \cdot \left(1 - e^{-\frac{t}{T_1}}\right)$$

$$M_{xy}(t) = M_0 \cdot e^{-\frac{t}{T_2}}$$

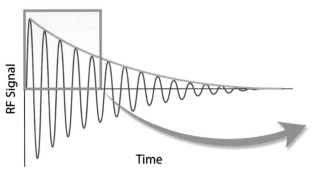

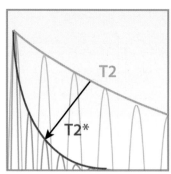

FIG. 6.13 ● **The comparison of T2 versus T2* decay.** Reprinted with permission from Huda W. *Review of Radiologic Physics.* 4th ed. Philadelphia, PA: Wolters Kluwer; 2016.

Transverse relaxation

For $\vec{M}_{xy}$, once the RF field is turned off, it will decrease toward zero because of the loss of phase coherence among proton spins. The relaxation process is often called spin-spin relaxation, because it is fundamentally caused by interactions among proton spins. The mechanism of this process is explained as follows:

Recall that spins precess at Larmor frequency, which is determined by the magnetic field they experience. In tissue, the magnetic field that each nucleus experiences is not exactly equal to the externally applied magnetic field B0. This microscopic neighborhood around a spin can cause the spin to experience a field slightly larger or smaller than B0. In addition, the spins in tissue are constantly in random thermal motion, so the microscopic neighborhoods of spins are continuously changing. The net result is that spins being tipped into the transverse plane progressively accumulate different amount of phase due to spatially variant and temporally changing precession frequencies. When the spins get out of synchronization with one another (losing coherence), the net transverse magnetization decays exponentially over time. The time it takes for the transverse magnetization to decrease to 37% of the initial magnetization is referred to as the T2 relaxation time (Figure 6.12).

Like T1, T2 also varies with the tissue type. However, its trend of variation differs from that of T1, which is described as follows (Figure 6.12 and Table 6.1):

- For tissues of solid type, there are a large number of interactions among adjacent proton spins at every moment, simply because

all the molecules are tightly bound to each other. The proton spins therefore get out of sync in their precession very rapidly, resulting in short T2.
- For tissues of liquid type, there are few interactions among proton spins at any moment, because the molecules are distant from each other. It therefore takes a long time for the proton spins to lose their coherence, resulting in a long T2.
- For tissues that exhibit both solid and liquid behaviors, intermediate T2 constants are expected.

T2, in theory, varies by B_0, but the variation is much smaller than that of T1. T2 is practically considered as constant with respect to B_0. In free induction decay (FID; Figure 6.13), the transverse magnetization diminishes much faster than would be predicted by natural atomic and molecular mechanisms (measured by T2). The factors that exacerbate the decay include B_0 inhomogeneity, susceptibility-induced field distortions produced by the tissue, velocity distribution, etc. The decay due to these macroscopic field disruption factors may be recovered with special designed pulse sequence. The time constant that characterizes the decay from all factors is T2* (T2* < T2).

Signal detection

The precessing transverse component of the magnetization (M_{xy}) can be detected using a receive coil oriented perpendicular to the direction of the main magnetic field (Figure 6.14). They can be the same coil used for producing $\vec{B}_1$, or a dedicated receiving coil. According to Faraday's Law of Induction, when

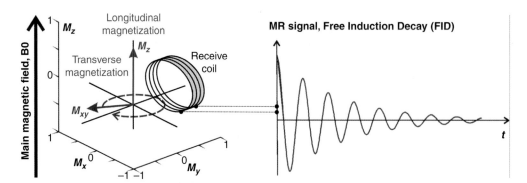

FIG. 6.14 ● **Spin magnetization and signal reception.** Radiofrequency excitation tips a fraction of the equilibrium magnetization into the transverse (x-y) plane. The resulting transverse magnetization $\vec{M}_{xy}$ rotates around the main magnetic field $\vec{B}_0$ at the Larmor frequency. This rotation and thus temporal change in magnetization direction induce a detectable magnetic resonance (MR) signal in a receive coil surrounding the object or patient. Relaxation effects and inhomogeneity within the imaged sample result in a signal reduction over time, leading to a characteristic MR signal, also referred to as the free induction decay. Reprinted with permission from Bammer R. *MR and CT Perfusion and Pharmacokinetic Imaging: Clinical Applications and Theoretical Principles.* Philadelphia, PA: Wolters Kluwer; 2016.

a changing magnetic field induces a voltage in a nearby conductor, the precessing magnetization induces an electrical current in the receive coil. This signal is then amplified, digitized, filtered, and stored as MR signal that will later be used for image reconstruction. The produced signal at any time point is a function of both the magnitude and the phase (or the direction) of $\vec{M}_{xy}$ at the time point.

Signal localization

The formation of images requires spatial localization of the acquired signals so that each voxel of the image volume has the correct signal for its location. Voxels are small unit cubes that make up the entire 3D volume.

Spatial localization on clinical MR systems are accomplished with three sets of gradient coils, which can produce gradient magnetic fields in three different directions. A gradient magnetic field is one with a linearly varying field strength along a certain direction. The gradient magnetic field is characterized by the change of the field strength per unit distance. The gradient magnetic field used on clinical scanners is typically on the order of a few thousandths of a Tesla per centimeter, so the unit mT/cm is used to describe the magnitude of a gradient magnetic field.

There are two basic methods for spatial location of MR signals, selective excitation and spatial encoding. Clinical imaging techniques use a mix of the two methods.

Any 3D image volume can be viewed as a stack of 2D image slices; for the simplicity of understanding, it is assumed in the following discussions of this section that the slices are in the transverse plane, ie, the x to y plane, and they stack up along the longitudinal, or z-direction. To achieve the goal of localization, the three aforementioned sets of gradient magnetic fields are

used, including the slice selection gradient (SSG), the frequency-encoding gradient (FEG), and the phase-encoding gradient (PEG). The three fields are orthogonal to each other, with SSG aligned with the z-direction and FEG and PEG inside the x to y plane (typically, FEG is along the x-direction and PEG along the y-direction).

SSG is used to selectively excite one slice of the image volume at a time. By turning on SSG, each slice in the image volume will experience a different magnetic field, and, therefore, requires an RF pulse of a unique frequency for its excitation. In fact, the RF pulse used on clinical scanners includes a band of frequencies, rather than a single frequency. By setting the band of frequencies of the RF pulse, one may excite only a slab of tissues whose Larmor frequencies lie within the band of frequencies of the RF pulse (Figure 6.15). The central frequency of the RF pulse determines the location of the slice. The thickness of the excited image slab may be controlled by both the magnitude of SSG and the bandwidth (BW) of the RF pulse (Figure 6.16). For the same SSG magnitude, shorter BW of the RF pulse results in thinner slices. Similarly, for the same BW of RF pulse, a larger SSG gradient results in thinner slices.

After a single image slice (a slab, more precisely) is excited, FEG and PEG are applied for spatial encoding of the proton spins within the slice. Instead of selectively imaging one pixel at a time within the slice, one always acquires signals collectively from all voxels from the slice but alters the relative contribution of each voxel to the total signal by having different FEGs and PEGs for each such measurement. Once the acquisition is over, the signal of each voxel can be solved mathematically through a reconstruction process. This spatial encoding process can be made efficient if each acquired signal corresponds to a data point in the k-space domain of the image slice through a

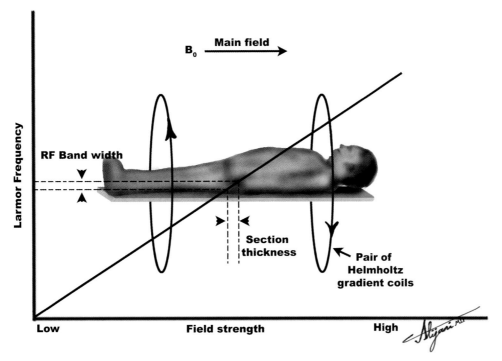

FIG. 6.15 ● **The principle of slice selection through the use of a set of gradient coils.** Reprinted with permission from Huda W. *Review of Radiologic Physics.* 3rd ed. Philadelphia, PA: Wolters Kluwer Health/ Lippincott Williams & Wilkins; 2010.

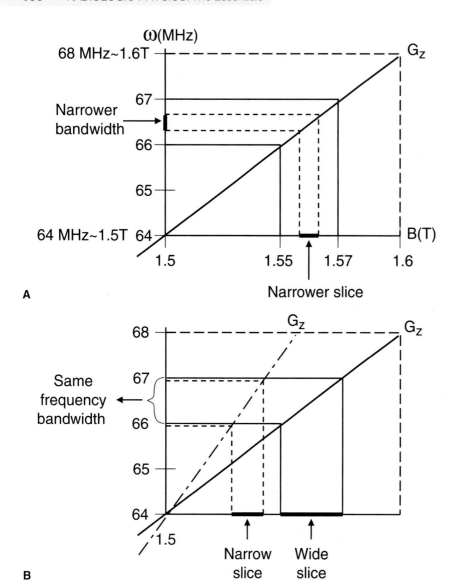

FIG. 6.16 ● A, B, The control of slice thickness through the use of different gradient and radio-frequency bandwidth. Reprinted with permission from Hashemi RH, Lisanti CJ, Bradley W. *MRI: The Basics.* 4th ed. Philadelphia, PA: Wolters Kluwer; 2018.

well-designed pulse sequence. For more details on k-space and image reconstruction, refer to the following section on image reconstruction.

IMAGE RECONSTRUCTION AND K-SPACE

An important concept in the understanding of MR image reconstruction is k-space. k-Space is a spatial frequency domain linked to the spatial domain. An object can be mathematically represented in any well-defined domain. In the spatial domain, an object is represented as its signal values as a function of spatial location. This is the domain we understand by intuition. Likewise, the same object can be represented as its signal values as a function of spatial frequency in the k-space. The underlying assumption is that any object can be viewed as a summation of many basic objects, each of which has its values oscillating at a certain combination of frequencies (one frequency for each dimension of the domain); the k-space representation of the object is therefore the entire collection of weightings for each combination of spatial frequencies.

As previously described, the signal read out at each time point of MR image acquisition is collectively from all proton spins within the excited slice; each proton spin is at its own phase of precession because of the application of the PEG and FEG fields. Each such signal essentially represents a point in the k-space. By deliberate manipulation of the PEG and PEG fields, all the points in the k-space can be acquired and the image can then be reconstructed using standard mathematical methods. A common acquisition scheme in covering all the necessary data points in the k-space is as follows: within a single time of repetition (TR), one horizontal line of k-space, whose k_x varies while k_y stays constant, is acquired; then during each of the next TRs, k_y changes to a different value by altering the PEG such that a different line of k-space is covered (Figure 6.17).

For a data point in the k-space counterpart of an image, its contribution to the image varies by its position in the k-space (Figure 6.18). If the point is near the center of the k-space, it carries mostly information from low-spatial-frequency, or slowly varying, components of the image, which primarily determines the contrast observed in an image. If the point is far from the center of k-space, it carries mostly information from

FIG. 6.17 ● Illustration of how a pulse sequence works to fill the data points in k-space. MR, magnetic resonance; PEG, phase-encoding gradient; RF, radiofrequency; TR, time of repetition. Reprinted with permission from Bushberg JT, Seibert JA, Leidholdt EM, Boone JM. *Essential Physics of Medical Imaging.* 3rd ed. Philadelphia, PA: Wolters Kluwer Health/Lippincott Williams & Wilkins; 2012.

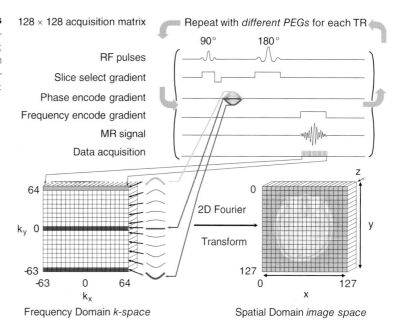

high-spatial-frequency, or rapidly changing, components of the image, which accounts for sharply transitioning boundaries and small-sized features in the image.

PULSE SEQUENCES

A pulse sequence is a time series of events comprising RF pulses, magnetic field gradients, and data acquisition. Variant pulse sequences have been designed to produce desired signal and contrast by manipulating the magnetization. Three basic pulse sequences used in clinical imaging are discussed here (Figure 6.19). SE and GE, aka gradient recalled echo (GRE), are two pulse sequences that form the foundation of the majority of clinical pulse sequences. IR sequences introduce an extra inversion pulse to achieve the goal of selective enhancement or suppression of certain tissues.

FIG. 6.18 ● A chest image viewed in both the spatial domain and the k-space domain, and the roles of low-frequency and high-frequency k-space data points. Reprinted with permission from Garcia MJ. *Noninvasive Cardiovascular Imaging: A Multimodality Approach.* Philadelphia, PA: Wolters Kluwer Health/Lippincott Williams & Wilkins; 2010.

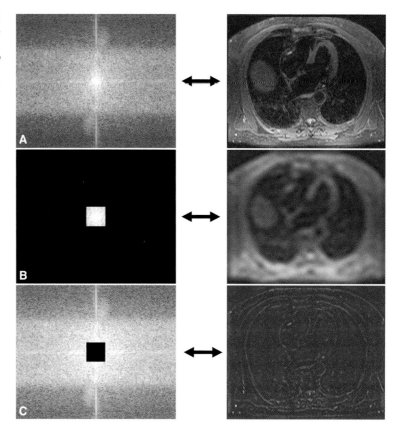

Spin Echo

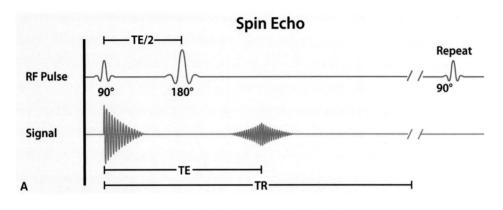

A

Gradient Recalled Echo

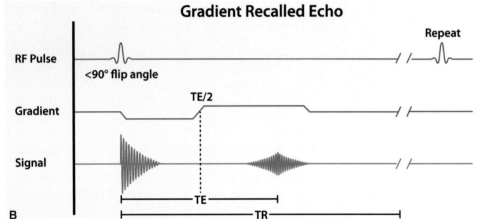

B

Inversion Recovery

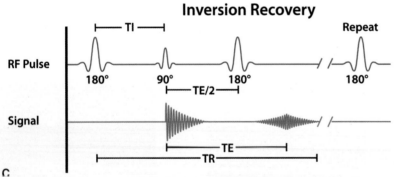

C

FIG. 6.19 • Illustrations of three magnetic resonance (MR) pulse sequences: (A) spin echo, (B) gradient echo (aka gradient recalled echo), and (C) inversion recovery. Spin-echo pulse sequence starts with a 90° radiofrequency (RF) pulse, followed by a 180° refocusing RF pulse at time TE/2 resulting in an echo at time TE. In a gradient echo sequence, there is a single RF pulse with a flip angle typically <90°, and an echo is created at time TE by reversal of a dephasing gradient at time TE/2. An inversion recovery sequence adds a 180° inversion pulse some time before a regular pulse sequence (it is a spin-echo sequence in this illustration). Reprinted with permission from Huda W. *Review of Radiologic Physics.* 4th ed. Philadelphia, PA: Wolters Kluwer; 2016.

Spin echo

In an SE pulse sequence, a 90° RF pulse is first applied, and is then followed by a 180° refocusing RF pulse sometime later. The 90° RF pulse synchronizes the precessing motion of all spins within a voxel, but, once it is over, the spins begin to dephase, or lose their coherence in phases. The dispersion of the spins is due to several reasons: magnetic field inhomogeneity, random interactions among spins, and others. At the application of the refocusing pulse, the spins will be rotated about an axis in the transverse plane and the phase dispersion is reversed; as a result, an echo peaks at the so-called time of echo (TE). If the 90° pulse marks the starting point, the time of the 180° refocusing pulse application is at exactly TE/2, halfway between the 90° pulse and the peak of the echo (Figure 6.20). The phase dispersion due to macroscopic field inhomogeneity will be fully recovered at TE. But the dephasing caused by the random spin-spin interactions cannot be refocused by the refocusing pulse. Therefore, the

decay of signal in an SE pulse sequence follows the time constant of T2 instead of T2*.

The magnitude of transverse magnetization, $\vec{M}_{xy}$, in an SE pulse sequence can be expressed as

$$M_{xy} = M_0(1 - e^{-\text{TR}/\text{T1}})e^{-\text{TE}/\text{T2}},$$

where M_0 is the magnitude of the net magnetization vector when only the static magnetic field is present, TR is the time of repetition, TE is the time of echo, T1 is the time constant of spin-lattice relaxation, and T2 is the time constant of spin-spin relaxation.

As can be seen from the given equation, the signal is a function of three tissue-specific parameters: proton density (the major factor affecting M_0), T1, and T2. Through the manipulation of TR and TE, two key acquisition parameters of an SE sequence, one may selectively highlight one of the three parameters in the acquired signal for optimized differentiation (Table 6.2 and, Figures 6.21-6.23).

FIG. 6.20 ● **Illustration of the principle of spin-echo pulse sequences in a rotating frame of reference.** The starting 90° pulse produces a free induction decay (FID) that decays according to T2* relaxation. After a delay time TE/2, a 180° radiofrequency pulse inverts the spins that reestablishes phase coherence and produces an echo at a time TE. Inhomogeneities of external magnetic fields are canceled, and the peak amplitude of the echo is now determined by T2 decay instead of T2* decay. The sequence is repeated for each repetition period, TR. Reprinted with permission from Bushberg JT, Seibert JA, Leidholdt EM, Boone JM. *Essential Physics of Medical Imaging.* 3rd ed. Philadelphia, PA: Wolters Kluwer Health/Lippincott Williams & Wilkins; 2012.

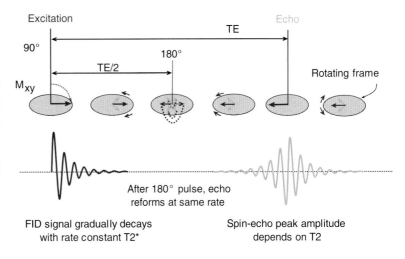

FID signal gradually decays with rate constant T2*

Spin-echo peak amplitude depends on T2

Table 6.2 **THE RATIONALES OF MRI IMAGE WEIGHTING THROUGH THE ADJUSTMENT OF SCAN PARAMETERS**

Weighting in Images	TR Setting	TE Setting	Rationale
T1 weighted	Short	Short	With short TE, there is nearly no T2-decay and therefore no T2 weighting in the formed images. Short TR ensures that each repetition starts with a signal showing significant T1 dependence.
T2 weighted	Long	Long	With long TR, each repetition starts with a signal complete its T1 relaxation and therefore with no T1 dependence. Long TE ensures that there is just enough T2 decay to introduce T2 weighting in the formed images.
Proton density weighted	Long	Short	With long TR and short TE, there is neither T2 nor T1 weighting in the formed images. All there is left in the images are proton density differences for different pixels.

Abbreviations: MRI, magnetic resonance imaging; TE, time of echo; TR, time of repetition.

FIG. 6.21 ● **Illustration of T1 relaxation and the effect of imaging timing on image contrast.** Reprinted with permission from Leyendecker JR, Brown JJ. *Practical Guide to Abdominal and Pelvic MRI.* Philadelphia, PA: Lippincott Williams & Wilkins; 2004.

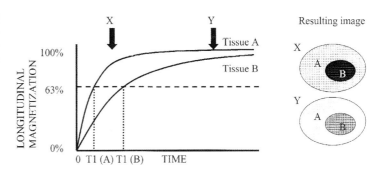

FIG. 6.22 ● **Illustration of T2 relaxation and the effect of imaging timing on image contrast.** Reprinted with permission from Leyendecker JR, Brown JJ. *Practical Guide to Abdominal and Pelvic MRI.* Philadelphia, PA: Lippincott Williams & Wilkins; 2004.

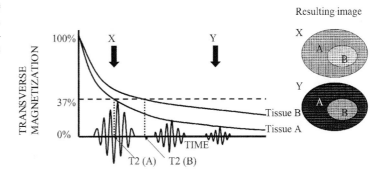

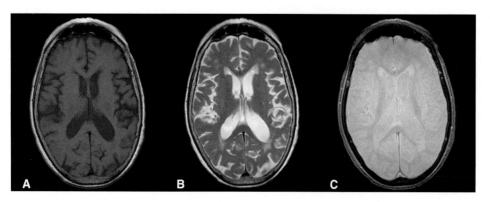

FIG. 6.23 ● A-C, T1-, T2-, and proton-density-weighted brain images (from left to right).

Note that the selection of "long" and "short" in the setting of TR or TE is a relative concept. The selection for TR is relative to T1; it is considered long if TR is several times of T1 and short if TR is only a small fraction of T1. The same applies to TE relative to T2.

Gradient echo

A GE pulse sequence differs from an SE pulse sequence (Figure 6.24) in that there is no 180° refocusing pulse, and the formation of an echo is based on the reversal of a gradient field (usually the frequency encoding). Echo time (TE) is when the area under the prephasing and rephasing gradient lobes is equal.

Mechanisms such as field inhomogeneity or susceptibility are not refocused at TE so GE signal intensity decays much faster and TE has to be shorter as for SE imaging.

Fast GRE are sequences with TR shorter than T2. The transverse magnetization does not fully decay prior to each new RF pulse and after several repetitions reaches a steady state. The signal at steady state might contain FID, SE, and stimulated echo (STE). By carefully structuring of the gradients and phases of the RF pulses variant fast GRE sequences have been developed to handle these signals for certain use, one may choose to kill all the SE and STE signals by applying a spoiler gradient, or constructively add the two echoes together, or just keep one of them; each resulting pulse sequence has its unique weighting and tissue contrast. Benefits of these types of pulse sequences include new contrast mechanisms, high SNR, and fast acquisition time (through the use of very short TRs).

Inversion recovery

IR sequences put a 180° RF pulse (also called IR module) before the excitation RF pulse with a time delay. The inversion RF pulse flips the longitudinal magnetization from the +z to −z axis. The time between the 180° inversion pulse and the 90° RF pulse is called the time of inversion (TI). TI allows the inverted magnetization to recover toward its equilibrium value. Starting with the excitation RF pulse, a host pulse sequence (SE, GE, or echo planar imaging [EPI]) will be played out and form an image. The definitions of TR and TE remain the same as those in a generic SE pulse sequence, with TR being the time between two successive inversion pulses and TE the time between the RF pulse and the peak of the echo. By varying TI, TR, and TE, a range of image contrast can be produced by an IR pulse sequence.

The 180° inversion pulse is often timed specifically to null signals from a certain type of tissue for improved contrast among tissues of clinical interest. When it is applied, the longitudinal magnetization vector $\vec{M}_z$ of the affected tissue is turned from $\vec{M}_0$ by 180° to $-\vec{M}_0$, and then starts its relaxation back to $\vec{M}_0$, following a temporal behavior governed by T1 of the tissue. If a 90° RF pulse is applied at exactly the time when $\vec{M}_z = 0$ for a particular type of tissue (this time, relative to the inversion pulse, is called the bounce point or null point) no transverse magnetization will be produced for this tissue, whereas other tissues have nonzero transverse magnetization produced from their $\vec{M}_z$ at the moment (Figure 6.25).

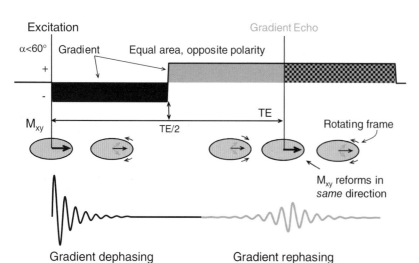

FIG. 6.24 ● **Illustration of the principle of gradient pulse sequences in a rotating frame of reference.** Transverse magnetization spins are dephased with an applied gradient of one polarity and rephased with the gradient reversed in polarity; this produces a "gradient echo." Extrinsic inhomogeneities like those originated from nonuniform static field B_0 are not canceled, and the resulting signal follows a T2* decay. Reprinted with permission from Bushberg JT, Seibert JA, Leidholdt EM, Boone JM. *Essential Physics of Medical Imaging*. 3rd ed. Philadelphia, PA: Wolters Kluwer Health/Lippincott Williams & Wilkins; 2012.

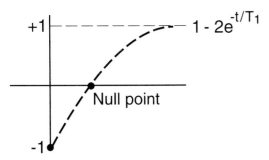

FIG. 6.25 ● **The null point following a 180° inversion pulse.** If an excitation RF pulse is applied right at the null point for a specific tissue, there will be no flipping of magnetic vectors, and therefore it produces no signal from the particular tissue. Reprinted with permission from Hashemi RH, Lisanti CJ, Bradley W. *MRI: The Basics.* 4th ed. Philadelphia, PA: Wolters Kluwer; 2018.

Short tau inversion recovery (STIR) and fluid-attenuated inversion recovery (FLAIR) are two important applications of IR used clinically for selectively nulling signals from tissues with short and long T1 values, respectively (Figures 6.26 and 6.27). STIR is often used for suppressing signals from fat (TI is about

FIG. 6.26 ● **Fat suppression by short tau inversion recovery.** Time of inversion is chosen so that the T1 recovery curve for fat crosses zero at the time of the 90° pulse. In the remaining part of the pulse sequence, only other tissues will produce nonzero signals. WM, water molecule. Reprinted with permission from Hashemi RH, Lisanti CJ, Bradley W. *MRI: The Basics.* 4th ed. Philadelphia, PA: Wolters Kluwer; 2018.

FIG. 6.27 ● **Suppression of cerebral spinal fluid (CSF) by fluid-attenuated inversion recovery (FLAIR).** The same lesion on T2-weighted (A) and FLAIR (B) images. The conspicuity of the lesion in the vicinity of CSF is substantially improved with the application of FLAIR. Reprinted with permission from Engel J, Pedley TA, Aicardi J, et al. *Epilepsy.* 2nd ed. Philadelphia, PA: Wolters Kluwer Health/Lippincott Williams & Wilkins; 2008.

160-180 ms at 1.5 T), whereas FLAIR is used for reducing signals from cerebrospinal fluid (TI about 2200 to 2500 ms at 1.5 T).

FAST MRI

In the early days of MRI, the acquisition time for a study is typically long, which greatly limited the value of MRI in medical applications. It is the continued technical innovations in the following years that have made MRI both valuable and sufficiently fast in a great many applications. Techniques and methods used in MRI to shorten acquisition time are discussed as follows.

Acquisition time of standard 2D spin-echo sequences

The acquisition time of an MR image is the time it takes to acquire all data points in the k-space counterpart of the image. For a standard SE pulse sequence, the acquisition time of an image slice can be expressed as

$$\text{Acquisition Time} = TR \times \# \text{ PEG steps} \times NEX$$

where TR is the time of repetition, # PEG steps is the number of steps in the phase-encoding direction, and NEX is the number

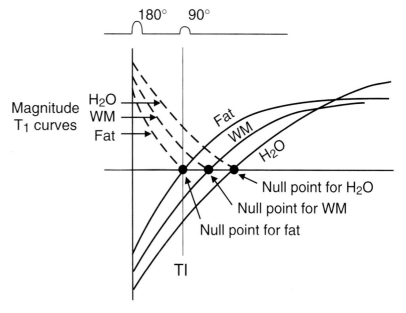

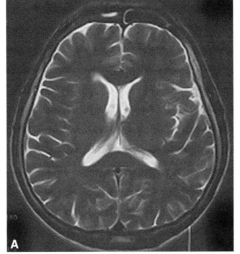

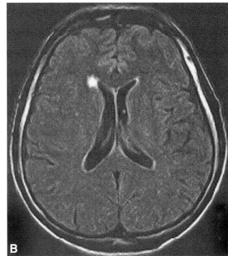

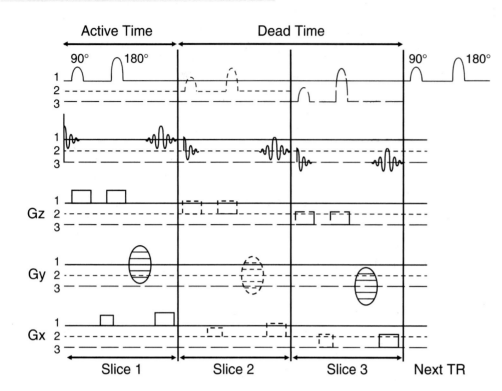

FIG. 6.28 ● **Illustration of multislice acquisition.** Within each time of repetition cycle, when there is sufficient "dead time" where the system would otherwise just wait for recovery of the slice, other slices may be acquired for time savings and shorter total scan. TR, time of repetition. Reprinted with permission from Hashemi RH, Lisanti CJ, Bradley W. *MRI: The Basics*. 4th ed. Philadelphia, PA: Wolters Kluwer; 2018.

of excitations. One can estimate the acquisition time of a standard SE sequence with some realistic assumptions. Assume that # PEG steps is 128 and NEX is 1. To acquire a T2- or proton-density-weighted image, TR is required to be much longer than T1 of protons in water and a typical choice is 2.5 seconds; the acquisition time of a single slice is therefore $2.5 \times 128 \times 1 = 320$ seconds, or about 5 minutes. To acquire a T1-weighted image, a reasonable TR setting is 500 ms; the acquisition time of a single slice is $0.5 \times 128 \times 1 = 64$ seconds, or about 1 minutes. One can easily see that the acquisition of multiple slices in this manner to cover a 3D volume requires scan time on the order of hours. It is therefore necessary to shorten MR acquisition time to a much more acceptable range for clinical use.

Multislice acquisition

For SE sequences with long TR, much time is "wasted" in waiting for the longitudinal recovery of proton spins. Instead of idling, another slice can be excited during the recovery time so that the total acquisition time for the desired number of slices can be reduced (Figure 6.28). The acceleration factor is essentially the number of slices that can be excited during a single TR.

Fast pulse sequences

MR pulse sequences capable of faster acquisition of k-space signals than the standard SE have been developed to meet the demand for faster MR scan time.

Fast spin echo

Fast spin echo (FSE) is an extension of the standard SE featured by the use of multiple 180° refocusing pulses within a single TR (Figure 6.29). The number of echo signals produced within each TR is called the echo train length (ETL), and, because each echo signal fills one k-line in the k-space, multiple k-lines are filled within each TR, resulting in an acceleration of acquisition time equal to ETL. Each echo has its own TE value, resulting in k-space data with nonuniform T2 weighting. Because the image contrast

is predominantly determined by the low-spatial-frequency data in k-space, the TE of FSE sequence is defined as the TE when the central k-space line is acquired. This TE is called the effective TE. To produce a T1-weighted or proton-density-weighted image, earlier echoes in the echo train are used to sample the central k-space data so that TEeff takes its minimal value. To minimize the blurring effect from later echoes, ETL is kept low (typically 3-7 for 2D). For T2-weighted imaging, a later echo can be assigned to the central k-space data while the peripheral k-space (high spatial frequency) is acquired earlier with less decayed signal. ETL is typically long (16-22 for 2D) with long TR and long TEeff. There are some differences between conventional SE and FSE in tissue contrast. Fat although having long T2 is abnormally dark in T2-weighted SE images due to J-coupling. However, in FSE, fat is shown bright secondary to disruption of J-coupling. FSE also shows diminished sensitivity to susceptibility that makes the FSE the sequence of choice whenever metal objects are present, significantly reducing artifacts.

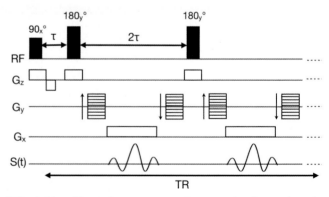

FIG. 6.29 ● **The pulse sequence diagram of a fast spin echo sequence.** Multiple 180° refocusing pulses are applied within each time of repetition (TR) to acquire multiple k-space lines. Reprinted with permission from Atlas SW. *Magnetic Resonance Imaging of the Brain and Spine*. 5th ed. Philadelphia, PA: Wolters Kluwer; 2017.

Gradient echo

GE acquisitions can be fast because the flip angle of the excitation pulse is typically less than 90. Therefore, no lengthy period of time is required for T1 recovery, and short TR can be used. A TR of 50 ms or less in a GE sequence means 10 times or more time reduction in the acquisition of a single slice compared to an SE sequence using a TR of 500 ms.

As discussed earlier, when TR becomes so short that transverse magnetization has not fully diminished before the next RF, the residual transverse magnetization needs to be carefully handled to avoid any unwanted disruption by stimulated echoes. Some pulse sequences apply a spoiler gradient before the end of each TR to eliminate the residual transverse magnetization, whereas others utilize these residual signals in the next TR to form coherent images together with the echo produced by the next RF.

Echo planar imaging

EPI can achieve extremely fast acquisition time by acquiring all k-lines within a single or a few TR intervals. EPI employs a series of bipolar readout gradients (Figure 6.30) to generate a train of GEs and multiple k-space lines can be sampled under the envelope of an FID or a SE. Because GEs can be produced at a much faster rate than SEs, EPI generates an image in a considerably shorter time. A single 2D image can be acquired with one RF excitation (single-shot EPI) or multiple RF excitations (segmented EPI). High demands are placed on hardware including fast data sampling, rapid reversal of gradient fields, and others. EPI is prone to a variety of artifacts like ghosting from system imperfections, displacement from chemical shift, off-resonance effects from magnetic susceptibility variations, and distortion from field inhomogeneities. T2* decay also causes image blurring. EPI proves to be a valuable tool in diffusion imaging,

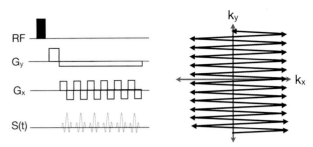

FIG. 6.30 ● **The pulse sequence diagram of an echo planar imaging sequence.** The rapid change of the polarity of frequency-encoding gradient makes possible the acquisition of the entire k-space within one or just a few time of repetitions. Reprinted with permission from Atlas SW. *Magnetic Resonance Imaging of the Brain and Spine.* 5th ed. Philadelphia, PA: Wolters Kluwer; 2017.

perfusion imaging, functional MRI, dynamic studies, and real-time imaging.

Parallel imaging

In parallel imaging, the spatial dependence of the B1 field of each channel in the phased array coil is used to assist spatial localization of the MR signal. Therefore, a reduction in the number of phase-encoding steps that is required for aliasing free image reconstruction can be achieved (Figure 6.31). Parallel imaging methods can be generally categorized as either k-space based (eg, GRAPPA) or image space based (eg, SENSE). The coils must have some sensitivity difference in the phase-encoding direction in order to provide additional spatial information for reconstruction. Parallel imaging although accelerates the scanning time also has SNR penalty. The acceleration factor applied clinically is about 2-4 depending on the anatomy and coil placement.

FIG. 6.31 ● **Illustration or example of parallel imaging.** Data acquisition is accelerated by skipping data lines in k-space, resulting in aliasing artifacts in the image (eg, point P contains signals from two points in the original). The folded image pixel can be resolved by exploiting differences in coil sensitivity of antenna elements (eg, coil #1 and coil #2) placed around the object (ie, point P and the point P′ folded upon it are "seen" differently by coil #1 and coil #2). Reprinted with permission from Higgins CB, de Roos A. *MRI and CT of the Cardiovascular System.* 3rd ed. Philadelphia, PA: Wolters Kluwer Health/ Lippincott Williams & Wilkins; 2013.

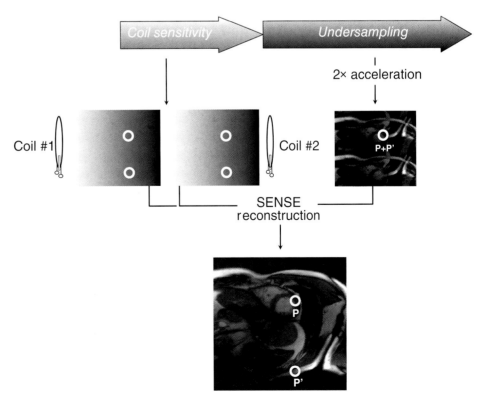

IMAGE QUALITY

The SNR is an important quantity used to describe the performance of an MRI system. It is a measure of true signal to noise (eg, random quantum mottle). The main source of noise in the image is the patient's body (RF emission due to thermal motion). The whole measurement chain of the MR scanner (coils, electronics, etc.) also contributes to the noise. A lower SNR generally results in a grainy appearance to images. For any pulse sequence, the SNR of an MR image can be expressed as a function of a number of variables, as shown here:

$$SNR \propto I \times voxel_{x,y,z} \times \sqrt{\frac{NEX}{BW}} \times f(QF, B, \text{slice gap, reconstruction}),$$

where I is the signal intensity specific to the pulse sequence, $voxel_{x,y,z}$ is the volume of the voxel, NEX is the number of excitations, BW is RF bandwidth, and $f(QF, B, \text{slice gap, reconstruction})$ is a function of coil quality factor (QF), static magnetic field strength (B), slice gap, and the reconstruction algorithm.

Voxel size

MR signal comes from excited spins of each voxel; therefore, it is linearly related to the voxel size. Increasing FOV, decreasing matrix size, and increasing slice thickness can all increase voxel size. Larger voxels contain more spins and result in more signal and higher SNR in general (Figure 6.32).

Number of excitations

NEX describes the number of repeated RF excitations used to generate multiple signals for each desired data point. By averaging the acquisitions, the signal remains constant, but the noise goes down with the square root of the number of excitations. So the doubling of NEX results in about 40% increase in SNR.

Bandwidth

BW refers to the frequency bandwidth used by the receiving coils in acquiring the echo signals during the readout. The use of a narrower BW reduces the amount of electronic noise that is detected by the receiving coils and contributes to an increase in SNR proportional to

its square root. A narrower RF BW, however, requires a smaller readout gradient field, which may lead to more pronounced chemical shift artifacts, and place a limit on the minimum TE that can be used.

f factor

The QF of an RF coil refers to its ability of electrical signal production in response to magnetic signals coming from the patient. The tuning of the coil is necessary to ensure the resonance frequencies specific to the patient are most efficiently detected. Its positioning is also crucial for high SNR. Various designs and configurations of RF coils have been devised to ensure high SNR in a variety of applications.

The static magnetic field strength (B) affects the SNR as a power function, which accounts for the improvement of SNR from 1.5 T magnets to 3 T magnets and the motivation of stronger magnets for MRI. New acquisition techniques such as parallel imaging and reconstruction techniques and filters can affect not only the level but also the statistical distribution of image noise.

ARTIFACTS

Artifacts represent incorrect information regarding the underlying truth about the object of interest.

Motion artifacts

MR images are often affected by artifacts because of patient motion, including both voluntary and involuntary movements of body parts, blood flow, and others. Typical appearances of motion artifacts are multiple copies of the image superimposed onto the original at various locations along the phase-encoding direction. Such artifacts are also called ghost artifacts. The reason why they are much more pronounced in the phase-encoding direction is as follows: the time separation between any two neighboring k-lines, equal to TR, is on the order of seconds, much longer than the time of acquire a single k-line; therefore, motion causes more inconsistency and artifacts between k-lines than within each k-line. Examples of these artifacts on clinical MR images are given in Figures 6.33 to 6.35.

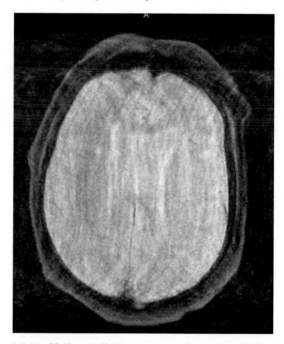

FIG. 6.33 ● **Motion artifacts on magnetic resonance brain images.** Head movement during the scan gives rise to "ghosts" in the phase-encoding direction.

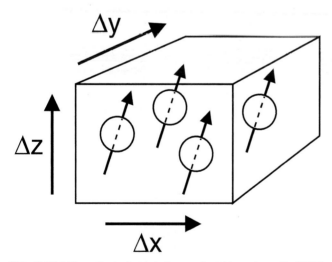

FIG. 6.32 ● **The effect of voxel size on signal-to-noise ratio (SNR) of magnetic resonance imaging images.** The more spins in a voxel, the more is the signal. Therefore, increasing voxel size increases SNR. Reprinted with permission from Hashemi RH, Lisanti CJ, Bradley W. *MRI: The Basics.* 4th ed. Philadelphia, PA: Wolters Kluwer; 2018.

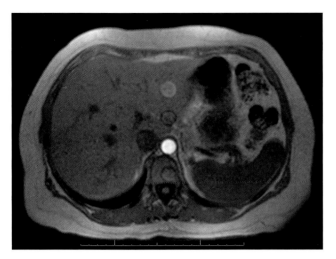

FIG. 6.34 ● **Motion artifacts on magnetic resonance abdomen images.** The pulsating motion of the aorta gives rise to replicated aorta "ghosts" in the phase-encoding direction.

Field-inhomogeneity-related artifacts

Ideally, a uniform external magnetic field is desired to make every proton inside the field at the same precessional frequency; in doing so, gradient fields may be applied later to introduce frequency differences encoded by spatial locations. This is, however, not realistic because there are inevitably variations in the field strength across the FOV. Such field inhomogeneity causes geometric distortions, due to its interference with spatial localization, and loss of signal, due to more rapid dephasing of proton spins. GE sequences are more prone to field inhomogeneity–related artifacts, for example, zebra banding artifacts (Figure 6.36). When chemically selective fat saturation technique is used, field

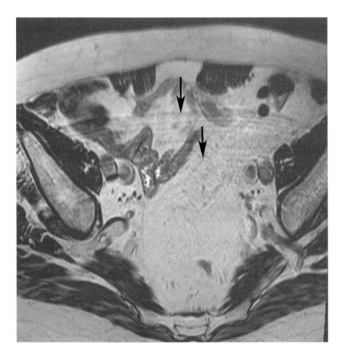

FIG. 6.35 ● **Motion artifacts on magnetic resonance pelvis images.** Respiratory motion related abdominal organ movement led to the observed artifacts (arrows). Reprinted with permission from Berquist TH. *MRI of the Musculoskeletal System.* 6th ed. Philadelphia, PA: Wolters Kluwer Health/Lippincott Williams & Wilkins; 2013.

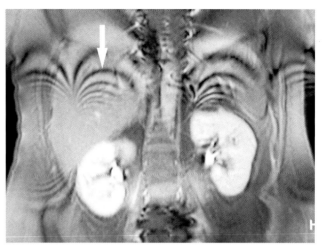

FIG. 6.36 ● **Field inhomogeneity artifacts.** The artifacts on this set of images (arrow) have appearances of "zebra stripes" and are attributed to local field inhomogeneity. Such artifacts are more often seen with gradient echo sequences, because of the lack of refocusing echoes to mitigate field inhomogeneity effects. Reprinted with permission from Leyendecker JR, Brown JJ. *Practical Guide to Abdominal and Pelvic MRI.* Philadelphia, PA: Lippincott Williams & Wilkins; 2004.

inhomogeneity will cause insufficient fat saturation due to spatially dependent fat frequency (Figure 6.37). Field inhomogeneity is usually worse close to the magnet bore; therefore, artifacts are more common with big FOV. In addition, the higher the field strength is, the more challenging it becomes to ensure field homogeneity.

Susceptibility artifacts

When a material is placed in a magnetic field, it interacts with the externally applied field through induced internal magnetization and alters the local field surrounding it (Figure 6.5). Susceptibility refers to the way and the extent of a material in altering a local magnetic field. Susceptibility differences cause the local magnetic field experienced by the tissue to be substantially different from those by neighboring tissues. Susceptibility artifacts often manifest as geometric distortions and/or local signal loss. They most often occur near metal objects (Figure 6.38) or interfaces like the junction of the front lobe and sinus, and junction of the pons and sphenoid sinus (Figure 6.39).

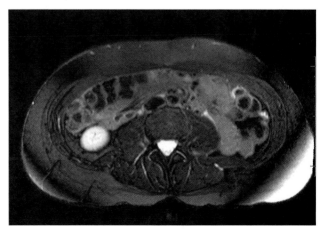

FIG. 6.37 ● Insufficient fat saturation due to field inhomogeneity.

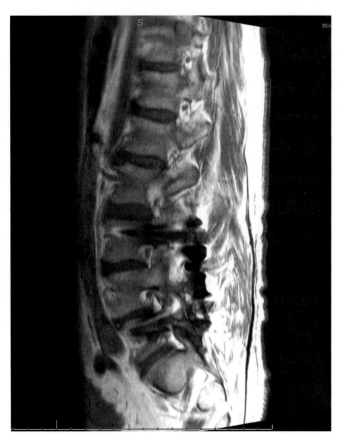

FIG. 6.38 ● **Susceptibility-induced distortion and signal loss in a sagittal spin image due to metal implants.**

Chemical shift artifacts

Owing to the impact of magnetic shielding by electron clouds, protons of fat molecules precess at a slightly different frequency from those of water molecules. The relative difference between the precessional frequencies of fat and water, defined as the ratio of their absolute difference relative to the frequency of water protons, is about 3.5 parts per million (ppm). At 1.5 T, when the Larmor frequency of water protons is 63.27 MHz, the absolute difference is 220 Hz; at 3 T, it is twice as much. This difference mainly leads to two types of chemical shift artifacts.

Chemical shift artifacts of the first kind occur regardless of the use of SE or GE sequences, manifesting as paired bright-dark boundaries near certain fat-containing organs. MRI assumes a uniform Larmor frequency everywhere in the image in the absence of gradient fields and that, when the readout gradient is applied, the protons' precessional frequency varies across the FOV for spatial localization. When the system detects the signal produced by fat, it thinks the signal is produced by water at a different spatial location and leads to the shift of the pixels. Usually, this produces a bright boundary on one side of the organ and a dark one on the other side. This chemical shift artifact is most commonly seen around water-containing structures (liver, kidneys, optic nerves, thecal sac, muscles, nerve fascicles) surrounded by fat. A clinical example is shown in Figure 6.40.

Chemical shift artifacts of the second kind occurs exclusively in GE imaging. The artifacts look like organs and muscle bundles have been outlined with a black pen. Owing to the difference in their Larmor frequencies, the water and fat molecules have a specific difference in their frequency; and at specific time points, protons in these two molecules experiencing the same magnetic field may come to be in phase (same phase) or out of phase (180° apart in phase). At 1.5 T, with 220 Hz being their absolute difference, protons of water and fat molecules will be in phase and produce bright signals when TE is equal to the

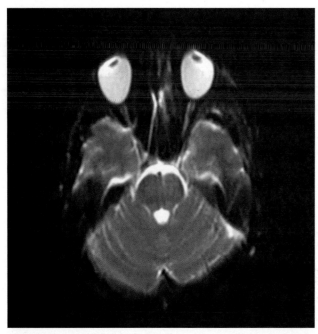

FIG. 6.39 ● **Susceptibility artifacts on magnetic resonance brain images.**

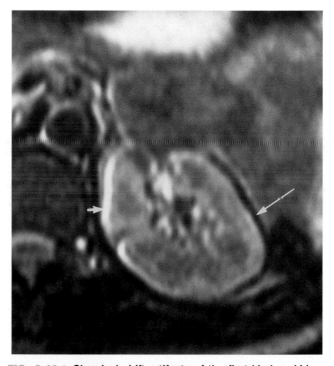

FIG. 6.40 ● **Chemical shift artifacts of the first kind on kidney images.** Misregistration between fat and kidney tissue caused by chemical shift produces a high-density band (short arrow) on the medial aspect of the left kidney and a low-density band (long arrow) on its lateral aspect. Reprinted with permission from Brant WE, Helms CA. *Fundamentals of Diagnostic Radiology*. 3rd ed. Philadelphia, PA: Lippincott Williams & Wilkins; 2007.

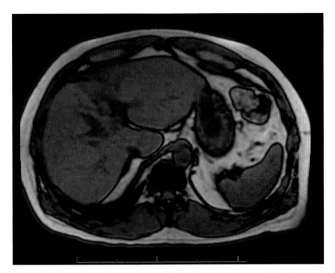

FIG. 6.41 • **Chemical shift artifacts of the second kind on abdomen images.** Note the black lines surrounding the organs, often referred to as Indian ink or black line artifacts.

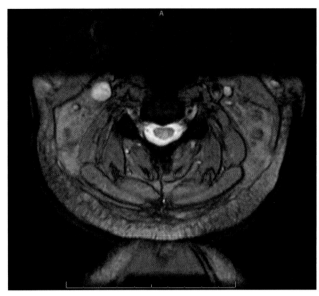

FIG. 6.43 • Wraparound artifacts on magnetic resonance brain images.

multiples of 4.5 ms, and will be opposite in their phases and produce dark signals when TE is at odd multiples of 2.25 ms. As a result, voxels with mixed fat and water, typically on boundaries of organs, look bright when they are in phase and dark when out of phase. Since this second type of artifact is due to a phase cancellation effect, it is not limited to the frequency-encode direction (as is the chemical shift artifact of the first kind), but may be seen in all pixels along a fat-water interface where both fat and water exist in each voxel (Figures 6.41 and 6.42). This type of artifact can be reduced by applying fat suppression technique (Figure 6.42).

Wraparound artifacts

The wraparound artifact is generally easily recognized as a folding over of anatomic parts into the area of interest (Figure 6.43). They are caused by the undersampling of the k-space signal (the dimensions of an object exceed the defined FOV) along the direction(s) of anatomy wrapping around (Figure 6.43). Wraparound artifacts can be eliminated by oversampling. In the frequency-encoding direction, oversampling does not incur a penalty in regard to acquisition time and is inherently applied by all vendors. In phase-encoding

FIG. 6.42 • **Chemical shift artifacts of the second kind for a patient with Crohn disease.** These are coronal gradient echo images without (A) and with (B) fat saturation. In voxels where both water and fat protons coexist, there is signal cancellation seen as a dark thin line (arrows) known as black boundary or chemical shift artifact. The artifacts and the fatty tissue that is causing them are eliminated by acquiring fat-saturated images (B). Reprinted with permission from Shirkhoda A. *Variants and Pitfalls in Body Imaging.* 2nd ed. Philadelphia, PA: Wolters Kluwer Health/Lippincott Williams & Wilkins; 2011.

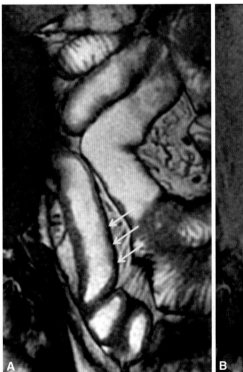
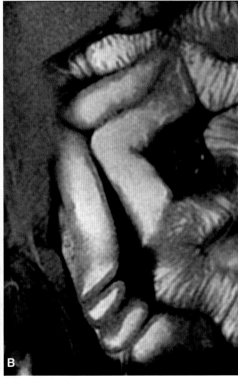

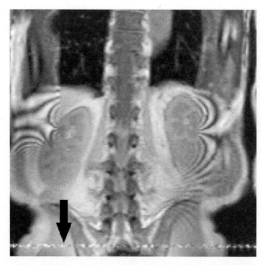

FIG. 6.44 ● **Zipper artifacts caused by radiofrequency leak.** For this case, the frequency encoding is in the cranial-caudal direction, perpendicular to the horizontal direction of the zipper artifacts (arrow). Reprinted with permission from Leyendecker JR, Brown JJ. *Practical Guide to Abdominal and Pelvic MRI*. Philadelphia, PA: Lippincott Williams & Wilkins; 2004.

direction, oversampling increases acquisition time proportionally. Using oversampling may affect spatial resolution and SNR depending on the matrix size.

RF leak artifacts

In the environment near an MR scanner, there are easily common RF sources whose signals, when leaked into an MR room and detected by the RF coils, cause artifacts on patients' images. Noise with a narrow RF distribution presents as "zipper" artifacts in the direction of phase encoding (Figure 6.44). The most common origin of this RF noise is an extraneous source that reaches the receiver coil due to defective shielding. A second common cause is RF emission from anesthesia monitoring equipment (eg, pulse oximeters) used within the scanner room.

MR SAFETY
MR safety aspects

MRI safety includes several aspects of an MRI system. They are projectile effect, sound effect, and heat effect.

Projectile effect

The "projectile effect" refers to the capability of the fringe field of an MR system to attract a ferromagnetic object, drawing it rapidly into the scanner by considerable force. The projectile effect can pose significant risk to the patients inside the bore and anyone in the path of the projectile. The force increases with ferromagnetic composition, total mass, and the gradient of the magnetic field strength at its location. Oxygen tanks, wheelchairs, and other objects have been reported to cause severe damage. To prevent a ferromagnetic object entering the scanner room and become projectile, all patients and individuals must be carefully screened to identify any problematic objects. Medical equipment and devices need to be identified as MR safe or MR conditional to be brought into the scanner room.

Peripheral nerve stimulation and acoustic injury

During MRI examinations, the time-varying gradient magnetic fields may stimulate nerves or muscles in patients by inducing electrical fields. The risk of peripheral neurostimulation is dictated by the rate of change of the magnetic field over time, termed dB/dt and expressed in Tesla per second (T/s). MR imaging studies that pose the greatest risk of peripheral neurostimulation are those that involve high-bandwidth readouts and/or rapid gradient switching, such as echo planar imaging. Reducing the read bandwidth or increasing the repetition time can reduce dB/dt.

The quickly switching gradients are also responsible for the high acoustic noise. Hearing protection such as head phones and earplugs is essential to avoid hearing damage in anyone in the scanner room during scanning.

Heat effect

The majority of the RF power transmitted during MRI procedures is transformed into heat within the patient's tissue as a result of resistive losses. The dosimetric term used to describe the absorption of RF radiation is the SAR. SAR is the mass-normalized rate at which RF power is coupled to biologic tissue with units of watts per kilogram (W/kg). The U.S. Food and Drug Administration sets the SAR limits for whole body weight, partial body, and head. SAR is a complex function of numerous variables such as RF frequency, flip angle, transmit RF coil, tissue volume contained within the transmit RF coil, TR, as well as other factors. Thermophysiologic response to MR-induced heating depends on the duration of exposure, the rate at which energy is deposited, the response of the patient's thermoregulatory system, and the presence of an underlying health condition, although with MR procedures conducted within SAR limit, many incidents of excessive heating have been reported. In many of these cases, positioning of the patients played an important role. Body parts in direct contact with transmit RF coils or skin-to-skin contacts form closed loops for electric current conduction. Other mechanisms like electrically conductive materials (ECG leads, electrodes, etc.), clothing containing metallic fabric, and monitoring devices contacting defects could also contribute to cause excessive heating. Specific guidelines to prevent excessive heating and burns associated with MR procedures have been published by the IMRSER (Institute for Magnetic Resonance Safety, Education, and Research) and shall be practiced regularly.

Implant safety

Medical devices and implants contain varying amounts of ferromagnetic material and can be subject to translational force and/or torque. The force is proportional to the mass of the ferromagnetic materials in the implant. The potential for injury is also related to the proximity of the implant to vital vascular, neural, or soft-tissue structures.

Certain metallic devices (electrically conductive implants such as wires or leads) can act as an "antenna" and concentrate RF energy, which leads to excessive local heating, especially at the tip of these devices.

Active implants can interact in several ways with the RF and gradients and may cause excessive heating and/or device malfunction. For example, cardiac pacemakers were originally an absolute contraindication to MR imaging because there was risk for radiofrequency pulses causing inappropriate asynchronous pacing and risk for burns from atrial and ventricular leads.

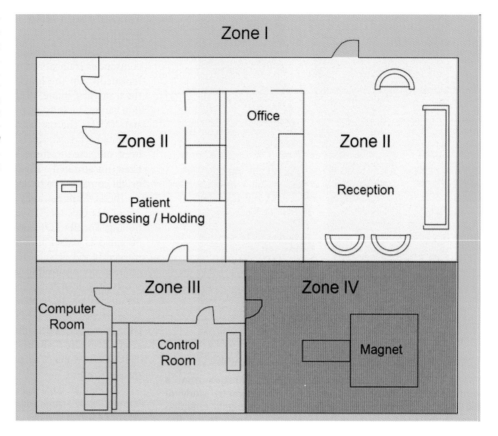

FIG. 6.45 ● **Example of magnetic resonance zoning for a typical layout.** Reprinted with permission from Bushberg JT, Seibert JA, Leidholdt EM, Boone JM. *Essential Physics of Medical Imaging.* 3rd ed. Philadelphia, PA: Wolters Kluwer Health/Lippincott Williams & Wilkins; 2012; Adapted from Kanal E, Barkovich AJ, Bell C, et al. ACR guidance document for safe MR practices: 2007. *Am J Roentgenol.* 2007;188:1447–1474. Copyright © 2007, American Roentgen Ray Society

The terminology for MR safety of implant or device is "MR safe," "MR unsafe," or "MR conditional." MR-safe devices are nonhazardous in all MR imaging environments, whereas MR-unsafe devices are considered to be contraindicated in any MR imaging environment. An MR-conditional device is MR imaging–compatible only in specific operating conditions. MR safety information shall be acquired through manufacturer or several online catalogues give model information.

MR zoning

MR safety zones are categorized from zone 1 to zone 4. The definitions of the four zones are as follows (example shown in Figure 6.45):

- Zone 1: all areas that are open to public access
- Zone 2: a buffer zone between zones 1 and 3, typically referring to the reception area where the patients get registered and go through MR safety screening before entering the next zone

- Zone 3: an area where the access is restricted to MR personnel, the screened patient, and other ancillary medical staff
- Zone 4: the MR scanner room

ADVANCED APPLICATIONS
MR angiography

Magnetic resonance angiography (MRA) may be performed with or without enhancement by gadolinium-based contrast agents. Contrast-enhanced MRA (CE-MRA) is the most commonly used clinical imaging technique, whereas noncontrast-enhanced MRA has been a hot topic of research for its potential clinical benefits.

Contrast-enhanced MRA

Over the last decade, CE-MRA has become the method of choice for evaluating most of the vascular systems within the body due to its intrinsically high signal to noise, short acquisition time, and relative freedom from flow-related artifacts (Figures 6.46 and 6.47).

FIG. 6.46 ● Contrast-enhanced magnetic resonance angiography of lower extremities in the coronal plane (A) with digital subtraction (B). There are multiple superficial femoral artery aneurysms (arrow) in the right lower extremity and a femoral to below-the-knee bypass graft in the left lower extremity. Reprinted with permission from Geschwind J, Dake M. *Abrams' Angiography.* 3rd ed. Philadelphia, PA: Wolters Kluwer Health/Lippincott Williams & Wilkins; 2014.

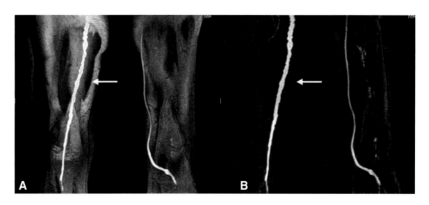

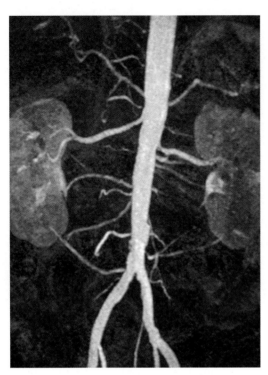

FIG. 6.47 ● **Maximum intensity projection images from a contrast-enhanced magnetic resonance angiography study of the aorta and renal arteries showing excellent signal retention through the aorta into the distal renal arteries and into the iliac arteries.** Reprinted with permission from Higgins CB, de Roos A. *MRI and CT of the Cardiovascular System.* 3rd ed. Philadelphia, PA: Wolters Kluwer Health/Lippincott Williams & Wilkins; 2013.

CE-MRA uses the gadolinium-based contrast agent injected intravenously to dramatically shorten the T1 of blood. By implementing a T1-weighted imaging sequence during the first pass of the contrast agent, images can be produced that show arteries with striking contrast relative to surrounding stationary tissues and veins.

Vascular signal intensity of CE-MRA is determined principally by the concentration of gadolinium within the vessel. Flow-related phenomena (eg, velocities, flow direction, turbulence)—factors that play dominant roles in the appearance of vessels on noncontrast MRA studies—have little or no effect on CE-MRA.

Synchronizing the acquisition with the arrival of the contrast agent is critical to image quality. If the time of the peak bolus is misjudged, the MRA may be ruined with inadequate arterial filling or contaminating contrast present in the venous system or urinary tract.

Noncontrast-enhanced MRA

Noncontrast-enhanced MRA provides alternative techniques of vascular imaging by MRI and offers benefits compared to contrast-enhanced MRA in certain applications. One of the benefits comes when imaging patients with impaired renal functions or certain vascular diseases that would contraindicate the use of gadolinium-based agents. Although noncontrast-enhanced MRA techniques are, in general, limited by longer acquisition time, recent advances in technology have spurred new interests in them. A brief description of two methods of noncontrast-enhanced MRA, time-of-flight (TOF) MRA and phase-contrast (PC) MRA, is provided as follows.

Time-of-Flight MRA

TOF MRA is based on the principle of flow-related enhancement. Tissues contained within an imaging volume are subjected to a continuous train of radiofrequency (RF) pulses. These RF pulses repeatedly flip the longitudinal tissue magnetization (Mz) into the transverse plane. With short TR, the longitudinal magnetization cannot be fully recovered and evolves to a new lower steady state (Mss). The tissues within the imaged volume are partially saturated. "Fresh" blood flowing into the imaged slab has not been subjected to these RF pulses and is therefore fully magnetized (unsaturated). The signal from inflowing blood thus appears bright compared to background tissue.

The TOF angiography can be implemented with a conventional 2D or 3D GE (GRE) sequence with optional gradient-moment nulling. For 2D TOF, multiple thin (1- to 2-mm thick) slices are obtained as a stack in a plane perpendicular to the course of the imaged blood vessels. The slices in 2D TOF MRA are acquired sequentially; a traveling saturation band is generally placed on the upstream side of each slice to suppress contaminating signal from venous inflow. 2D TOF offers short imaging times with excellent sensitivity to slow flow. However, it is insensitive to in-plane flow and, therefore, is best suited for straight vessels such as the carotid arteries (Figure 6.48) or the vessels in the lower extremities. 2D TOF is also subject to patient motion artifacts that may create misregistration.

3D TOF is used for more compact anatomic regions with various flow directions, for example, intracranial arteries (Figure 6.49) and renal arteries. A slab (or multiple thin slabs) is oriented perpendicular to the vessels at the entry. Small flip angle is used to prevent blood signal saturation. 3D TOF offers higher SNR and high spatial resolution; however, it is insensitive to slow flow and saturation effects that limit maximum slab thickness of each acquisition.

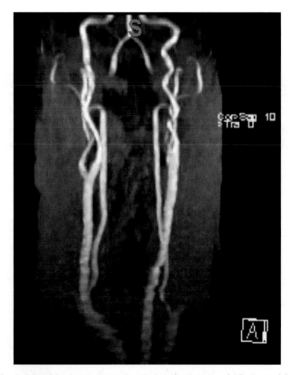

FIG. 6.48 ● Maximum intensity projection image of 2D time-of-flight magnetic resonance angiography of carotid artery.

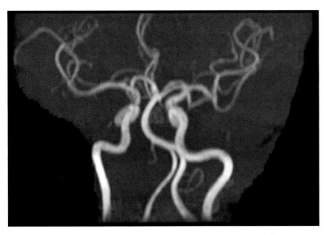

FIG. 6.49 ● Maximum intensity projection image of a 3D time-of-flight magnetic resonance angiography study of intracranial arteries.

Phase-Contrast MRA

Phase-contrast MR angiography uses pairs of bipolar gradient pulses to generate flow-sensitive phase image. A stationary spin subjected to such a gradient pair will experience no net phase shift, but a moving spin (with motion in the same direction the gradient is applied) will have a net phase shift proportional to its velocity. Two spins flowing at the same speed but in opposite directions will have equal but opposite phase shifts. The phase data are used to reconstruct either velocity-encoded flow quantification images or MR angiographic images (Figure 6.50). The maximum measurable velocity that corresponds to a phase shift of 180° is a user-defined parameter, referred to as encoding velocity, or Venc. For flow quantification applications, where velocities exceed the Venc, velocity aliasing will occur.

Phase-contrast MR angiography has the advantage of high sensitivity to turbulent flow and inherently low background signal. However, its use has been limited by its long acquisition time. The most commonly used applications today for phase-contrast imaging are: 1) vascular scout image; 2) quantification of blood flows within the heart and great vessels; 3) qualitative or quantitative CSF flow measurements; 4) intracranial MR venography.

Diffusion MRI

Diffusion refers to the random motion of the molecules driven by thermal energy. In a perfectly homogeneous medium, diffusion is random and isotropic. But in a human body, diffusion within the tissue is influenced by cellular architecture and pathology. Diffusion-weighted imaging (DWI) provides qualitative and quantitative information about the diffusion properties.

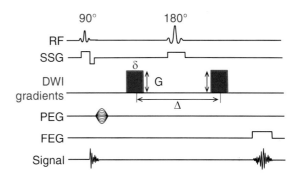

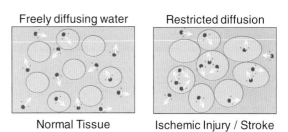

FIG. 6.51 ● **Pulse sequence diagram of diffusion-weighted imaging (DWI).** The effect of diffusion weighting, that is, the degree of signal loss due to the diffusion process, is closely related to the magnitude of the gradients, *G*, the duration of the gradients, δ, and the time interval between the gradients, Δ. FEG, frequency-encoding gradient; PEG, phase-encoding gradient; RF, radiofrequency; SSG, slice selection gradient. Reprinted with permission from Bushberg JT, Seibert JA, Leidholdt EM, Boone JM. *Essential Physics of Medical Imaging.* 3rd ed. Philadelphia, PA: Lippincott Williams & Wilkins, a Wolters Kluwer business; 2012; Adapted from Kanal E, Barkovich AJ, Bell C, et al. ACR guidance document for safe MR practices: 2007. *Am J Roentgenol.* 2007;188:1447–1474.

In a DWI sequence, a bipolar gradient is applied after excitation and before signal sampling (Figure 6.51). The parameter "b value" decides the diffusion weighting and is expressed in s/mm². It is proportional to the square of the amplitude and duration of the gradient applied. The bipolar gradient has zero net effect on static spins, because the phase due to the positive gradient will be fully recovered by the negative gradient (positive after 180° RF). When diffusion is present, spins within the voxel experience different phases due to movement and lose coherence.

Diffusion is qualitatively evaluated on trace images (Figure 6.52) where tissues with restricted diffusion are bright. A parameter called apparent diffusion coefficient (ADC) also gives quantitative measurement of the diffusion property that removes

FIG. 6.50 ● Phase-contrast magnetic resonance angiography study with both anatomy and blood-flow images.

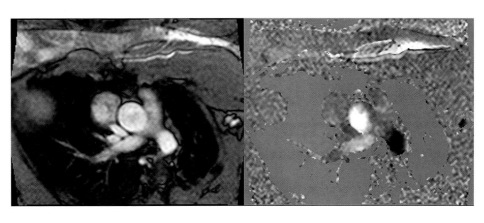

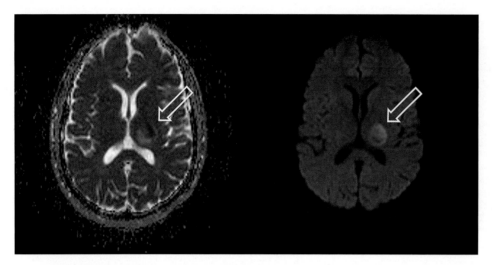

FIG. 6.52 ● **Magnetic resonance brain diffusion study.** Left: T2-weighted image (b=0); Right: diffusion trace image (b=1000). Note the relative enhancement of the lesion from left image to right image (arrows) due to restricted diffusion within the lesion.

the T2 effects. The signal intensity of each voxel in a trace image is inversely related to its ADC value. Acute brain ischemia has been the most successful application of DWI. The use of DWI in combination with perfusion MRI outlines salvageable areas of ischemia.

Diffusion tensor imaging measures the degree of anisotropy and structural orientation. White matter tracts with tightly packed coherently oriented fiber bundles hinder water displacement perpendicular to the direction of the fibers.

The 3D pattern of diffusion anisotropy of white matter tracts can be modeled by the diffusion tensor, a 3×3 symmetric matrix. By acquiring sets of diffusion-encoded images with more than six noncollinearly oriented diffusion gradients, the tensor can be mathematically resolved for each voxel. A number of diffusion tensor metrics are used to characterize the dimensions and shape of the diffusion ellipsoid associated with the microstructure of a particular voxel. The three principal axes of the diffusion tensor, termed the "eigenvectors," can be calculated by diagonalizing the diffusion tensor. The fractional anisotropy (FA) index measures the degree of directionality of intravoxel diffusivity. The value of FA varies between 0 and 1. For perfect isotropic diffusion, three eigenvalues are equal and FA = 0. With progressive diffusion anisotropy, the eigenvalues become more unequal, the ellipsoid

becomes more elongated, and FA → 1. The fiber orientation information inherent in the primary eigenvector can be visualized on 2D images (called colored FA map) by assigning a color to each of three mutually orthogonal axes (Figure 6.53), typically red to left-right, green to anteroposterior, and blue to superior-inferior.

Fiber tracking is a technique to visualize the entire white matter tracts in 3D for presurgical planning purpose. In each brain voxel, the dominant direction of axonal tracts can be assumed to be parallel to the primary eigenvector of the diffusion tensor. Fiber tracking uses the diffusion tensor of each voxel to follow an axonal tract from voxel to voxel through the brain.

Perfusion MRI

Perfusion refers to the delivery of blood to tissues through capillary beds. The values of perfusion MRI have been well demonstrated in the imaging of stroke and intracranial tumors. Three methods are commonly used for perfusion MRI: Dynamic Susceptibility Contrast (DSC), Dynamic Contrast Enhanced (DCE), and Arterial Spin Labeling (ASL). Both DSC and DCE require bolus administration of exogenous gadolinium-based contrast agent, while ASL is performed without exogenous contrast.

DSC-MRI begins with a bolus of gadolinium chelate injected intravenously. As the gadolinium first passes through the regional

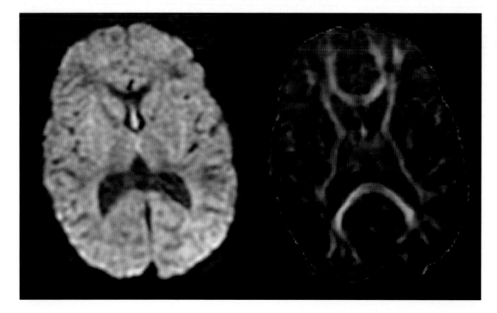

FIG. 6.53 ● Diffusion tensor imaging: Diffusion-weighted raw image (left), color fractional anisotropy map (right).

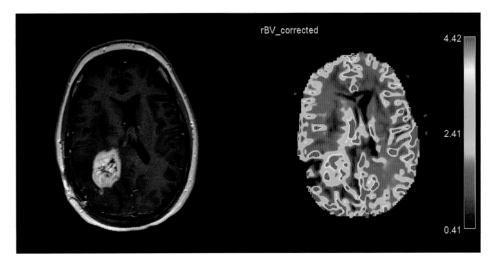

FIG. 6.54 ● MR brain dynamic susceptibility contrast perfusion study: T1-weighted postcontrast image (left), relative cerebral blood volume map (right).

circulation, it remains largely confined to the intravascular space. Due to its paramagnetic properties, gadolinium alters the local magnetic field and causes T2 (T2*) dephasing and loss of signal as the bolus passes. Following the injection, a series of T2- or T2*-weighted images are acquired by SE or GE sequence over the organ of interest. By measuring signal intensity as a function of time and fitting to a mathematical model, various perfusion parameters (eg, blood volume, blood flow, mean transit time) can be extracted (Figure 6.54).

DCE-MRI acquires T1-weighted images (mostly with GE sequence) over a period of 5-10 minutes following contrast administration. During this time frame, gadolinium contrast accumulates within the extracellular extravascular space and causes T1 shortening. Signal enhancement in T1-weighted images can be related to tissue contrast agent concentration. Several physiologic parameters can then be derived from the signal-time function, including the transfer constant (Ktrans), fractional plasma volume (vp), and fractional volume of the tissue extracellular space (ve).

ASL does not require the administration of gadolinium contrast. Instead, the water molecules in proximal blood vessels are "magnetically labeled" (saturated or inverted) by radiofrequency pulses (Figure 6.55). As these molecules flow into the organ of interest, the tissue signal intensity will be modified in proportion to perfusion. In the typical ASL pulse sequence, images are acquired both with and without labeling pulses, then subtracted. By applying a mathematical model, various perfusion parameters (principally blood flow) can be obtained.

MR spectroscopy

MR spectroscopy (MRS) is an analytical method that quantifies metabolites in tissues of interest. MR spectra may be obtained from different nuclei. Protons (1H) are the nuclei most used for clinical applications, mainly because of their high sensitivity and abundance. In clinical practice, 1H-MRS is mostly used for detailed analysis of tumors and metabolic diseases.

1H-MRS is based on the chemical shift properties of the atom. As was discussed previously, when placed in a static magnetic field, protons precess at the Larmor frequency, which is proportional to the magnitude of the local field. Protons inside the molecules of different metabolites have different electron cloud distributions surrounding them, and the shielding effect of these electrons gives rise to different magnitudes of local magnetic field and therefore different shifts in frequency (a phenomenon called

chemical shift). The value of frequency shift gives information about the molecular group carrying 1H and is expressed in parts per million (ppm).

The MR spectrum (Figure 6.56) is represented by the x-axis that corresponds to the metabolite frequency in ppm according to the chemical shift and the y-axis that corresponds to the peak amplitude. The relative areas under each peak are roughly proportional to the quantity of nuclei in each molecule.

In conventional MRI, frequency differences between voxels are used for spatial encoding. This is typically accomplished by applying a frequency-encoding gradient during signal evolution. In MRS, however, frequency-encoding gradient is not played during readout. The frequency information contained in the time domain signal is decoded by Fourier Transform to identify chemical shifts between molecular species.

The 1H-MRS acquisition usually starts with anatomic images, which are used to select a volume of interest (VOI), where the spectrum will be acquired. The voxels can either be isolated by

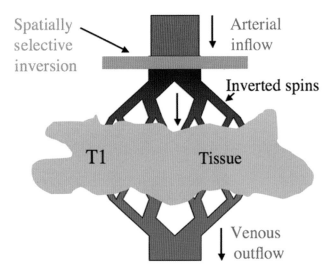

FIG. 6.55 ● **Illustration of arterial spin labeling perfusion techniques.** Inflowing arterial spins are inverted with spatially selective radiofrequency pulses. The inverted spins then flow into the tissue, where they attenuate the signal slightly. The degree of attenuation is a measure of perfusion. Reprinted with permission from Atlas SW. *Magnetic Resonance Imaging of the Brain and Spine.* 5th ed. Philadelphia, PA: Wolters Kluwer; 2017.

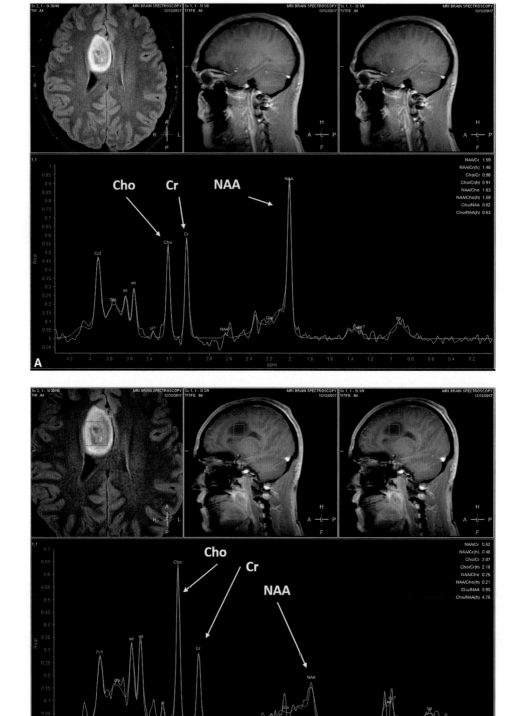

FIG. 6.56 ● The comparison of spectra from two voxels, one within the lesion (A) and the other within normal tissue (B). In the voxel within the center of the lesion, there is elevation of the choline peak (Cho), decreased but present *N*-acetylaspartate (NAA) peak, evaluation of the Cho/NAA and Cho/creatine (Cr) ratios.

single-voxel-spectroscopy (SVS) or spatially encoded by multiple-voxel-spectroscopy imaging.

In SVS, a single voxel is selected by a combination of slice-selective excitations in three dimensions in space. It results in three orthogonal planes whose intersection corresponds to the VOI.

The same sequences used for SVS are used for the signal acquisition in multivoxel MRS imaging. The main difference is that, after the excitation, PEGs are used in one, two, or three dimensions (1D, 2D, or 3D) to encode the signal.

The majority of metabolites of clinical interest have frequency shifts between 0 and 5 ppm, indicating that the differences in their frequencies are only a few hertz. Excellent shimming is required to ensure homogeneity of the magnetic field.

It is also crucial to achieve a high SNR in order to distinguish peaks for different metabolites on the acquired spectrum. Signals from protons in water and fat molecules must be effectively suppressed; it is typically achieved by the application of specific saturation techniques.

Suggested Readings

Andolina VF, Lillé SL. *Mammographic Imaging*. 3rd ed. Philadelphia, PA: Wolters Kluwer Health; 2011.

Atlas SW. *Magnetic Resonance Imaging of the Brain and Spine*. 5th ed. Philadelphia, PA: Wolters Kluwer; 2017.

Bammer R. *MR and CT Perfusion and Pharmacokinetic Imaging: Clinical Applications and Theoretical Principles*. Philadelphia, PA: Wolters Kluwer; 2016.

Berquist TH. *MRI of the Musculoskeletal System*. 6th ed. Philadelphia, PA: Lippincott Williams & Wilkins, a Wolters Kluwer business; 2013.

Bushberg JT, Seibert JA, Leidholdt EM, Boone JM. *Essential Physics of Medical Imaging*. 3rd ed. Philadelphia, PA: Lippincott Williams & Wilkins, a Wolters Kluwer business; 2012.

Garcia MJ. *Noninvasive Cardiovascular Imaging: A Multimodality Approach*. Philadelphia, PA: Lippincott Williams & Wilkins; 2010.

Geschwind J, Dake M. *Abrams' Angiography*. 3rd ed. Philadelphia, PA: Lippincott Williams & Wilkins, a Wolters Kluwer business; 2014.

Hashemi RH, Lisanti CJ, Bradley W. *MRI: The Basics*. 4th ed. Philadelphia, PA: Wolters Kluwer; 2018.

Higgins CB, de Roos A. *MRI and CT of the Cardiovascular System*. 3rd ed. Philadelphia, PA: Lippincott Williams & Wilkins, a Wolters Kluwer business; 2013.

Huda W. *Review of Radiologic Physics*. 4th ed. Philadelphia, PA: Wolters Kluwer; 2016.

McRobbie DW, Moore EA, Graves MJ, Prince MR. *MRI from Picture to Proton*. 2nd ed. Cambridge, UK: Cambridge University Press; 2007.

Shirkhoda A. *Variants and Pitfalls in Body Imaging*. 2nd ed. Philadelphia, PA: Lippincott Williams & Wilkins, a Wolters Kluwer business; 2011.

CHAPTER SELF-ASSESSMENT QUESTIONS

1. Gradients are turned on to perform _____ in an MR sequence.

   A. slice selection
   B. spatial encoding
   C. diffusion weighting
   D. All of these

2. Field inhomogeneity can cause _____ artifacts, which is _____ when magnet field is higher.

   A. distortion, improved
   B. aliasing, worse
   C. distortion, worse
   D. aliasing, improved

3. Contrast-enhanced MRA injects Gd-based contrast agents to ___ T1 of blood. To limit the acquisition window in arterial phase, _____ sequence is usually used.

   A. increase, SE
   B. decrease, SE
   C. increase, GE
   D. decrease, GE

4. SNR of image can be improved by _____.

   A. higher bandwidth
   B. higher spatial resolution
   C. higher magnet field strength
   D. higher gradient strength

5. EPI is most commonly used in ____.

   A. diffusion imaging
   B. BOLD imaging
   C. vascular imaging
   D. A and B
   E. A, B, and C

Answers to Chapter Self-Assessment Questions

1. **D** Gradient fields can be applied for all listed purposes.

2. **C** Spatial encoding in MRI is done by superimposing gradient fields on the ideally homogeneous static field. Inhomogeneity in the static field will be confused with the effect from the superimposed gradient fields and lead to signals being misplaced during reconstruction, eventually causing image distortion. Homogeneity is generally more difficult to achieve in higher strength magnetic field.

3. **D** The use of gadolinium as MRI contrast is primarily based on its T1 shortening effect. GE pulse sequences are usually used to acquire the arterial phase because of its fast speed.

4. **C** Both higher bandwidth and higher spatial resolution are associated with increased noise, and therefore lower SNR. SNR is not dependent on gradient strength.

5. **D** Faster acquisition time of EPI has made it a valuable tool in applications like diffusion imaging and functional imaging. Poor SNR, low spatial resolution, and artifacts have limited the use of EPI in vascular imaging and many other applications.

Ultrasound Imaging

7

Ryan Christopher Sieve, MD

LEARNING OBJECTIVES

1. Understand the properties of ultrasound waves and the interactions sound waves have with human tissue.
2. Identify the different types of transducers used in diagnostic imaging and the benefits and limitations of each.
3. Describe the different fields and properties within an ultrasound beam.
4. Understand how ultrasound images are acquired and processed.
5. Understand how the Doppler effect is utilized in ultrasound imaging.
6. Identify common ultrasound artifacts and how these affect diagnostic interpretation.
7. Know how to apply quality assurance and quality control (QC).
8. Understand the potential biologic effects caused by ultrasound.

ULTRASOUND CHARACTERISTICS

Ultrasound: A special sound wave

Sound waves are a form of mechanical energy that propagates through an elastic medium via pressure disturbances. This leads to compression and rarefaction of the particles that compose it. Pressure changes are created by forces acting on the molecules within the medium. A simple model to illustrate this is a spring (Figure 7.1). Mechanical deformation induced by an external force (eg, plane piston) causes compression, which leads to an increase in pressure of the medium, and subsequently rarefaction. The force is reversed by the backward motion of the piston, which causes the compressed particles to transfer their energy to adjacent particles, ultimately leading to a reduction in the local pressure amplitude (rarefaction). The compression continues to travel forward while the section of spring contacting the piston becomes stretched. A series of longitudinal compressions and rarefactions propagate through the medium with the continued back-and-forth motion of the piston. The vibrations of longitudinal waves occur along their travel direction, whereas those of transverse waves are perpendicular to the travel direction.

An additional method of producing acoustic energy involves short bursts, which equate to a small pulse traveling through a medium by itself. Reflections of the incident energy pulse result from differences in the elastic properties of the medium. Multiple pulses of ultrasound that are reflected back to the receiver from the tissue interfaces form the image. The pulse emitted by a transducer is approximately 1 ms or less. As the pulse propagates through the tissue, signals are reflected back to the transducer. A formula relates the depth at which the returning echo signal is formed with the time delay between the pulse emission and echo reception:

$$D = vt/2$$

where D is depth, v is the velocity of sound, and t is the echo reception time. The time delay includes the round trip of the sound—from transducer to the reflector and back to the transducer.

Amplitude, wavelength, frequency, and velocity

The amplitude of a sound wave equals the degree of pressure change from equilibrium. Larger amplitudes lead to denser compressions, which create sound with higher intensities. The wavelength (λ) of an ultrasound is the distance (in millimeter or micrometer) between compressions or rarefactions. Wavelength can also be measured between two repeating points on a sinusoidal wave of pressure amplitude (successive wave crests) (Figure 7.2). Frequency (f) is the number of times the wave oscillates during a cycle per second (sec). Frequency also refers to the number of wavelengths passing a specific point per second. The unit of measurement is in hertz (Hz), given that 1 Hz equals one oscillation per second. Sound waves with frequencies between 15 and 20 000 Hz (20 kHz) compose the audible acoustic spectrum. Sound waves with frequencies below 15 Hz are called infrasound, whereas those with frequencies above 20 kHz are called ultrasound. Medical ultrasound typically uses frequencies between 2 and 15 MHz (15 000 000 Hz); however, specialized applications can use frequencies as high as 50 MHz. The period of a sound wave represents the time duration of one wave cycle and is equal to $1/f$. The speed of sound, which is the distance traveled by the wave per unit of time, is equal to the wavelength divided by the period. Because period and frequency are inversely proportional (period = $1/f$), the relationship between velocity, wavelength, and frequency can be represented as

$$v = \lambda f$$

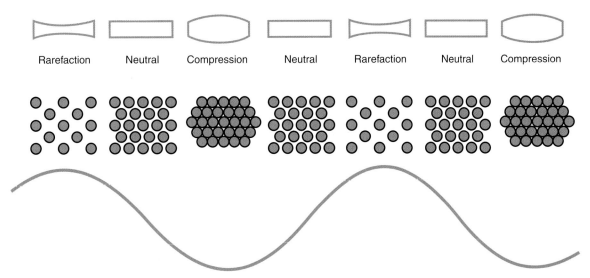

Rarefaction   Neutral   Compression   Neutral   Rarefaction   Neutral   Compression

FIG. 7.1 ● **As ultrasound travels through soft tissue, alternative regions of high pressure and low pressure are produced.** Those regions of high pressure, aka compressions, result from molecules being squeezed together, whereas those of low pressure, aka rarefactions, are created when molecules are pulled apart. Pressure change as a function of location can often be approximated as a sinusoidal curve. Reprinted with permission from Knight KL, Draper DO, *Therapeutic Modalities.* 2nd ed. Philadelphia, PA: Lippincott Williams & Wilkins, A Wolters Kluwer business; 2012.

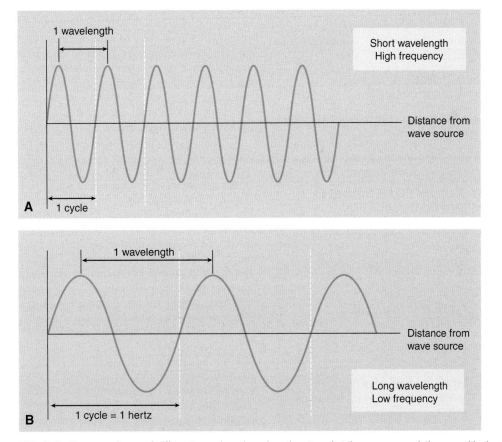

FIG. 7.2 ● Two waveforms of different wavelengths; when they travel at the same speed, the one with shorter wavelength (A) needs more vibrations to travel the distance of a wavelength within the same time (i.e., higher frequency) than the one with longer wavelength (B) does. Wavelength is the distance between two successive peaks at any time point. Reprinted with permission from Fosbinder RA, Orth D. *Essentials of Radiologic Science.* 1st ed. Philadelphia, PA: Lippincott Williams & Wilkins, A Wolters Kluwer business; 2011.

where v is the velocity of sound (m/s), λ is the wavelength (m), and f is the frequency (cycles/s).

The velocity of sound depends on the medium in which the wave is propagating through, and this is highly variable between different materials. The speed of the wave depends on two factors—the bulk modulus (B) and the density (ρ) of the medium. The bulk modulus is a measurement of the stiffness of a medium and how well it resists compression. Relating speed of sound in a medium with bulk modulus and density can be represented as

$$v = \sqrt{B/\rho}$$

where the SI units are as follows: v (m/s), B (kg/ms^2), and ρ (kg/m^3). A highly compressible medium (eg, air) has a low speed of sound, whereas a less compressible medium (eg, bone) has a higher speed of sound. The density and speed of sound for relevant materials in medical imaging are listed in Table 7.1. The varying speeds of sound modulated at the boundaries of tissues provide the fundamental reason for contrast in ultrasound imaging.

Within a given tissue medium, ultrasound frequency is independent of changes in sound speed. Hence, the wavelength is determined by frequency and the propagation medium. Wavelength depends on the compressibility of the material the sound wave is propagating through. An ultrasound transducer with a frequency of 2 MHz will result in a wavelength of 0.77 mm in soft tissue, 0.17 in air, and 1.7 mm in bone.

Given that the speed of sound in soft tissue is approximately 1540 m/s (equal to 1.54 mm/μs), the wavelength (in mm) within soft tissues can be calculated as follows:

$$\lambda = v/f = 1.54 \text{ mm/μs}/f \text{ (MHz)} = 1.54 \text{ mm}/10^{-6} \text{ s}/f$$
$$(10^6/\text{s}) = 1.54 \text{ mm}/f \text{ (MHz)}$$

The wavelength changes at the boundaries of two different media due to the change in sound speed.

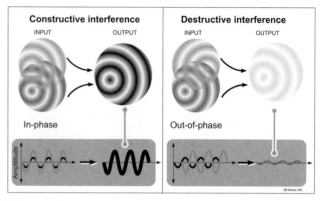

FIG. 7.3 ● When two ultrasound waves interact with each other, the output may be a constructive interference (left), destructive interference (right), or a complex interference pattern. Reprinted with permission from Savage RM, Aronson S, Shernan SK. *Comprehensive Textbook of Perioperative Transesophageal Echocardiography.* 2nd ed. Philadelphia, PA: Lippincott Williams & Wilkins, A Wolters Kluwer business; 2010.

The wavelength and frequency determine the spatial resolution of the image and the attenuation of the ultrasound beam energy. An ultrasound beam with high frequency, and hence a small wavelength, provides superior resolution and image detail than does a low-frequency beam. However, a high-frequency beam is limited in the depth it can penetrate. Ultrasound beams with a low frequency provide lower resolution and image detail; however, they can penetrate to a much deeper depth. Consequently, the choice between using a higher or lower frequency ultrasound beam depends on the particular clinical application. Lower frequency waves (3.5-5 MHz) are used for thicker body parts (eg, abdominal imaging), whereas higher frequency waves (7.5-10 MHz) are used for smaller body parts or when the target is close to the skin (eg, thyroid, breast).

Ultrasound machines contain acoustic transmitters, which produce different independent sound beams. These unique beams can interact with one another, leading to constructive or destructive wave inference or complex interference patterns (Figure 7.3). Interactions of two ultrasound waves that have the same frequency and phase result in a beam with increased amplitude (constructive interference). Interactions of two ultrasound waves that are 180° out of phase with one another result in an output wave with a lower amplitude (destructive interference). Interactions between ultrasound waves of slightly different frequencies result in waveforms of varying amplitudes (complex interference). The two most important factors determining the degree of interference include the phase of the sound wave and the amplitude of the interacting beams.

Pressure, intensity, and the dB scale

Acoustic energy causes displacement of particles and variations in local pressure as it propagates through a medium. The variations in pressure are referred to as pressure amplitude (P). Pressure amplitude is equal to the difference between the peak maximum value or peak minimum value and the average pressure within a medium. The peak maximum (positive pressure amplitude) and the peak negative (negative pressure amplitude) values are equal when a symmetrical waveform is present. However, the compressional amplitude typically exceeds the rarefactional amplitude to a large degree in most diagnostic ultrasound applications. The SI unit of pressure is the pascal (Pa), which equals one newton per

Table 7.1	**DENSITY AND SPEED OF SOUND IN TISSUES AND MATERIALS FOR MEDICAL ULTRASOUND**		
Material	*Density (kg/m^3)*	*c (m/s)*	*c (mm/s)*
Air	1.2	330	0.33
Lung	300	600	0.60
Fat	924	1450	1.45
Water	1000	1480	1.48
"Soft tissue"	1050	1540	1.54
Kidney	1041	1565	1.57
Blood	1058	1560	1.56
Liver	1061	1555	1.55
Muscle	1068	1600	1.60
Skull bone	1912	4080	4.08
Lead-zirconate-titanate	7500	4000	4.00

Reprinted with permission from Bushberg JT, Seibert JA, Leidholdt EM, Boone JM. *Essential Physics of Medical Imaging.* 3rd ed. Philadelphia, PA: Wolters Kluwer Health/Lippincott Williams & Wilkins; 2012.

square meter (N/m^2). Most diagnostic ultrasound beams deliver peak pressure levels of approximately 1 MPa (megapascal), which exceeds the earth's atmospheric pressure 10-fold.

Power refers to energy per unit time. Intensity (I) is the amount of power per unit area. Intensity is proportional to the pressure amplitude squared ($I \propto P^2$). Therefore, doubling the pressure amplitude leads to a quadruple increase in intensity. The units of intensity in medical diagnostic ultrasound are milliwatts per centimeter square. Relative intensity is defined in units of the decibel (dB) and calculated using the following equation:

$$\text{Relative intensity (dB)} = 10 \log (I_2/I_1)$$

Alternatively, relative pressure (also defined in units of dB) can be calculated as follows:

$$\text{Relative pressure (dB)} = 20 \log (P_2/P_1)$$

In these equations, I_1 and I_2 refer to intensity levels and P_1 and P_2 refer to pressure amplitude values. The base 10 logarithm ("log") is used to compress the large potential variance in intensity ratios between the incident pulse and the returning echoes. Every 10 unit change in the dB scale represents a change in intensity to the order of 10 times the magnitude, which means a 20 dB change equates to a change in 100 times the magnitude. An intensity value of 60 dB is equivalent to an incident intensity that is 10^6 (ie, 1 million) times that of the returning echo. The dB levels are positive when the incident ultrasound intensity is greater than that of the returning echo (ie, intensity ratio > 1). Alternatively, the dB levels are negative when the incident ultrasound intensity is less than that of the returning echo (ie, intensity ratio < 1). Furthermore, a decrease of 3 dB equals a 50% loss of signal intensity. The thickness of tissue required to reduce the intensity of the ultrasound by 3 dB is referred to as the half-value thickness (HVT).

Distance, area, and volume measurements

Measurements of distance, area, and volume during ultrasound examinations are possible because the speed of sound in soft tissues is nearly constant (1540 ± 15 m/s). Calibration of the instrument is readily determined depending on the round-trip time of the pulse and the echo. Careful selection of the reference points is necessary to ensure measurement accuracy. Selecting points along the direction of the ultrasound beam typically yields measurements more reliable than points measured in the lateral plane given the improved spatial resolution. Furthermore, measuring the distance between the leading edges of two objects lying in the axis of the beam is reliable because these points are less affected by variations in echo signal amplitude. The circumference of a circular object can be calculated using the measured radius (r) or diameter (d) with $2\pi r$ or πd. The area of an object or region of interest is calculated using distance measurement and by assuming a specific geometric shape. The area of a region of interest in a single image plane can be extended to 3D volume measurements by estimating the slice thickness (elevational resolution).

Ultrasound interactions

Several interactions occur between the ultrasound and the matter it propagates through, including reflection, refraction, scatter, absorption, and attenuation. The difference of acoustic impedance between two materials at a tissue boundary leads to reflection. When an incident beam is directly perpendicular to a boundary, some of the beam returns to the transducer (reflected) while a portion of the beam continues straight through the medium. Refraction occurs when the incident beam interacts with a boundary with nonperpendicular angles. Scattering refers to diffusion of the beam in multiple directions within a medium, which leads to texture and gray scale. Absorption is the process whereby acoustic energy is converted into heat energy. Absorption and scattering within a medium leads to loss of intensity (attenuation) of the ultrasound beam.

Acoustic impedance

The acoustic impedance of a material or tissue describes its stiffness and flexibility to the ultrasound beam. In essence, it describes the degree to which particles within a medium will react and change in response to mechanical vibrations. The acoustic impedance (Z) of a material is the product of the density (ρ) and the velocity of the sound wave (v) within the material:

$$Z = \rho \times v$$

with the units of kg/m^3 for density and m/s for velocity. The units of acoustic impedance (kg/m^{2}s) are expressed as the SI units of rayls (1 kg/m^{2}s = 1 rayl). A tissue medium's ability to resist change because of mechanical stimulation increases as the density of the medium increases. Large differences in acoustic impedance between two adjacent media lead to a large reflection in energy, whereas small differences allow for continued propagation of energy with little reflection. The lung, for example, has low acoustic impedance because of pockets of air within alveoli, which scatter the sound wave. The adjacent soft tissues have a relatively large acoustic impedance. This results in near-complete reflection of the incident sound waves when propagating to the soft tissue-lung interface. Minor reflection occurs between tissues that have similar acoustic impedances. Of tissues in the body, bone has the highest acoustic impedance (7.8 × 10^6 rayls), whereas air has the lowest (0.0004 × 10^6 rayls). Table 7.2 lists the relative acoustic impedances of tissues in the body relevant to diagnostic ultrasound imaging. Piezoelectric crystals have a very high acoustic impedance, much greater than that of bone.

As mentioned earlier, ultrasound energy that is perpendicular to a tissue boundary results in a portion returning directly to the source (as echoes) and the other portion being transmitted directly through the medium. Sound waves experience an 180° phase shift in pressure amplitude as they propagate from a medium of lower acoustic impedance into a medium of higher acoustic impedance.

Table 7.2 **RELATIVE IMPEDANCES OF MATERIALS OF INTEREST IN ULTRASOUND IMAGING**	
Material	*Acoustic Impedance Relative to Soft Tissue*
Air	<0.01
Fat	0.9
Soft tissue (average)	1
Bone	5
PZT (piezoelectric crystal)	20

Abbreviation: PZT, lead-zirconate-titanate.
Reprinted with permission from Huda W. *Review of Radiologic Physics*. 3rd ed. Philadelphia, PA: Wolters Kluwer Health/Lippincott Williams & Wilkins; 2010.

Reflection

The difference in the acoustic impedances of two tissues at a boundary results in reflection of the ultrasound beam. Reflection, which is also known as backscatter, is the principle tissue interaction of sound waves to produce an ultrasound image. Approximately 1% of the intensity of an ultrasound is reflected at a typical muscle-fat interface, resulting in nearly 99% propagation of the beam through the boundary. The energy reflected back from an interface is known as an echo. Nearly 100% of the ultrasound energy is reflected at muscle-air interfaces, which essentially leads to nonvisualization of the deeper anatomy. This explains the need to apply acoustic coupling gel in the transducer-skin interface during an examination. Any air pockets between the transducer and the skin lead to degradation of the image because of reflective interactions. Values of reflected intensities for several interfaces commonly encountered in medical diagnostic ultrasound are listed in Table 7.3. The posterior shadowing caused by bowel gas often leads to nonvisualization of certain organs in abdominal imaging, in particular the pancreas and appendix. A large fraction of the incident beam energy is reflected at bone-tissue interfaces given the significant difference between acoustic impedances. It is essentially impossible to image through bone or air given the extensive shadowing, leading to a void of echoes.

Scattering

Scatter is the redirection of acoustic energy in numerous directions, which results in the production of a weak signal. The interactions between sound waves and individual molecules, particularly at small interfaces or large rough surfaces, will result in scatter. There are two general types of reflector surfaces—nonspecular and specular. A nonspecular surface does not follow the typical rules of reflection and reflects ultrasound echoes in all different directions, a phenomenon known as acoustic scattering (Figure 7.4). This occurs at irregular interfaces possessing wavelengths that are equal to or smaller than the incident ultrasound beam (typically 1 mm or less). Only a small amount of the transmitted energy reaching a nonspecular reflector returns to the transducer. The amplitudes of returning scattered echoes are much lower than those of specularly reflected echoes. However, this usually does not pose an issue because modern ultrasound receivers have a dynamic range capable of utilizing information obtained from a wide range of amplitudes. Scattered echoes originate from small, poorly reflective objects that are less angle

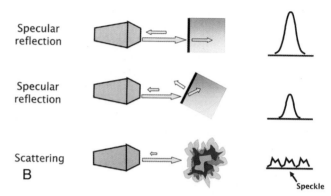

FIG. 7.4 ● Ultrasound scattering is caused by small reflectors within a tissue. The characteristics of a particle in a specific tissue or organ lead to unique scatter patterns. Interactions at boundaries can also result in scatter, especially at higher frequencies. Reprinted with permission from Feigenbaum H, Armstrong WF, Ryan T. *Feigenbaum's Echocardiography*. 6th ed. Philadelphia, PA: Lippincott Williams & Wilkins, A Wolters Kluwer business; 2004.

dependent (eg, blood cells). Specular reflection occurs at large, smooth surfaces that are regularly shaped (eg, valves). For specular reflection, the angle of incidence (i) is equal to the angle of reflection (r) (Figure 7.5). As the angles i and r decrease, the chance that the reflected beam will return to the transducer and be detected as an echo increases.

The dynamic range indicates how wide a spectrum of echo signals the ultrasound system can accept without distortion. Echo signals below the dynamic range are regarded as noise, whereas signals above the range are regarded as saturated and set to the maximum level. The dynamic range is an adjustable setting in real time. Smaller ranges create a steeper gradient, which provides for more contrast on the display. This is useful in improving the appearance of a low-contrast structure, such as a mass. The downside to increasing the contrast is the production of a less clear, coarse image. Alternatively, larger dynamic ranges generate less contrast, but smoother images.

Several factors influence the amplitude of the ultrasound signal returning from the insonated tissues, including the acoustic impedance differences at the scatterer interfaces, the number of scatterers present, the size of each scatterer, and the frequency of

Table 7.3 **REFLECTION INTENSITIES AT AN INTERFACE BETWEEN SOFT TISSUE AND THE SPECIFIED MATERIAL**

Material Adjacent to Soft Tissue	Reflected Intensity (%)
Air	>99
Lung	50
Bone	40
Fat	0.8
Muscle	<0.1

Reprinted with permission from Huda W. *Review of Radiologic Physics*. 3rd ed. Philadelphia, PA: Wolters Kluwer Health/Lippincott Williams & Wilkins; 2010.

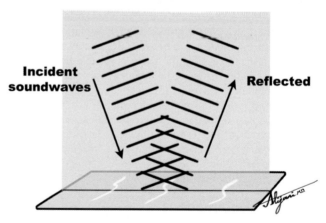

FIG. 7.5 ● Specular reflection occurring from a smooth reflector. The angle of incidence is equal to the angle of reflection. Reprinted with permission from Huda W. *Review of Radiologic Physics*. 3rd ed. Philadelphia, PA: Lippincott Williams & Wilkins, a Wolters Kluwer business; 2010.

the ultrasound. Objects described as *hyperechoic* have a higher scatter amplitude in comparison to the background signal, whereas *hypoechoic* objects demonstrate a relatively low-scatter amplitude.

Acoustic scattering from nonspecular surfaces increases proportionally with increasing ultrasound frequencies. Most organs of the body give rise to a characteristic scatter "signature" due to the inherent tissue properties (see Figure 7.4). Specular reflection occurs at smooth interfaces that have dimensions larger than the incident ultrasound wavelength. Specular reflection is not affected by changes in frequency. The echoes from specular reflector surfaces are used to create ultrasound images.

Refraction

Reflection occurs when the incident beam is at an angle perpendicular to the tissue boundary. Interactions occurring at nonperpendicular angles result in *refraction* of the ultrasound energy. Refraction refers to the change in direction of an ultrasound beam when moving between two tissues that have different speeds of sound (acoustic velocities). The frequency of the sound wave remains constant between the two tissue media; however, the wavelength changes to accommodate the different velocity in the second tissue. The wavelength shortens if the velocity is decreased, and vice versa. The sound pulse is refracted as it enters the second medium as a result of the change in wavelength. The angle of refraction depends on the change in the velocity of sound occurring at the tissue boundary. This is determined by Snell's law:

$$\sin\theta_i/\sin\theta_t = v_2/v_1$$

where θ_i is the angle of incidence, θ_t is the transmitted angle, v_1 is the velocity of sound in medium 1, and v_2 is the velocity of sound in medium 2. When the velocity of sound is greater in tissue 2 compared to tissue 1, the angle of transmission is greater than the angle of incidence, and vice versa (Figure 7.6). If the velocity of

sound between the two tissue media is the same, then no refraction occurs. Refraction also does not occur with perpendicular incidence. The velocity of sound is relatively low in compressible tissues, such as fluid, lung, and fat, and high in less compressible issues, such as bone.

The ultrasound machine assumes that sound waves propagate in a straight line. Any refraction results in image artifacts. Examples include the misplacement of an object within an image and an artifact known as edge shadowing, which occurs beyond a curvilinear interface. Total refraction is a phenomenon in which $v_2 > v_1$ and the angle of incidence of the propagating sound beam at a tissue interface is greater than the critical angle. The critical angle, designated as θ_c, is the angle that creates an angle of refraction of 90° when a wave moves from a material with a slower speed of sound into a material with a faster speed of sound. By setting the angle of incidence (θ_t) to 90° and plugging it into Snell's law, the critical angle can be calculated as

$$\sin\theta_c = v_1/v_2$$

Attenuation/Intensity

Attenuation describes the energy loss (ie, change in wave amplitude) of an ultrasound beam as it propagates through a tissue medium. This occurs because of several factors, including reflection, refraction, scatter, and absorption. The amplitude decay model is calculated as

$$A = A_0 e^{-\mu z}$$

where A is the reduced amplitude of the sound wave, A_0 is the amplitude of the unattenuated wave, e refers to Napier's constant (which is rounded to 2.71828), μ is the attenuation coefficient (expressed in decibels per cm: dB/cm), and z is distance traveled. The attenuation coefficient is the loss of intensity (dB) per centimeter that a sound wave travels through a medium. The amount of attenuation depends on the frequency of the ultrasound beam and the properties of the propagating medium. Water, for example, results in the least attenuation of an ultrasound beam. Thus, it serves as a good conductor for deeper structures. A diagnostic scenario exemplifying the good conducting property of simple fluid (eg, water, urine) is the transabdominal portion of a pelvic ultrasound examination (Figure 7.7). The urinary bladder is ideally filled before scanning to allow for a "diagnostic window" to

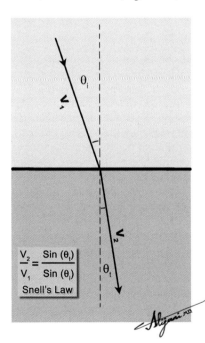

FIG. 7.6 ● **Refraction of an ultrasound beam.** The angle of transmission (θ_t) is smaller than the incident angle (θ_i) when $v_2 < v_1$. Reprinted with permission from Huda W. *Review of Radiologic Physics.* 3rd ed. Philadelphia, PA: Lippincott Williams & Wilkins, a Wolters Kluwer business; 2009.

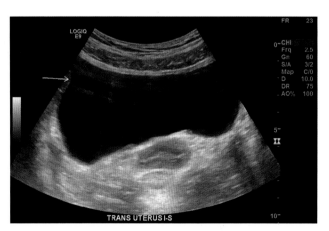

FIG. 7.7 ● The distended bladder (arrow) serves as a "diagnostic window" to the uterus during the transabdominal portion of a pelvic ultrasound due to the low attenuation of simple fluid.

Table 7.4	ATTENUATION COEFFICIENTS FOR SELECTED TISSUES AT 1 MHZ
Tissue Composition	**Attenuation Coefficient (1-MHz Beam, dB/cm)**
Water	0.0002
Blood	0.18
Soft tissues	0.3-0.8
Brain	0.3-0.5
Liver	0.4-0.7
Fat	0.5-1.8
Smooth muscle	0.2-0.6
Tendon	0.9-1.1
Bone, cortical	13-26
Lung	40

Reprinted with permission from Bushberg JT, Seibert JA, Leidholdt EM, Boone JM. *Essential Physics of Medical Imaging*. 3rd ed. Philadelphia, PA: Wolters Kluwer Health/Lippincott Williams & Wilkins; 2012.

the uterus. Ultrasound attenuation occurring in a homogeneous tissue is exponential. Tissues and fluids each possess a characteristic attenuation coefficient, and these vary widely (Table 7.4). Another way to calculate the rate of attenuation is as follows:

$$\text{Attenuation (dB)} = \mu \times f \times x$$

where μ is the attenuation coefficient (in dB/cm at a frequency of 1 MHz), f is the ultrasound frequency (in MHz), and x is the tissue thickness (in cm). The attenuation coefficient for soft tissues (0.3-0.8) can be rounded to approximately 0.5 dB/cm per MHz of frequency (0.5 × [dB/cm]/MHz). Multiplying the ultrasound frequency for a given sound wave with (0.5 × [dB/cm]/MHz) provides the approximate attenuation coefficient in units of dB/cm. This demonstrates that attenuation increases linearly with increasing frequencies. A 2 MHz wave will experience twice the attenuation of a 1 MHz wave per unit distance (in cm), a 5 MHz will suffer 5 times the attenuation of a 1 MHz wave, and so on. It is important to note, however, that the dB scale increases logarithmically. Thus, a linear increase of attenuation is observed with increasing frequencies, whereas the ultrasound beam intensity is accentuated exponentially with distance (Figure 7.8). The

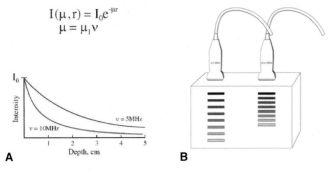

FIG. 7.8 • Ultrasound attenuation is an exponential function of depth and frequency (A). A higher frequency ultrasound wave undergoes higher attenuation within the same medium than a lower frequency wave (B). Reprinted with permission from Bigeleisen PE, Gofeld M, Orebaugh SL. *Ultrasound-Guided Regional Anesthesia and Pain Medicine*. 2nd ed. Philadelphia, PA: Lippincott Williams & Wilkins, a Wolters Kluwer business; 2015.

HVT refers to the thickness of a particular tissue medium required to attenuate the ultrasound beam intensity by 50%, which results in a 3 dB reduction in intensity. A 3 dB intensity reduction is of special importance because this equates to an absolute reduction in intensity by two. The equation for intensity in decibels is given as follows:

$$\text{dB} = 10 \log_{10} (I/I_0)$$

where I is intensity and I_0 is the reference intensity. The HVT decreases as the ultrasound beam frequency increases. Ultrasound is attenuated to a much greater degree than is audible sound given its high frequency.

Ultrasound intensity is the amount of energy (joules) flowing through a unit cross-sectional area (cm^2) per a unit of time (seconds). Joules (J) are related to watts via the following equation: 1 watt (W) = 1 J/s. The intensity is typically expressed as W/cm^2 (or mW/cm^2). The power of an ultrasound beam is a measure of the total energy passing through the whole area of the beam per unit time. In other words, total power is the product of ultrasound intensity and the beam area:

$$\text{Power} = \text{intensity (mW/cm}^2\text{)} \times \text{area (cm}^2\text{)}$$

This equation assumes that intensity is uniform. The product of total power and the amount of time the beam is on gives the total energy.

As previously mentioned, relative sound intensity is measured on a logarithmic scale and expressed as decibels (dB). Keeping in mind the relative intensity equation of 10 log$_{10}$ (I/I_0), dB values will be positive if the intensity of interest (I) is greater than the relative intensity (I_0), which represents signal amplification. Negative values occur if I is less than I_0, which represents signal attenuation. The levels of intensity in ultrasound imaging are very low, which makes the logarithmic decibel relative intensity scale useful practically. A reduction in intensity to 10% corresponds to −10 dB; a reduction to 1% corresponds to −20 dB; etc.

Absorption

Absorption is the conversion of acoustic energy to other forms of energy, namely, heat. This energy is transferred to the propagating medium, which "absorbs" it. Absorption of ultrasound energy by the tissue medium is one of the most important determinants of attenuation. Three main factors influence the extent of absorption—beam frequency, the viscosity of the tissue medium, and the relaxation time of the medium. Higher frequencies lead to increased absorption because the particles within the medium travel past each other faster, generating more heat. The absorption of ultrasound in soft tissues demonstrates a proportional increase with higher frequencies. Alternatively, minimal absorption occurs in fluids. Viscosity is a measure of the friction between particles traveling past one another within a tissue medium. Greater frictional forces lead to more heat generation. Thus, ultrasound absorption increases with higher viscosity. Relaxation time refers to the length of time for particles within a medium to revert to their original positions after being displaced by an ultrasound pulse. A longer relaxation time means that displaced particles have a higher probability of encountering the next ultrasound pulse before fully relaxing. The particles may be moving in an opposite direction than the new compression pulse, which results in increased dissipation of energy from the ultrasound beam. Therefore, increases in all three factors—frequency, tissue viscosity, and tissue relaxation time—lead to increases in heat generation, and hence, absorption of the ultrasound beam.

ULTRASOUND IMAGE ACQUISITION

A knowledge of the production, propagation, and interaction of ultrasound waves is needed to understand the formation of ultrasound images. Using a pulse-echo approach, each ultrasound pulse is transmitted into the patient, undergoes partial reflections from tissue interfaces creating echoes, which then return to the transducer. Several hardware components are required to create an image using a pulse-echo approach, including the beam former, pulser/transmitter, receiver, amplifier, scan converter, and display system. This section begins with a discussion on different transducers used in ultrasound imaging.

Transducer

A transducer converts one type of energy into another by way of piezoelectric material. The piezoelectric material converts electrical energy into mechanical energy to produce ultrasound. The mechanical energy is converted back to electrical energy for ultrasound detection. Modern-day transducers contain a broadband array of hundreds of individual elements. A transducer is composed of several major elements, including the matching layer, piezoelectric material, damping block, acoustic absorber, insulating cover, sensor electrodes, and the housing unit (Figure 7.9).

Piezoelectric material

The functional component of the transducer is made of the piezoelectric material. This material exhibits the piezoelectric effect; that is, when mechanical stress is applied, the net polarization of the material changes as a result of the changes in the alignment of the molecular dipoles inside the material (a molecular dipole is a molecule whose center of positive charge is spatially separate from its center of negative charge), leading to electrical charges generated on the surface of the material. The piezoelectric effect is a reversible process; when an external electric field is applied, the material experiences mechanical stress and undergoes physical deformation. Such interesting characteristics of the piezoelectric material have made it useful in both generation and detection of ultrasound.

An imbalance in the charge distribution occurs when an external pressure is applied, which creates a potential difference (voltage) across the element. The voltage, which is measured by surface electrodes, is proportional to the incident mechanical pressure amplitude.

Ultrasound transducers use a synthetic piezoelectric ceramic, most commonly lead-zirconate-titanate (PZT). A multistep process gives the ceramic its piezoelectric characteristics, which begins with molecular synthesis and heating. Next, an external applied voltage orients the internal dipole elements. The orientation is permanently maintained via cooling. Finally, the material is cut and molded into a specific shape. No piezoelectric properties are exhibited by PZT in its natural state. The dipoles align in the material once heated beyond its "Curie temperature" (328°C-365°C) and an external voltage is applied. The dipoles retain their alignment once the material has cooled. No net charge is present on ceramic surfaces at equilibrium. A voltage is produced between the surfaces when compressed. Mechanical deformation occurs when a voltage is applied between electrodes attached by both surfaces (see Figure 7.10).

Resonance transducers

Resonance transducers used for pulse-echo ultrasound operate in "resonance" mode, in which a voltage of very short duration (~1 μs) is applied. The piezoelectric material contracts and then subsequently vibrates at a natural resonance frequency (f_0), which is determined by the thickness cut. Ultrasound waves with a wavelength twice the thickness of the piezoelectric material are preferentially emitted. The operating frequency depends on the thickness and speed of sound within the piezoelectric material. The speed of sound within PZT is approximately 4000 m/s. Using this speed of sound, the wavelength can be calculated for a given frequency. As an example, a 5-MHz transducer will have a wavelength of

$$\lambda = c/f = 4000 \text{ m/s}/5 \times 10^6/\text{s}$$

$$\lambda = 8 \times 10^{-4} \text{ m} = 0.80 \text{ mm}$$

Damping block

The damping block, which is typically composed of tungsten or rubber in an epoxy resin, absorbs the ultrasound energy that is transmitted to the back of the crystal in addition to stray ultrasound signals from the housing unit. The damping material is located behind the piezoelectric element of the transducer. It also serves to dampen the transducer vibration to create an ultrasound pulse that has a short spatial pulse length (SPL). This is necessary to maintain the detail along the beam axis, the axial resolution. The damping block must be composed of a material that has the same acoustic impedance as the crystal. This prevents the unwanted production of echoes from a damping block-crystal interface, which would lead to reverberation artifact when the energy returns to the crystal. The damping block also serves as a mechanical pulse damper by limiting the SPL. The effect of dampening the transducer vibration, which is also known as "ring-down," is 2-fold. Firstly, the purity of the resonance frequency is lessened. Secondly, a broadband frequency spectrum is introduced. Frequencies higher and lower than the resonance frequency are introduced with ring-down, which increases the bandwidth (range of frequencies). The Q factor represents the bandwidth of the sound propagating from a transducer, where f_0 is the center (resonance) frequency and the bandwidth is the width of the frequency distribution:

$$Q = f_0/\text{Bandwidth}$$

A transducer that has a narrow bandwidth and a corresponding long SPL is known as a high Q transducer. Those that have a wide bandwidth and a short SPL are known as low Q transducers. Medical imaging applications require a transducer

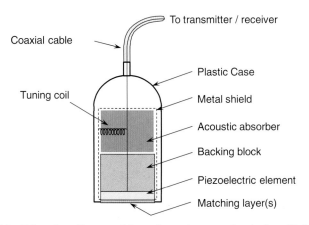

FIG. 7.9 ● An ultrasound transducer is comprised of multiple components. Reprinted with permission from Bushberg JT, Seibert JA, Leidholdt EM, Boone JM. *Essential Physics of Medical Imaging.* 3rd ed. Philadelphia, PA: Lippincott Williams & Wilkins, a Wolters Kluwer business; 2012.

To transmitter / receiver

Coaxial cable

Plastic Case

Tuning coil

Metal shield

Acoustic absorber

Backing block

Piezoelectric element

Matching layer(s)

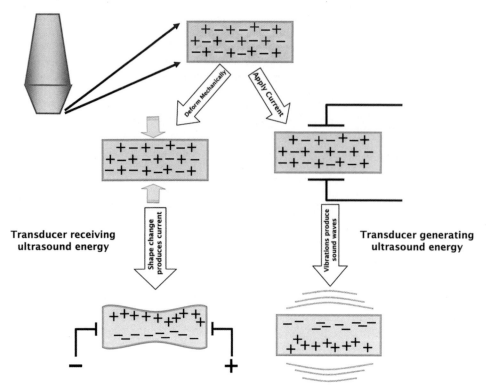

FIG. 7.10 • **Illustration of how a piezoelectrical crystal works as the detecting/receiving component of an ultrasound transducer.** When an electric current is applied to it, the crystal vibrates, resulting in the generation and transmission of ultrasound wave. When ultrasound wave is incident upon the crystal, it responds by producing an electrical impulse. Reprinted with permission from Penny SM. *Introduction to Sonography and Patient Care.* 1st ed. Philadelphia, PA: Lippincott Williams & Wilkins, a Wolters Kluwer business; 2015.

Transducer receiving ultrasound energy

Transducer generating ultrasound energy

with a broad bandwidth to achieve high spatial resolution along the direction of the beam. Figure 7.11 shows the examples of high and low Q transducers and their respective relationships with SPL.

Matching layer

Differences in the acoustic impedance of the transducer crystal and the surface of the patient's skin can prohibit adequate transmission of echoes into the patient. A layer of material (matching layer) placed on the front surface of the transducer increases the efficiency of energy transmission into and out of the patient. A matching layer has an intermediate impedance value, which is between that of the transducer and soft tissue. This serves to minimize the acoustic difference between the transducer and the patient. The ideal thickness of a matching layer is one-fourth of the wavelength of sound, which is determined from the center operating frequency of the transducer and the speed of sound within the matching layer. This is known as quarter-wave matching. The matching layer, in combination with acoustic coupling gel, improves the quality of the images obtained.

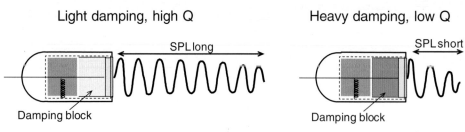

Light damping, high Q

SPL long

Damping block

Heavy damping, low Q

SPL short

Damping block

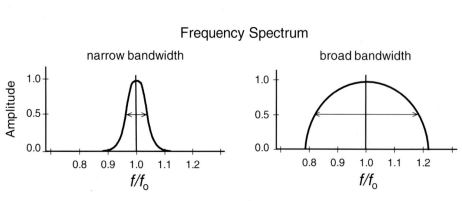

Frequency Spectrum

narrow bandwidth

broad bandwidth

Amplitude

f/f_0

f/f_0

FIG. 7.11 • **Damping block effect on the frequency spectrum.** The damping block is located at the back of the transducer behind the piezoelectric material. Light damping allows many cycles to occur, which results in an increase in the SPL and a narrow frequency bandwidth. Heavy damping decreases the SPL and broadens the frequency bandwidth. The Q factor refers to the center frequency divided by the bandwidth. Reprinted with permission from Bushberg JT, Seibert JA, Leidholdt EM, Boone JM. *Essential Physics of Medical Imaging.* 3rd ed. Philadelphia, PA: Lippincott Williams & Wilkins, a Wolters Kluwer business; 2012.

Transducer arrays

Most ultrasound transducers contain numerous piezoelectric elements (usually between 128 and 512), which are arranged in linear or curvilinear arrays. The length of each individual element is typically 2 to 3 mm. The multielement arrays used to produce a beam are normally either linear (sequential) or phased (Figure 7.12). Linear arrays contain between 128 and 512 elements. Linear array transducers activate a single group of approximately 20 adjacent elements to produce one line of sight. Each line of sight provides information for one line of an image. A large number of lines of sight are sequentially generated and combined to form the entire image. After the production of a line of sight, the grouped elements then listen for returning echoes. Grouped elements are used to increase the near field rather than a single element. Another line of sight (A-line) is generated by firing another group of elements that are displaced by one or two elements. With a linear array, a full rectangular field of view is produced by firing groups of elements along the entire length of the array. Curvilinear arrays produce diverging images, which result in a wider field of view than do linear arrays. Clinical applications of linear arrays include peripheral vascular ultrasound and the imaging of small body parts (eg, thyroid, scrotum). Curvilinear array transducers are used in abdominal ultrasound.

Phased arrays usually have between 64 and 128 elements, which are contained in a tighter package than those of linear arrays transducers. All of the elements are utilized during the production of an ultrasound beam. The elements are electrically activated at slightly different times, and this allows the ultrasound beam to be focused and steered through an arc without moving the transducer. Returning echoes are detected by each individual transducer element, which allows for the generation of images. Phased-array transducers are used in cardiac ultrasound because the smaller size allows for imaging between ribs.

Capacitive micromachined ultrasonic transducers

Capacitive micromachined ultrasonic transducers (CMUTs) are a relatively new method in medical imaging to produce high-frequency ultrasound energy. Rather than conventional piezoelectricity, which utilizes PZT complexes, CMUTs are silicon based and transduce energy via changes in capacitance. CMUTs have been heavily investigated since the 1990s and have proved to be useful within medical imaging and therapy.

CMUTs are formed with silicon using micromachining techniques. The capacitor cell of a CMUT consists of a fixed electrode, known as the backplate (or bottom electrode), and a free electrode, referred to as the membrane (also top electrode or top plate), which are separated by a vacuum gap. An alternating current applied between these two elements results in membrane vibration, which generates ultrasound energy. The top plate is attracted to the conductive substrate by electrostatic force. Therefore, this concept of operation is known as electrostatic transduction. The attraction is resisted by a mechanical restoring force due to the stiffness of the plate. The CMUT can also serve as a receiver of ultrasonic waves. If an incident ultrasound wave reaches the membrane, a change in capacitance is detected as a current or voltage signal. A direct current bias voltage needs to be applied for signal detection and for transmission.

There are several different ways in which micromachined transducers are fabricated, including sacrificial release surface methods, wafer bonding, and top-down processing. Sacrificial release surface micromachining involves the formation of a cavity beneath a thin plate after a sacrificial layer is deposited or grown on a carrier substrate. The sacrificial layer is then carefully removed with an etchant. Different combinations of the sacrificial layer, plate, and substrate material can be tried to fabricate CMUTs. A process known as deep reactive ion etching provides electrical connectivity to either end of the substrate. A limitation of the sacrificial release process is the relative lack of control of important factors of the deposited layers, such as the uniformity, absolute thickness, and mechanical properties.

Wafer bonding is a method of fabricating CMUTs, which improves upon the limitations of the sacrificial release process. There are several variations of the bonding process, including simple wafer bonding, local oxidation of silicon (LOCOS), and a thick-buried-oxide process. Simple wafer bonding utilizes two wafers—a prime quality silicon wafer and a silicon-on-insulator wafer. The advantage of this process is the improved control over the thickness, uniformity, and mechanical properties of the plate, which is due largely in part to the use of a single-crystal silicon device layer. Limitations include a reduced breakdown voltage and increased parasitic capacitance between the cells, in addition to the relative tendency of electrical short circuits due to contamination during packaging. LOCOS provides for an extended insulation layer structure in the post area, which improves the aforementioned limitations of the simple wafer bonding process. The thick-buried-oxide process is a newer method, which confines and isolates the CMUT bottom electrode to the specific area under the gap where a high electric field is desired. This minimizes the chance of dielectric breakdown and parasitic capacitance in the post region.

CMUTs have several advantages over conventional piezoelectric methods of transduction, including better acoustic

Linear array

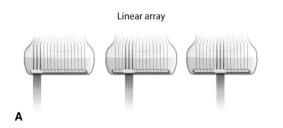

A

Phased array steering using time delays

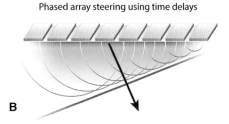

B

FIG. 7.12 • **Multielement transducer arrays.** A linear (or curvilinear) array generates a beam by firing a subset of the total number of transducer elements (A). A phased array produces a beam by firing all of the transducer elements with fractional time delays, which allow the beam to be steered and focused without moving the transducer (B). Reprinted with permission from Huda W. *Review of Radiologic Physics.* 4th ed. Philadelphia, PA: Lippincott Williams & Wilkins, A Wolters Kluwer business 2016.

matching with the propagation medium, which allows for greater bandwidth capabilities, potentially lower costs owing to improved fabrication methods, and the ability to have integrated circuits on the same "wafer." Because a wider pulse-echo bandwidth can be employed (typically >100%), the images obtained from CMUTs offer improved axial resolution, allowing for small targets to be resolved, and improved lateral resolution. State-of-the-art CMUT probes produce images that are comparable or even superior to those of conventional PZT probes. There is much promise surrounding 2D arrays in eventually leading to improvements in efficiency, speed, volumetric imaging, and multibandwidth operation. The 2D arrays of CMUTs offer the potential for real-time 3D imaging in harmonic imaging applications and in high-frequency applications, such as intravascular imaging.

Although CMUTs offer a better axial resolution, further improvements are needed in the sensitivity and resolution to match that of piezoelectric arrays, particularly in deeper depths of penetration. CMUTs are relatively new in the field of ultrasound. Although the potential for CMUTs in diagnostic imaging is wide, the therapeutic capabilities have not yet been fully explored.

Special purpose transducer assemblies

As previously discussed, different ultrasound transducers are employed for different purposes. For example, an ultrasound unit will typically come equipped with a linear array transducer of low frequency that provides good penetration. Such a transducer will optimize ultrasound imaging of the abdomen in which deep penetration of sound waves is needed. A separate phased transducer employing a high frequency is used for "small parts." Such a transducer will have low penetration, although it will provide high spatial resolution for objects of relatively low depth below the skin surface. Furthermore, there are a large number of special purpose transducers for more specific applications. Intracavitary transducers, for example, include transvaginal, transurethral, transrectal, and transesophageal devices. These allow for high-resolution, high-frequency imaging of structures that would otherwise be difficult to image using a standard transcutaneous approach given the depth and/or proximity to cavity wall. Intravascular transducers provide information on the morphology of a vessel wall, estimate the degree of stenosis, and assess for the efficacy of vascular intervention. The differences in the appearance of curvilinear arrays, phased arrays, and intracavitary ultrasound probes are shown in Figure 7.13.

Ultrasound beam properties

The near field and far field

An ultrasound beam propagates from the transducer surface into the propagation medium as a longitudinal wave with two different beam patterns—a slightly converging beam and a diverging beam. The converging beam extends to the "near field," which is adjacent to the transducer face. A diverging beam extends beyond this point into the "far field."

The length of the near field for an unfocused, single-element transducer is determined by the diameter of the transducer and the frequency of the transmitted sound (Figure 7.14). Ultrasound beams converge in the near field because of constructive and destructive interference patterns. The transducer diameter (and hence, the radius) and the wavelength of the propagating wavelength directly determine the length of the near field:

$$\text{Near field length} = r^2/\lambda$$

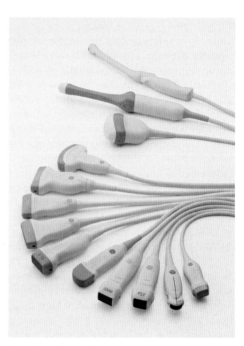

FIG. 7.13 ● **A variety of ultrasound transducers for different clinical applications.** The transducers shown in the picture are (from top to lower right): a 2D endocavity transducer, a 3D intracavity transducer, a transabdominal 3D/4D volume transducer, a curved array transducer, three linear transducers, followed by sector and tightly curved phased-array transducers for intercostal imaging. Reprinted with permission from Sanders RC. *Clinical Sonography: A Practical Guide*. 5th ed. Philadelphia, PA: Lippincott Williams & Wilkins, A Wolters Kluwer business; 2015.

where *r* is the radius of the transducer and λ is the wavelength. The near-field length increases 4-fold with a doubling of the transducer size. Doubling the frequency of the transducer halves the wavelength. This results in a doubling of the extent of the near field. Pressure amplitudes vary widely while in the near field. These variations decrease in a monotonic manner once in the far field.

The far field, also known as the Fraunhofer zone, is the location beyond the near field, in which the beam diverges. The angle of ultrasound beam divergence (θ) for a large-area single-element transducer depends on diameter and wavelength:

$$\sin \theta = 1.22 * \lambda/d$$

where *d* is the effective diameter of the transducer and λ is the wavelength (with the prerequisite that the diameter and wavelength have the same unit of distance). High-frequency, large-diameter transducers produce less beam divergence. Ultrasound intensity within the far field decreases monotonically with distance. Small ultrasound beams of minimal intensity are emitted at diverging angles from the primary beam. These are known as side lobes and result in imaging artifacts (to be discussed in more detail in a subsequent section).

Transducer array beam formation and focusing

The piezoelectric element width in a transducer array is narrow—usually less than one wavelength. This generates a diverging beam very close to the transducer face. The effective width of a transducer equals the sum of each simultaneously fired individual element. A collimated beam is produced via constructive and

Huygens' Principle and Transducer Beam Formation

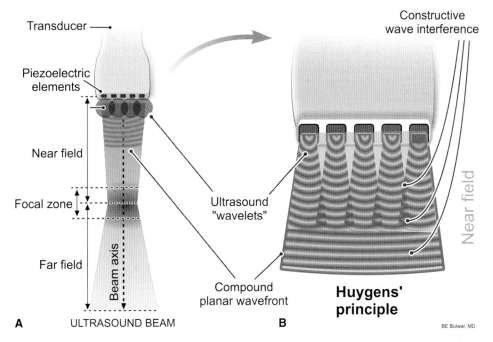

FIG. 7.14 ● **An ultrasound beam converges in the near field and diverges in the far field.** Pressure amplitude variations are complex and rapidly changing in the near field and monotonically decreasing in the far field. Reprinted with permission from Savage RM, Aronson S, Shernan SK. *Comprehensive Textbook of Perioperative Transesophageal Echocardiography.* 2nd ed. Philadelphia, PA: Lippincott Williams & Wilkins, A Wolters Kluwer business; 2010.

destructive interference from the interaction of individual beams. The properties of the collimated beam are similar to those of a single transducer with the same size. The beam of a phased-array transducer is produced from interactions of individual waves of each transducer.

The focal distance for a single transducer or a group of elements that are simultaneously produced in a linear array depends on several factors, two of which include the transducer diameter and the operating frequency. Furthermore, the focal distance of phased and many linear arrays can be adjusted to a certain depth. This is achieved via the application of time delays between transducer elements, which adjusts the converging distance of the beam. Reducing the time interval between transducer elements leads to greater focal distances because the beam converges distally. Focal zones closer to the transducer are created by pulsing the outermost elements before the innermost elements. Multiple focal zones can be generated to focus on several anatomic structures simultaneously. This is performed via the repeated acquisition of data with different phase timing of the elements. Phased-array transducers use every element to generate an ultrasound beam. Setting an adjustable time delay for the excitation of each individual element allows for beam focusing (Figure 7.15).

Side lobes and grating lobes

Unwanted ultrasound energy that spreads out from the transducer and is directed away from the main pulse is called side lobes. Radial expansion and contraction occur when a transducer of a multielement array generates the main ultrasound beam in thickness mode (Figure 7.16). These can occur in phased-array systems and conventional transducers. Side lobes result in artifacts when the transducer is in receive mode because

the echoes are mistakenly rerouted along the main beam. The side lobe energy composes a large amount of the total beam energy in continuous mode operation because of the relatively narrow frequency bandwidth of the transducer (high Q). The side lobe energy is diminished within pulsed mode operation as a spectrum of acoustic wavelengths is created by the low Q ultrasound beam. Side lobes are emitted in a forward direction for multielement arrays (see Figure 7.16B). Two approaches can be employed to reduce the degree of side lobes, including the use of small transducer elements (widths less than half the wavelength) and decreasing the amplitude of peripheral transducer element excitations compared to those of the center. Similar to side lobes, grating lobes are unwanted energy emitted far off-axis by multielement arrays. Side lobes are forward directed, whereas grating lobes are emitted from the array surface at large angles (Figure 7.17).

Spatial resolution

Spatial resolution is the ability of an ultrasound system to separate and distinguish between two objects that are in close proximity. A higher spatial resolution equates to distinguishing objects at smaller distances. The ability to resolve structures along the direction of the ultrasound beam is referred to as axial resolution. The returning echoes need to be distinct without overlap to achieve satisfactory axial resolution. Axial resolution occurs along the axis of the beam, is independent of depth, and is determined by the pulse length. The reason why the depth of imaging does not affect axial resolution is because the resolution is the same at any point along the beam axis. A minimum separation distance is necessary to avoid overlapping of returning echoes from two reflectors, which equals one-half of the SPL. This is because the

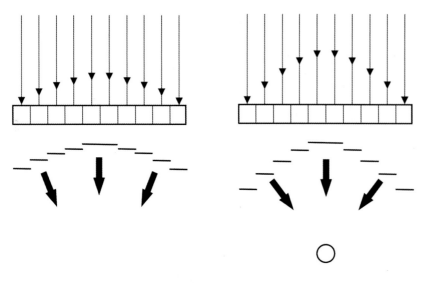

FIG. 7.15 ● **For phased-array transducers, beam focusing is achieved by delaying the energizing of the center elements.** Different amounts of delay result in variable focal distances in tissue. The outer elements in an array must be energized first prior to beam focusing. The phase differences of the ultrasound pulses result in a focal distance at predicable depths in tissue. Reprinted with permission from Siegel MJ. *Pediatric Sonography.* 5th ed. Philadelphia, PA: Wolters Kluwer; 2018.

distance traveled between two reflecting objects is twice the separation distance. Therefore,

$$\text{Axial resolution} = 1/2 \text{ SPL}$$

where the SPL represents the number of cycles in the pulse multiplied by the wavelength (Figure 7.18). Objects that are closer than one-half the SPL will result in overlapping of structures and will not be distinguished as unique entities. The lower the value of the axial resolution (typically in units of millimeter), the better the system is at resolving close objects. Therefore, improved axial resolution can be achieved by reducing the pulse duration, reducing

the number of cycles, or using a higher frequency (which reduces the wavelength). The pulse duration and number of cycles are reduced by further damping the transducer element. The typical pulse for ultrasound imaging purposes contains three cycles. At a frequency of 5 MHz, with a wavelength of 0.31 mm, the SPL is calculated as follows: $3 \times 0.31 = 0.93$ mm. The axial resolution would equal 1/2 of 0.93 or 0.47 mm. Axial resolution does not change with depth.

The ability to distinguish between adjacent objects that are perpendicular to the beam direction is the lateral resolution. This is also known as azimuth resolution. The main determinant

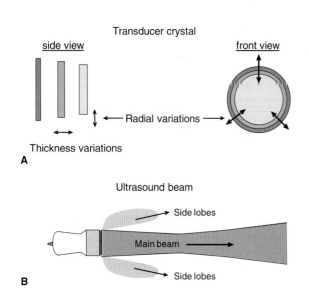

FIG. 7.16 ● A. Radial expansion occurs when a transducer in a multielement array generates the main ultrasound beam. B. Side lobes, which result from the radial transducer vibration, are directed away from the main beam. Reprinted with permission from Bushberg JT, Seibert JA, Leidholdt EM, Boone JM. *Essential Physics of Medical Imaging.* 3rd ed. Philadelphia, PA: Lippincott Williams & Wilkins, a Wolters Kluwer business; 2012.

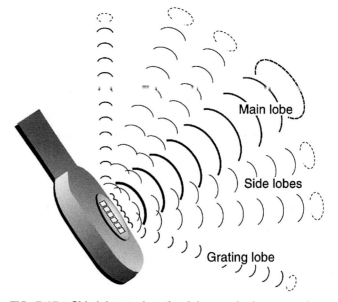

FIG. 7.17 ● **Side lobes and grating lobes are both unwanted energy emitted off-axis by linear and phased-array transducers.** Side lobes are directed forward whereas grating lobes are emitted at large angles from the surface of the array. Reprinted with permission from Perrino AC, Reeves ST. *Practical Approach to Transesophageal Echocardiography.* 1st ed. Philadelphia, PA: Lippincott Williams & Wilkins, A Wolters Kluwer business; 2003.

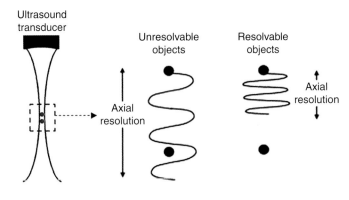

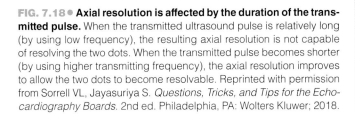

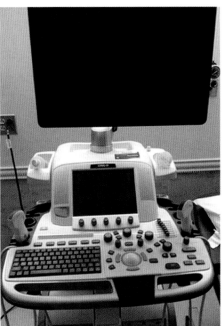

FIG. 7.18 ● **Axial resolution is affected by the duration of the transmitted pulse.** When the transmitted ultrasound pulse is relatively long (by using low frequency), the resulting axial resolution is not capable of resolving the two dots. When the transmitted pulse becomes shorter (by using higher transmitting frequency), the axial resolution improves to allow the two dots to become resolvable. Reprinted with permission from Sorrell VL, Jayasuriya S. *Questions, Tricks, and Tips for the Echocardiography Boards*. 2nd ed. Philadelphia, PA: Wolters Kluwer; 2018.

of lateral resolution is the transducer beam diameter, which is inversely related to frequency (Figure 7.19). In contrast to axial resolution, lateral resolution is depth dependent because the beam diameter varies with distance from the transducer in the near and far fields. The most optimal lateral resolution occurs at the boundary between the near and far fields (focal distance). The effective beam diameter is approximately one-half that of the transducer diameter at the near field-far field interface. The lateral resolution is markedly reduced in the far field where the beam diverges. Lateral resolution is also reduced when adjacent objects are within the same beam diameter because the returning echoes will overlap. This results in both objects erroneously being displaced as one on the display. An acoustic lens is employed on focused transducers to decrease the beam diameter at a specified distance from the transducer. The lateral resolution of an acoustic lens is better at shorter depths rather than at the interface of the near and far fields.

The ability of an ultrasound system to differentiate between closely spaced objects lying in the vertical axis of the ultrasound beam is known as elevational resolution. Lateral resolution is heavily dependent on the transducer element width, whereas elevational resolution is dependent on the transducer element height/thickness. It is also referred to as the slice-thickness dimension because of how important of a role the transducer height plays in image resolution. This is particularly true in regard to volume averaging that occurs close to the transducer and also in the regions deep to the focal zone (the far field). Slice thickness is generally a poor indicator of resolution for array transducers. Elevational resolution is improved using a fixed focal length lens along the surface of the array. The downside to this, however, is the decreased resolution secondary to partial volume averaging.

The ultrasound beam can be guided and focused in the elevational dimension when using multiple linear array transducers that have multiple rows. Typically, the transducers will contain between five and seven rows and are known as 1.5-dimensional transducer arrays. The slice-thickness dimension is minimized at a specified depth with phased excitation of the outer to inner arrays, which facilitates elevational focusing. A smaller slice thickness can be produced at different tissue depths using multiple excitations that differ in focusing distances. Two disadvantages of elevational focusing include the reduction in frame rate that is needed to build one image from multiple excitations and the inflexibility of positioning secondary to increased transducer thickness.

Beam former

The beam former generates the electronic delays for individual transducer elements in an array for transmit and receive focusing. It can be thought of as the engine of the ultrasound unit and has a primary role in image formation. In phased arrays, the beam former is responsible for beam steering. The majority of modern high-end ultrasound equipment has a digital beam former and digital electronics for transmitting and receiving. Digital beam formers control circuits that have several functions, including transmit and receive actions, preamplification, TGC, and digital-to-analog converters (DACs) and analog-to-digital converters (ADCs).

Pulser/Transmitter

A pulser (or transmitter) generates the electrical voltage needed to excite the piezoelectric transducer elements. By adjusting the applied voltage amplitude, the pulser also controls the output transmit power. The DACs used in digital beam former systems determine the amount of voltage applied. Increasing the transmit amplitude creates sounds of higher intensity. The echo detection from weaker reflectors is also improved with a higher transmit amplitude. This results in a higher signal-to-noise ratio in the images, but with the negative consequence of transmitting more power to the patient. The labels given to the output power vary between manufacturers and include "output," "power," "dB," and "transmit." In addition, methods of indicating output power in terms of a thermal index (TI) and mechanical index (MI) are typically provided. The components of an ultrasound unit are displayed in Figure 7.20.

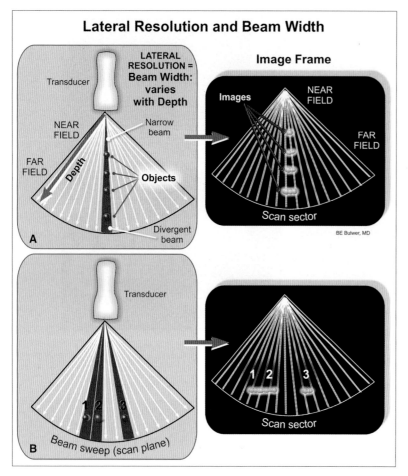

FIG. 7.19 ● **Lateral resolution refers to the ability to distinguish between objects that are perpendicular to the beam direction.** Lateral resolution is determined by beam diameter and varies with depth. Due to beam divergence, beam diameter increases proportionally with depth; as a result, the same object appears larger on the acquired image when it is at greater depth (A). At a certain depth, beam diameter at the depth determines lateral resolution (B): if the distance between two objects is longer than beam diameter, then the two can be resolved; if the distance is shorter than beam diameter, they cannot be resolved due to overlapping. Reprinted with permission from Savage RM, Aronson S, Shernan SK. *Comprehensive Textbook of Perioperative Transesophageal Echocardiography.* 2nd ed. Philadelphia, PA: Lippincott Williams & Wilkins, A Wolters Kluwer business; 2010.

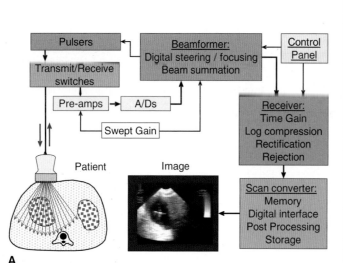

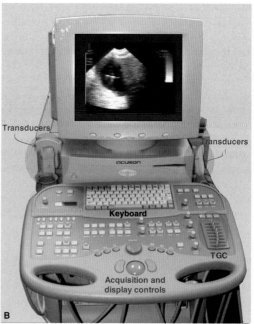

FIG. 7.20 ● A. Components of an ultrasound unit. Each transducer element in the array has a pulser, transmit-receive switch, preamplifier, and an analog-to-digital converter (ADC). The swept gain reduces the dynamic range of the signals prior to digital conversion. The beam former focuses, steers, and sums the beam. The receiver processes the data. B. An ultrasound unit is composed of a keyboard, various acquisition and processing controls, multiple transducer selections, and an image display monitor. Reprinted with permission from Bushberg JT, Seibert JA, Leidholdt EM, Boone JM. *Essential Physics of Medical Imaging.* 3rd ed. Philadelphia, PA: Lippincott Williams & Wilkins, a Wolters Kluwer business; 2012.

Pulse-echo operation

The ultrasound beam is intermittently transmitted in the pulse-echo mode. The transducer is listening for echoes the majority of the time. The pulser of the ultrasound system provides a short voltage waveform. The time delay between the transmitted pulse and the detection of the returning echo is directly proportional to the depth of the interface. Given a speed of sound of 1540 m/s (0.154 cm/µs), this time is calculated as follows:

$$\text{Time (µs)} = 2D\,(\text{cm})/c\,(\text{cm/µs}) = 2D\,(\text{cm})/0.154\,\text{cm/µs} = 13\,\text{µs} \times D\,(\text{cm})$$

$$\text{Distance (cm)} = c\,(\text{cm/µs}) \times \text{Time (µs)}/2 = 0.077 \times \text{Time (µs)}$$

where c = speed of sound (µs), D = distance from the transducer to the reflector (cm), and 2 is a constant representing the round-trip distance (µs). One amplitude-modulated (A-line) of image data is produced from a single pulse-echo sequence (Figure 7.21). Thus, an image composed of individual A-lines requires several pulse-echo sequences.

The pulse repetition frequency (PRF) refers to the number of times the transducer is pulsed per second. The PRF usually ranges from 2000 to 4000 pulses per second (2-4 kHz) for medical imaging purposes. Pulse repetition period (PRP) is the time between pulses and is inversely related to the PRF. Thus, the higher the PRF, the lower the PRP. Furthermore, increases in the number of transducer pulses per second equates to a decrease in echo listening time. Analogous to the rate-limiting step in a chemical reaction, the maximum PRF depends on the amount of time required for echoes to return to the transducer from the most distant structures. Artifacts may occur if a second pulse is transmitted before the detection of the most distant echo, which causes confusion for the transducer. An equation for the maximum range is as follows:

$$\text{Maximal range (cm)} = 154\,000\,\text{cm/s} \times \text{PRP}$$
$$\text{(s)} \times 1/2 = 77\,000 \times \text{PRP} = 77\,000/\text{PRF},$$

where 154 000 cm/s is the speed of sound, and the division by 2 accounts for round-trip distance. Ultrasound transducers with higher frequencies have limited penetration depth, which allows

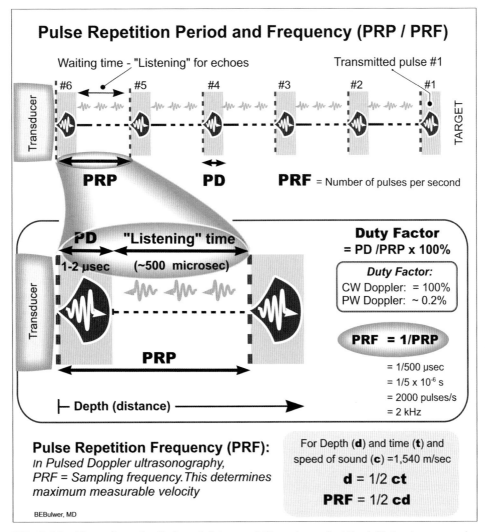

FIG. 7.21 ● **The pulse-echo timing of data acquisition shows that the initial pulse occurs in a very short time span.** The pulse duration is 1 to 2 µs and the time between pulses (pulse repetition period, PRP) is 500 µs in this example. The number of pulses per second is 2,000/s, equal to 2 kHz. Reprinted with permission from Savage RM, Aronson S, Shernan SK. *Comprehensive Textbook of Perioperative Transesophageal Echocardiography.* 2nd ed. Philadelphia, PA: Lippincott Williams & Wilkins, A Wolters Kluwer business; 2010.

for high PRFs. Using a lower frequency requires lower PRFs, however, because echoes will be returning from greater depths. It should be noted that transducer frequency is not the same as PRF and that the period of a sound wave (1/*f*) is not the same as the PRP (1/PRF).

The ratio of the number of cycles in a pulse to the transducer frequency is referred to as the pulse duration. This is equal to the amount of time that the pulse is firing (the "on" time). For example, a pulse composed of two cycles and a center frequency of 2 MHz will have a duration of 1 μs. The fraction of "on" time is known as the duty cycle and is calculated with the following equation:

$$\text{Duty cycle} = \text{pulse duration}/\text{PRP}$$

The duty cycle usually ranges between 0.2% and 0.4%, which means that the transducer is "listening" to returning echoes more than 99.5% of the time rather than producing echoes.

Preamplification and analog-to-digital conversion

Each preprocessing step is performed simultaneously in a multielement array transducer. A small voltage proportional to the pressure amplitude of the returning echoes is produced by every element with a multielement array transducer. These voltages are increased to useful levels by the process of preamplification. Because of the degree of attenuation that occurs with increasing distance, the initial preamplification is combined with a fixed swept gain to compensate (Figure 7.22). Each piezoelectric element in state-of-the-art ultrasound systems contains its own preamplifier and ADC. Units that digitize signals directly from the preamplification stage require ADCs with larger bit depths and

sampling rates. Ultrasound systems that digitize the signal after analog beam formation and summation usually have one, less powerful ADC.

Beam steering, dynamic focusing, and signal summation

Electronic delays are instituted in the echo reception process, which allows for the adjustment for beam direction. In addition, dynamic focusing aligns the phases of each detected echo as a function of echo depth. The signals from each active transducer element are summated after the phases are aligned. The resultant signal contains the acoustic information picked up during the PRP in a single-beam direction. The receiver processes this information further before the generation of a 2D image.

Receiver

Multiple signal processing steps occur once the receiver accepts data from the beam former during the PRP. These include, in order, gain adjustments and dynamic frequency tuning, dynamic range compression, rectification, demodulation, envelope detection, and the setting of amplitude thresholds.

Time gain compensation (TGC)

TGC, also known as depth gain compensation, time varied gain, and variable swept gain, is a technique which increases the signal gain of an echo as the return time increases. Consider the following example: an echo returning from a perfect reflector at the surface, such as an air bubble, will not undergo any attenuation because it is not traveling any distance. However, with the reflector at some depth (eg, 2 cm), the echo will undergo attenuation and become weaker because it will have traveled a total of 4 cm in the round trip. Echoes returning from deeper reflectors will undergo even greater attenuation. Compared to the reflector that is 2 cm deep, a reflector at 10 cm will return echoes that are extremely weak given the round trip of 20 cm. Left uncorrected, the images would display distant echoes as weaker compared to the more superficial echoes. Ultrasound scanners use TGC to amplify the signal of the distant echoes to create a more balanced image irrespective of the depth of the boundary. TGC is adjustable by the sonographer at the time of scanning. An ultrasound machine will typically have multiple slider knobs "at the fingertips" of the user, where each slider represents a certain depth in the image. Alternatively, a three knob system may be present, which controls the initial gain, slope, and far gain of the echo signals.

The spectrum between the threshold signal level and the maximum (saturation) level is known as the dynamic range. This encompasses the effective operational range of an electronic device. Put another way, the dynamic range refers to the range of ultrasound intensities displayed by the scanner. Dynamic range compression has a greater effect on the weaker echoes in comparison to the effect on stronger echoes. Following TGC, logarithmic amplification increases the smallest echo amplitudes and decreases the largest amplitudes. The output signal is proportional to the logarithm of the input signal. The end result is an appropriate display of the amplitude variations on the grayscale image. This is important in certain applications in which lower power setting are utilized, such as obstetrics, which require more gain to amplify weaker echo signals.

Echo display modes

A-mode (amplitude) displays the processed information from the receiver as a function of time. The transducer emits an ultrasound pulse, which produces echo signals along its path as it propagates

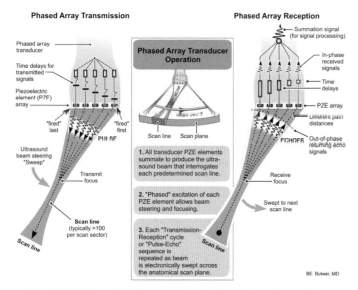

FIG. 7.22 ● The pulsed beam produced by a phased-array transducer is focused at a specified depth and receives echoes during the PRP. The figure demonstrates a digital beam former system, including the analog-to-digital converter (ADC), which converts the signals prior to beam focusing and steering. Timed delays align the phase of the echoes. The output is summed to produce the ultrasound echo train. Reprinted with permission from Savage RM, Aronson S, Shernan SK. *Comprehensive Textbook of Perioperative Transesophageal Echocardiography.* 2nd ed. Philadelphia, PA: Lippincott Williams & Wilkins, A Wolters Kluwer business; 2010.

through tissues. A digital signal proportional to the pulse amplitude is produced upon the return of echoes from tissue boundaries. The returning echo signals are amplified. A single "A-line" of data is generated per each PRP. Depth is plotted on the horizontal axis, whereas echo intensity (pulse amplitude) is plotted on the vertical axis. A-mode is primarily of historical interest. The only diagnostic application of A-mode imaging today is in ophthalmology to obtain precise measurements of the eye.

B-mode (brightness) electronically converts the A-line information obtained from many beams into pixels on the display monitor. The brightness of the pixels is generally proportional to the pulse amplitude. B-mode covers a plane of interest and generates a two-dimensional image. The echo signal amplitudes are plotted as a line with varying shades of gray, which allows for the visualization of subtle differences in signal. Structures that are more reflective appear brighter than those that are less reflective. B-mode display is utilized in M-mode and 2D grayscale imaging.

M-mode (motion) imaging uses B-mode data obtained from echoes returning from moving organs, including cardiac valve motion and myocardium. The data from a single ultrasound beam passing through a moving structure are displayed. Time is plotted on the horizontal axis and depth on the vertical axis. The echoes from sequential pulses are displayed next to one another, which allows for the visualization of the change of position of interfaces. Akin to B-mode imaging, the echo signal amplitudes are adjusted to varying brightness levels. These are plotted on a line with different shades of gray. Unlike the B-mode in which the transducer is swept across a region of interest, the ultrasound beam is stationary. Imaging is performed over a period of time to observe moving objects. Structures that are stationary are displayed as a straight trace, whereas moving structures generate wavy patterns. M-mode is also known as T-M (time-motion) as time-dependent motion is displayed.

Scan converter

Because image acquisition and image display are in different formats, a device known as a scan converter is needed to convert the data. The scan converter generates 2D images from echoes returning from multiple different directions. The images are converted into a data set that can be displayed on a monitor. Modern-day scan converters utilize digital technology to store and manipulate the data. Digital scan converters are very stable and have the ability to process images with a large number of different mathematical functions.

The digital information is configured as a matrix of pixels. Typical ultrasound machines use a matrix of approximately 500×500 pixels. Every pixel contains data that precisely localizes its position within the matrix. The correct pixel "addresses," or matrix coordinates, of each pixel depend on the transducer beam orientation and the delay times of the echoes.

ULTRASOUND IMAGE DISPLAY AND STORAGE

Electronic scanning and real-time display

The majority of modern ultrasound scanners use array transducers that contain several piezoelectric elements, which electronically sweep the ultrasound beam through the region of interest. Examples of array transducers include linear, curvilinear, and phased arrays. These arrays differ in how they produce the ultrasound beam and the configuration of the field of view coverage.

Linear array transducers produce images that are rectangular, whereas curvilinear array transducers produce trapezoidal

images (Figure 7.23). Linear and curvilinear array transducers typically employ 256 to 512 transducer elements that are each less than the width of a single wavelength. All of the elements are compacted into a 6- to 8-cm wide enclosure. The resulting beam propagates to the surface of the transducer at a perpendicular angle. A single line of acoustic data is obtained during the PRP. The next A-line of data is produced after a shift in one or more of the transducer elements and a repeat of the simultaneous excitation of the group. The linear array provides a wide field of view for the area near the transducer, which is an advantage over other arrays. Furthermore, its rectangular shape provides uniform data sampling across the image.

Phased-array transducers usually contain 64, 128, or 256 transducer elements, which are tightly grouped into a 3- to 5-cm wide enclosure. Each element actively contributes to the production of the ultrasound beam and recording of returning echoes. Varying time delays are applied to the transducer elements, which change the sweep angle across the field of view. A time delay is also used in processing the returning echoes to synchronize the echoes in space. The phased-array transducer elements are smaller in comparison to the linear and curvilinear array transducers. This relative small size allows for increased flexibility when scanning.

Image frame rate and spatial sampling

The PRF is equal to the number of pulses occurring in 1 second. PRF is measured in Hz and is calculated as follows:

$$PRF = 77\,000/\text{depth of view (cm)}$$

PRF is the reciprocal of the PRP:

$$PRF = 1/PRP$$

Recall that the PRP is the time interval between the onset of two different pulses. The equation of PRP is as follows:

$$PRP = 13 \text{ microseconds (µs)} \times \text{the depth of view (in cm)}$$

Hence, the PRP increases (and PRF decreases) as depth from the transducer increases. The PRP usually ranges from 100 µs to 1 ms. 2D images are created from multiple A-lines of data. Higher quality images are generated by combining more A-lines. The number of lines compiled is limited by the pulse-echo propagation time. The acquisition time for each A-line is as follows:

$$T_{\text{line}} = 13 \text{ µs/cm} \times D \text{ (cm)}$$

The time required per frame (T_{frame}) is calculated by N (the number of A-lines) $\times T_{\text{line}} = N \times 13 \text{ µs/cm} \times D$. The frame rate per second, which is the reciprocal of the time required for each frame, is

$$1/T_{\text{frame}} = 1/N \times 13 \text{ µs/cm} \times D =$$
$$0.77/\text{µs/N} \times D = 77\,000/\text{s/N} \times D$$

The maximum frame rate decreases if N or D is increased without a decrease in the other variable. Higher frame rates can be obtained via reductions in the imaging depth, number of lines, or the field of view. Transmit focusing is another factor that affects the frame rate.

Image display

Medical ultrasound systems generate highly complex transmit digital waveforms. A DAC is used to display the images on a monitor. The DAC translates the digital waveform into an analog video signal, which is compatible with specialized video monitors. The brightness and contrast of the digital data is modified with window and level adjustments before conversion. The analog

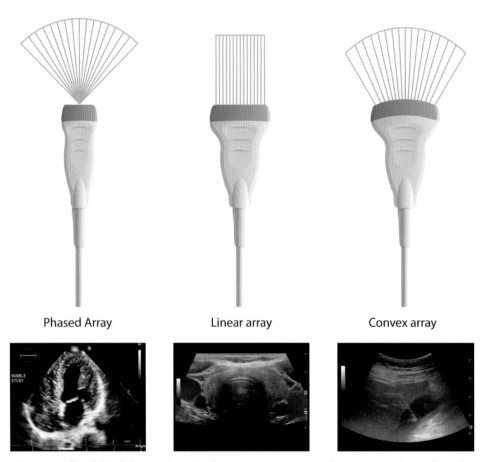

Phased Array   Linear array   Convex array

FIG. 7.23 ● The field of view produced by linear array transducers is rectangular in configuration while that of curvilinear array transducers is trapezoidal. Reprinted with permission from Huda W. *Review of Radiologic Physics*. 4th ed. Philadelphia, PA: Wolters Kluwer Health; 2016.

signal is then amplified by a linear high-voltage amplifier. DACs are typically only used in larger, expensive, less portable systems. As an alternative, many ultrasound systems utilize multilevel high-voltage pulsers to create the necessary signals.

The quality and resolution of images depend on the specifications of the display monitor, and in particular on the pixel density. Two types of zoom control are usually available for the operator to enlarge an image: write zoom and read zoom. Write zoom is a high-resolution zoom and is analogous to a digital zoom on a camera. When using write zoom, the operator must rescan the region of interest. Upon scanning, only the acoustic information from within the limited region is acquired and processed, which results in improved line density. Furthermore, all of the pixels obtained contribute to the displayed image. Read zoom, which is analogous to optical zoom on a camera, simply enlarges the selected region of interests and expands the displayed pixels. Image resolution is not affected when employing read zoom.

3D imaging

The major advantage of 3D ultrasound is that it overcomes limitations of traditional 2D imaging. For example, traditional ultrasound displays 3D anatomy in 2D, which forces the interpreter to synthesize the 3D anatomy in the mind while scrolling between scan planes. Another downside of 2D is that the images obtained are highly variable and operator dependent. The images

are acquired at arbitrary angles to the body, which leads to nonstandard and sometimes irreproducible, or at least difficult to reproduce, images.

The formation of 3D images first requires the acquisition of 2D image data in a series of individual scans for a given volume of tissue. Several volume sampling techniques are used to form the 3D data set from each individual 2D image, including linear translation, free-form motion, rocking motion, and rotation of the transducer (Figure 7.24). Surface display maximum intensity projection and multiplanar image reformation is possible if the volume data set acquisition geometry is known. A commonly known use of 3D imaging is within prenatal imaging (see Figure 7.24). One imaging protocol involves translating the transducer perpendicularly to the array direction, which produces a sequence of adjacent sectors scans over a 4- to 5-second period. Each sector scan produced serves as a single plane of the 3D volume data set. This stack of volume data is then sorted into image planes, thus providing alternate tomographic views. The computer calculates the 3D surface and integrates shading effects or false color to better delineate anatomy.

1D arrays provide an alternative method to using 2D arrays. A series of 2D images is acquired as the transducer scans over the region of interest. This data is then converted into a 3D image. Mechanical localizers can be used, which allow for precise position and angulation determination of each 2D image. The scanning time is reduced by adjusting the spatial interval between the images.

FIG. 7.24 ● Multiple techniques can be used to acquire 3D ultrasound images as depicted on the left. The top images on the right depict 4D acquisition of a fetus at two separate time points. The bottom image on the right depicts 3D surface evaluation of a fetus with cleft lip. From Bushberg JT, Seibert JA, Leidholdt EM, Boone JM. *Essential Physics of Medical Imaging.* 3rd ed. Philadelphia, PA: Lippincott Williams & Wilkins, a Wolters Kluwer business; 2012.

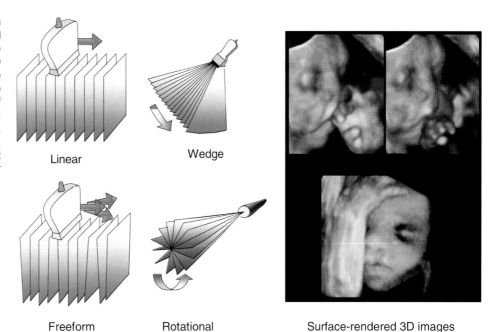

Linear

Wedge

Freeform

Rotational

Surface-rendered 3D images

Several different types of mechanical scanning approaches have been developed, which place the transducer on a rotating assembly. Integrated probes that are housed in the mechanical mechanism are easier to operate. However, these are larger and heavier and require the use of a special ultrasound machine, which limits their practicality in clinical practice. Transducers with external fixtures are generally bulky, although they can be affixed to conventional ultrasound machines.

3D reconstruction

Reconstruction of 2D data into 3D images has been briefly discussed previously. 3D images can be generated by one of two methods, including feature-based and voxel-based reconstruction. With feature-based reconstruction, the data within the acquired 2D images are segmented and outlined, which is done manually or with computer automation. The highlighted structures are integrated for display. Feature-based reconstruction is often used in echocardiographic imaging to display the surface of the heart chambers and left ventricular motion with a 3D model. An advantage of this type of reconstruction is the enhanced display of the surfaces of structures. Furthermore, the contrast between structures can be artificially increased to improve the appearance of the image. An important limitation of the feature-based approach is that tissue texture and other subtle features are lost because the reconstruction only takes into account the anatomic boundaries.

Voxel-based reconstruction is the most common method of generating 3D images in clinical ultrasound. A voxel is a 3D grid of picture elements. With this method of reconstruction, each pixel within an acquired 2D data set is localized into a 3D volume. All of the original information from the 2D images is preserved during reconstruction. However, gaps can be created between the pixels if the volume is not sampled properly during the scanning process. This leads to interpolation of data and introduction of potentially false data, which will inherently lead to artifacts and image degradation.

Image storage

The image data obtained by the ultrasound system is transcribed into a scan converter. A scan converter is a memory device that stores acquired acoustic information and translates it into data that can be displayed. The converter is a necessary component because the produced echo signals are of an entirely different format from that of the displayed data. The scan converter in effect serves as an interpreter between the produced (and received) echo data and the display format. Image data from every display type, including B-mode, M-mode, and Doppler mode, is capable of being stored by the converter. Not surprisingly, modern ultrasound systems store data in digital format rather than in the analog techniques used in the past.

The pixel depth in B-mode and M-mode imaging is typically 8 bits, which is composed of 256 gray levels, whereas that of color Doppler is usually 24 bits. Eight bits make up 1 byte. Thus, the pixel depth of an image in B-mode and M-mode is 1 byte and that of color Doppler is 3 bytes. The typical matrix size of an ultrasound image is 512×512, which describes the total number of pixels per image. The total image size is determined by the product of matrix size and pixel depth, while keeping in mind the pixel depth for B-mode and M-mode is 1 byte per pixel and that of color Doppler is 3 bytes per pixel. The unit of image size is megabytes (MB). One megabyte is equal to 2^{20} bytes.

Although ultrasound systems are digital and amenable to postprocessing techniques, the displayed images provide important feedback to the operator during real-time scanning. As previously discussed, the user has many controls and settings at his or her disposal to improve the quality of the image (focal zone, TGC, transducer frequency, etc). Postprocessing techniques can improve the images only to a certain degree. If the initially acquired images are suboptimal, the end product will be the same. It is of utmost importance that the user optimizes brightness and contrast during scanning.

DOPPLER ULTRASOUND

The common relatable example of the Doppler effect is the high-pitched sound the siren on a fire truck produces while approaching a listener standing on the side of the road, whereas a lower pitched sound is perceived after the truck passes by and continues away from the listener. The physics behind this phenomenon is based on the shift of frequency in a sound wave caused by a moving reflector. The Doppler effect is applied in

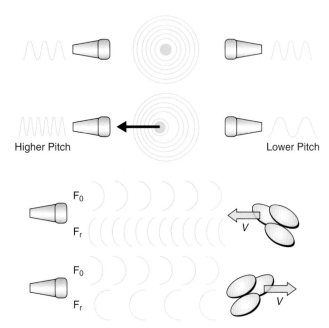

Higher Pitch

Lower Pitch

F_0

F_r

v

F_0

F_r

v

FIG. 7.25 ● **Illustrations of the Doppler effect.** First row: stationary source of sound produces waves at a given frequency. Second row: sound waves reflected from a moving object are compressed when moving toward the transducer, resulting in a higher frequency; sound waves are expanded when moving away from the transducer, resulting in a lower frequency. Third row: when red blood cells move towards the transducer, the reflected frequency will be higher than the emitted frequency. Fourth row: when red blood cells move away from the transducer, the reflected frequency will be lower than the emitted frequency. Reprinted with permission from Armstrong WF, Ryan T. *Feigenbaum's Echocardiography.* 8th ed. Philadelphia, PA: Wolters Kluwer Health; 2018.

ultrasound imaging to evaluate blood flow in vessels. This is based on the backscatter of blood cells, which serve as moving reflectors. Blood velocity can be measured by comparing the incident ultrasound frequency with the frequency reflected from the blood cells (Figure 7.25). The information acquired from these Doppler techniques is then extrapolated to create color blood flow maps. It should be noted that blood is a relatively weak scatterer, which leads to weak signals. This section explains the physical principles of Doppler ultrasound and how the extracted information from blood flow is formulated into data interpreted by the sonographer.

Doppler frequency shift

The Doppler shift is the change between an incident frequency and the reflected frequency. Blood moving toward the transducer will produce echoes with higher frequencies, whereas blood moving away from the transducer produces echoes with lower frequencies. Using our previous example, the sound waves from the fire truck siren are compressed (higher frequency) while approaching the listener and expanded when moving away (lower frequency). The difference between the incident and the returning frequencies is the Doppler shift frequency. The Doppler frequency shift (f_d) can be calculated using the following formula:

$$f_d = f_i - f_r = \text{reflector speed}/(\text{reflector speed} + \text{speed of sound}) \times 2 \times f_i$$

with the stipulation that the reflector is moving directly away from the source of sound. Within this formula, f_i is the frequency of the sound incident on the reflector and f_r is the frequency of the

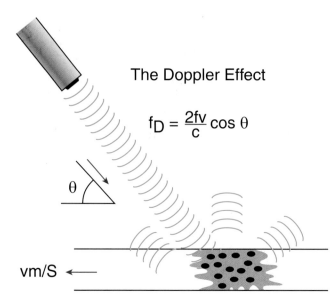

The Doppler Effect

$$f_D = \frac{2fv}{c} \cos \theta$$

θ

vm/S ←

FIG. 7.26 ● **The Doppler shift is dependent on the angle of the incident ultrasound pulse (θ) and the axis of the blood vessel at a fixed blood velocity, v.** The maximum Doppler shift occurs when the θ = 0. Reprinted with permission from Stephenson SR. *Obstetrics & Gynecology.* 3rd ed. Philadelphia, PA: Wolters Kluwer Health; 2015.

reflected sound. Because blood cells serve as the reflectors, this demonstrates that the Doppler shift is nearly proportional to the velocity of the cells. The equation needs to be modified to account for less Doppler effect if the sound waves and blood cells are not moving in parallel directions. The angle between the direction of the sound waves and the direction of the blood cells is represented by the Doppler angle θ (Figure 7.26). To calculate the velocity vector directed toward the transducer, the velocity along the axis of the vessels is multiplied by the cosine of the angle, cos θ. The Doppler shift underestimates the true blood velocity if this angular dependence is not corrected. A right triangle is created between the transducer and the blood velocity. The angle between the actual blood velocity and the adjacent side is the Doppler angle. The component of the blood velocity in the direction of the sound (adjacent side) is equal to the true blood velocity multiplied by the cos θ. A generalized equation can be used to calculate the Doppler frequency shift. Blood velocity can be neglected in the denominator because it is significantly less than the speed of sound (~200 cm/s vs 154 000 cm/s, respectively), which leaves the following equation:

$$f_d = 2 f_i \, v \cos \theta / c$$

where v is blood velocity, f_i is the frequency of the sound incident on the reflector, θ is the Doppler angle, and c is the speed of sound in the soft tissue. By rearranging this equation, the velocity of blood can be calculated:

$$v = f_d \, c / 2 f_i \cos \theta$$

To achieve accurate velocity measurements, the Doppler shift at a given angle θ is adjusted by 1/cos θ. Selected cosine values include cos 0° = 1, cos 30° = 0.87, cos 45° = 0.707, cos 60° = 0.5, cos 90° = 0. The ideal Doppler angle is between 30° and 60°. Using angles above 60° yields an apparent Doppler shift that is too small. Minor errors in angle accuracy can lead to significant errors in velocity (Table 7.5). If the angle is too small (below 20°), refraction and critical angle interactions can lead to aliasing of the signal in pulsed Doppler studies.

Table 7.5 **DOPPLER ANGLE AND ERROR ESTIMATES OF BLOOD VELOCITY FOR A +3° ANGLE ACCURACY ERROR**

Angle (°)	Set Angle (°)	Actual Velocity (cm/s)	Estimated Velocity (cm/s)	Percent Error (%)
0	3	100	100.1	0.14
25	28	100	102.6	2.65
45	48	100	105.7	5.68
60	63	100	110.1	10.1
80	83	100	142.5	42.5

Reprinted with permission from Bushberg JT, Seibert JA, Leidholdt EM, Boone JM. *Essential Physics of Medical Imaging*. 3rd ed. Philadelphia, PA: Wolters Kluwer Health/Lippincott Williams & Wilkins; 2012.

Continuous and pulsed mode doppler operation

Two transducers are required for a continuous-wave Doppler system, which is the most commonly used device for measuring blood velocity given its simplicity and cost-effectiveness. One transducer transmits the incident ultrasound while the other transducer detects the resultant continuous echoes (Figure 7.27). A resonant frequency, produced by an oscillator, powers the transmit transducer. The demodulator receives the same frequency signal by the oscillator and then compares the returning frequency to the incident frequency. The returning signal is amplified by a receiver, which then utilizes a "low-pass" filter to remove high-frequency oscillations. Very low-frequency signals from vessel walls are selectively removed by a wall filter. The Doppler signal is amplified to an audible sound level by an amplifier and then plotted as a function of time. A main advantage of continuous Doppler operation is the high accuracy of the Doppler shift measurement, which is a reflection of the narrow frequency bandwidth used. Secondly, no aliasing occurs during this mode of operation with high velocities. A vulnerability of continuous

mode is depth sensitivity with resultant degradation of accuracy by object motion in the beam path.

Pulsed Doppler operation uses the strength of continuous-wave Doppler (velocity determination) and combines that with the strength of pulse-echo imaging (range discrimination). The SPL in pulsed mode is longer, which results in a higher Q factor. This improves the measurement accuracy of the frequency shift. An electronic time gate circuit helps achieve depth selection by only accepting the echo signals falling within the gate window.

Duplex scanning

B-mode ultrasound imaging provides information on stationary reflectors. Doppler scanning utilizes flow information within a selected region of interest. Duplex scanning combines 2D B-mode imaging with pulsed Doppler data acquisition. By operating in 2D B-mode, a duplex scanner creates a real-time image and selects the Doppler gate window position. The scanner is then switched to Doppler mode to align the ultrasound beam at a certain orientation to obtain Doppler information. Because the velocity of sound and the transducer frequency are known, flow velocity can be estimated

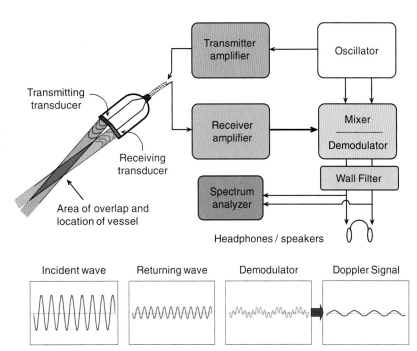

FIG. 7.27 ● **Diagram demonstrating a continuous wave Doppler system.** One transducer serves as a transmitter while the other receives. The overlapping signal determines the position of the blood velocity measurement. A low-pass filter selectively removes the highest frequencies while a high-pass filter (Wall filter) selectively removes the lowest frequencies. Reprinted with permission from Bushberg JT, Seibert JA, Leidholdt EM, Boone JM. *Essential Physics of Medical Imaging*. 3rd ed. Philadelphia, PA: Lippincott Williams & Wilkins, a Wolters Kluwer business; 2012.

directly from the Doppler shift frequency. The Doppler angle is estimated from the B-mode image and entered into the scanner computer. Flow (cm^3/s) is then estimated by multiplying the vessel's cross-sectional area (cm^2) and the velocity (cm/s).

Doppler spectral interpretation

Doppler spectral analysis relates frequency shift as a function of time, which provides information about blood flow. Spectral Doppler operation uses a single transducer, which alternates between transmitting pulsed waves and receiving returning echoes. The Doppler signal composes a spectrum of frequencies captured within a sampling gate at a given point in time. Because of the variations in the velocities of blood flow, a spectrum of Doppler shift frequencies is generated as opposed to a single frequency. A Doppler gate encompassing the entire lumen of a vessel will result in a larger range of blood velocities than does a gate encompassing the center of a vessel. This is because blood flowing in the center of the vessel is relatively fast with a narrow range of velocities, whereas blood flowing along the vessel wall is slower due to frictional forces. The spectrum of velocities within the sampling gate is displayed on a graph as a function of time. The three typical blood flow patterns observed in vessels are laminar, blunt, or turbulent flow. The type of flow within a given vessel depends on the size and shape of the vessel, the characteristics of the vessel wall, and the flow rate. Positioning a Doppler gate near a stenosis, such as one caused by plaque buildup, will result in the largest measured range of velocities. An important advantage of spectral Doppler is its high range resolution and specificity, which occurs because echoes are arising only from the preselected sample volume. Pulsed wave Doppler also allows for the analysis of multiple vessels and vessels that are at different depths. One notable limitation is its susceptibility to aliasing artifact.

Doppler ultrasound uses transducers with the same frequencies as those used in grayscale imaging. The frequencies typically range between 1 and 10 MHz. The process of demodulation describes the extraction of Doppler frequency, which is low, from the transducer frequency, which is high.

The fast Fourier transform is used to interpret the frequency shifts and direction of blood flow. This is a mathematical system that generates a Doppler spectrum by analyzing the detected signals. The Doppler spectrum is a distribution profile relating amplitudes versus frequencies and is continuously updated in a spectral Doppler display at real time (Figure 7.28). The information is typically displayed below the 2D B-mode image on the video monitor as a moving trace. Blood velocity is placed on the vertical axis and time is placed on the horizontal axis. The brightness of each point on the display changes to reflect Doppler signal intensity for a given frequency and time. Velocities in one direction are displayed as positive values above the x-axis while velocities in the opposite direction are designated as negative values below the x-axis. The standard practice is to display blood flowing toward the transducer as positive values above baseline (designated by the color red) and blood flowing away from the transducer as negative values below baseline (designated by the color blue). However, this setting can be switched on the ultrasound computer. The video monitor plots a color scale showing which color (red or blue) is being used for positive and negative values. It is important for the interpreting sonographer to confirm how the examination is set up, because confusion could lead to drastic interpretive errors.

In addition to providing information on the direction of flow, the spectral display allows for the determination of flow characteristics. The absence of flow can also be ascertained via the spectral display. This may prove difficult, however, because other factors, such as a technical problem in the acoustic or electric

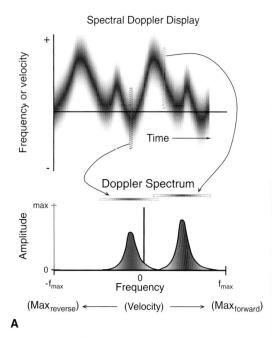

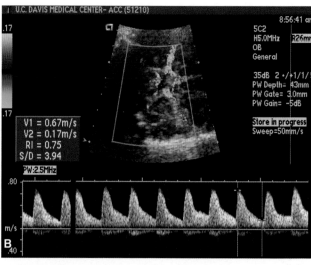

FIG. 7.28 ● A. The spectral Doppler display plots the Doppler shift frequency. The amplitude of the shift frequency is shown as gray-scale color variations. The bottom graph demonstrates two Doppler spectra as discrete points in time. B. Color flow image, which shows active color area and the corresponding spectral Doppler display (below) obtained from a sample gate in a vessel. Reprinted with permission from Bushberg JT, Seibert JA, Leidholdt EM, Boone JM. *Essential Physics of Medical Imaging.* 3rd ed. Philadelphia, PA: Lippincott Williams & Wilkins, a Wolters Kluwer business; 2012.

system, could lead to the false suggestion that flow is absent. The optimal Doppler angle for determining the direction of flow is about 30°. Normal flow in each vessel in the body has its own characteristic waveform. Disease processes have the potential to alter the vessel's normal waveform, which allows for interpretation for that particular disease. Vascular stenosis, for example, may cause disturbed and turbulent flow, leading to a wide distribution of velocities. Certain quantitative measures provide information about vascular impedance and pulsatile velocity changes, including resistive index (RI) and pulsatile index (PI):

$$RI = (maximum\ velocity - minimum\ velocity)/(maximum\ velocity)$$

$$PI = (maximum\ velocity - minimum\ velocity)/(average\ velocity)$$

Aliasing

Aliasing is an error caused by having a sampling frequency which is not sufficient relative to the high-frequency Doppler signals generated from fast moving blood. High velocities are displayed as negative, which leads to inaccurate measurements. To determine the corresponding velocity, at least two samples per cycle of Doppler shift frequency are required. Aliasing manifests on the spectral Doppler display by wrapping the signal to a negative amplitude (Figure 7.29). The highest positive frequency shift is displayed in the color that corresponds to the highest negative frequency shift. Consequently, this can lead to the false interpretation of reversed flow, when, in fact, the flow velocity is above the selected sampling range. Aliasing artifact occurs when the Doppler shift is higher than a threshold described by the Nyquist frequency:

$$Nyquist\ limit\ (kHz) = 1/2 \times pulse\ repetition\ frequency\ (PRF)$$

The easy solution for this problem is to simply increase the range of the velocity scale, which increases the PRF. If already set at the maximum sampling rate, the spectral baseline (representing zero velocity) can be adjusted to allocate a larger sampling range for blood flowing in that particular direction (toward or away from the transducer). A lower frequency transducer can be used to decrease the Doppler shift. Selecting a sample volume at a lesser depth can reduce aliasing via an increase in PRF with decreasing depth. Finally, by choosing a Doppler angle closer to 90°, the Doppler shift will decrease, which will reduce or eliminate aliasing.

Doppler imaging is susceptible to several additional artifacts. The tissues adjacent to the sampled vessels are prone to vibration,

which may be detected as a Doppler frequency shift. This leads to the display of a mixture of red and blue colors. Color and spectral Doppler are susceptible to mirror image artifact. These artifacts can occur with vessels adjacent to highly reflective surfaces, such as sub-diaphragmatic hepatic vessels. Twinkle artifact refers to the artifactual fluctuating appearance of red and blue colors that occurs at strongly reflective surfaces, such as calcifications. Pseudoflow (or pseudoblood) artifact results from the flow of substances other than blood, including ureteral jets, ascites, and amniotic fluid. Color may extend beyond the wall of the vessel on the display monitor, which can artifactually disguise a thrombus. One way to mitigate this artifact, known as color bleed, is to decrease color gain.

Color flow imaging

Color Doppler imaging provides a 2D visual display of blood moving within vessels. The Doppler frequency shifts are encoded as colors, which are superimposed on a grayscale image. The advantage of color Doppler is the ability to obtain information about velocity and position simultaneously. Using typical convention, red represents blood flowing toward the transducer and blue represents blood flowing away from the transducer. Green or yellow may be used to demonstrate turbulent flow. The colors intensify with increasing flow velocities, while the B-mode image displays the absence of movement. Flow information is obtained by averaging the values obtained from each pixel within a selected location. The direction and magnitude of flow in the region of interest is provided by color Doppler. Another advantage of color Doppler is the ability to detect flow within vessels that otherwise would be under the resolution of conventional imaging. However, the spatial resolution of a color Doppler image is lower than that of the B-mode image. 2D color flow imaging systems utilize phase-shift autocorrelation or time domain correlation techniques rather than using the full Doppler shift information.

Phase-shift autocorrelation measures the similarity of one scan line measurement with another during the time of maximum correlation. The echo pulse of an A-line is compared with that of a previous echo which is separated by a time equal to the PRP. The phase changes between two A-lines of data, which occur because of a Doppler shift over a given time interval, are detected by the system (Figure 7.30). The computed correlation is proportional to the phase change, which is proportional to the velocity at that point along the echo pulse trace. The direction of the moving object is maintained via phase detection of the echo amplitudes. The flow information must be integrated with the grayscale B-mode image because these are being acquired at the same time. The color flow data is then superimposed on the grayscale

FIG. 7.29 ● **Aliasing of the spectral Doppler display is characterized by "wrap-around" of velocities above the sampling gate (left image).** The aliased vessels are incorporated within the spectrum of displayed velocities when the spectral baseline is shifted (right image). Reprinted with permission from Bushberg JT, Seibert JA, Leidholdt EM, Boone JM. *Essential Physics of Medical Imaging.* 3rd ed. Philadelphia, PA: Lippincott Williams & Wilkins, a Wolters Kluwer business; 2012.

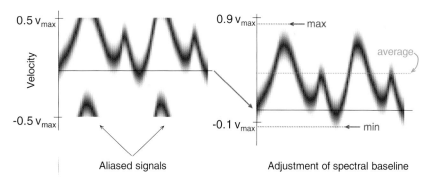

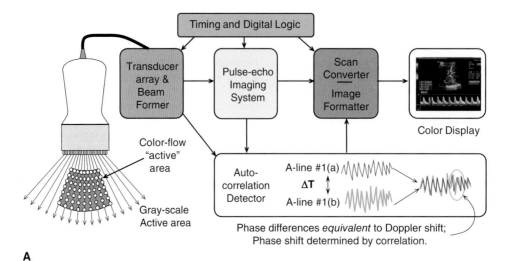

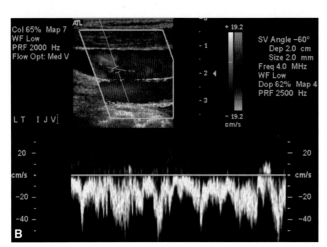

FIG. 7.30 ● A. Dynamic gray-scale B-mode images with color-encoded velocity displays are produced by color flow acquisition. Autocorrelation rapidly determines phase changes in areas of motion from consecutive A-lines of data moving in the same direction. B. Arterial and venous flow with color designations depicting the direction of blood flow (red towards the transducer; blue away from the transducer). Reprinted with permission from Bushberg JT, Seibert JA, Leidholdt EM, Boone JM. *Essential Physics of Medical Imaging.* 3rd ed. Philadelphia, PA: Lippincott Williams & Wilkins, a Wolters Kluwer business; 2012.

image along with a color scale map. An alternative technique for obtaining color flow information is time domain correlation. This method measures the reflector motion between consecutive pulse-echo acquisitions over a given time interval.

Power doppler

Power Doppler refers to a processing method which relies entirely on the total strength (amplitude) of the Doppler signal. The information obtained in the power Doppler is similar to that obtained in color Doppler. Unlike color flow imaging, however, directional information is ignored in the power Doppler. Quantitative flow is also spared because the amplitude of all Doppler signals is acquired, regardless of the frequency shift. To put it another way, the positive and negative velocities within a region of interest are summed with the power Doppler, but would cancel each other out with the color Doppler. The consequence of this system is the markedly improved sensitivity of motion compared to standard color flow imaging. This allows for the detection of very slow blood flow. The power Doppler is not affected by changes in Doppler angle. Furthermore, the system is immune to aliasing because

the strength of the frequency-shifted signals are analyzed, not the phase. However, the power Doppler is not without its own artifacts and issues. Because the power Doppler uses slower frame rates, a large number of motion artifacts may occur because of color signals emanating from transducer motion, patient motion, or moving tissues. These motion artifacts are known as "flash artifacts" in power Doppler imaging. A comparison between images obtained with color Doppler and power Doppler is shown in Figure 7.31.

ADVANCED ULTRASOUND IMAGING

Harmonic imaging

Harmonic imaging is used in ultrasound to improve the quality of images that would be obtained with conventional techniques. Harmonic frequencies are integral multiples of the fundamental ultrasound frequencies of the initial pulse. A high-frequency harmonic may be twice that of the fundamental frequency. Harmonic imaging takes advantage of the nonlinear propagation of

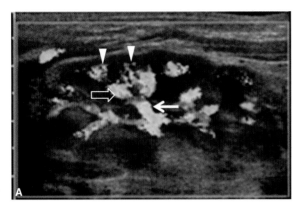
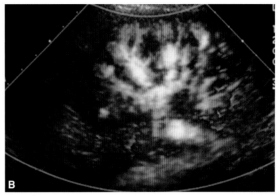

FIG. 7.31 ● **Color Doppler vs Power Doppler.** A is a Color Doppler images demonstrating the segmental artery in the renal hilum (arrow), interlobar arteries (open arrow), and arcuate arteries around the corticomedullary junction (arrowheads). B is a Power Doppler image with enhanced visualization of the vascular tree. Compared to Color Doppler, Power Doppler has increased sensitivity for flow detection, but it is not able to provide information about flow direction. Reprinted with permission from Siegel MJ. *Pediatric Sonography.* 4th ed. Philadelphia, PA: Wolters Kluwer; 2018.

the ultrasound wave through tissue, which leads to an asymmetric and distorted ultrasound wave shape. The high-pressure component of the wave travels faster than the low-pressure component. This discrepancy and distortion between the two components increases with depth. Harmonic imaging selects for the high frequencies. The first harmonic, which is twice the fundamental frequency, is often used because higher frequency harmonics suffer from too much attenuation. By filtering out the lower frequency echoes, the scatter and reflections from adjacent tissues and objects adjacent to the transducer are eliminated. Additional advantages of harmonic imaging include a reduction in reverberation and side lobe artifacts, improvement in the axial and lateral resolution, and increased signal-to-noise ratio. Furthermore, better resolution is obtained in patients with a large body habitus, which is often a severe limitation with conventional techniques. Harmonic imaging is most advantageous when imaging with lower frequencies (and hence longer wavelengths) that are able to penetrate to greater depths. This is typical of abdominal imaging. To characterize tissue or a mass deep within the abdomen, the lower frequency may be switched to a higher harmonic, which will improve the quality and resolution by eliminating noise adjacent to the transducer.

Contrast agents

Ultrasound contrast agents are being used in certain vascular and perfusion imaging protocols. These agents, which are intravenously administered, are encapsulated microbubbles (3-6 μm) containing air, nitrogen, or insoluble gases (perfluorocarbons). Human albumin is often used to contain the encapsulated gas for an amount of time that will be useful and practical for targeted vascular imaging. The microbubbles may perfuse into tissues given their small size; however, this requires the agent to remain extremely stable. Microbubble contrast agents create a large difference in the acoustic impedance between the gas, fluids, and tissues. The bubbles produce reflections in all directions because of the relatively small size in comparison to the wavelength of the ultrasound beam. These agents also produce harmonic frequencies because of their compressibility causing shifts in the returning frequency. Pulse inversion harmonic imaging is a technique to improve the utilization of ultrasound contrast agents. The sensitivity for the microbubbles is increased, while the signal from the surrounding tissues is reduced. Two excitation pulses, standard

and inverted (phase-reversed), are sent sequentially along the same beam direction. These pulses cancel out for soft tissues because positive and negative pressures of equal but opposite amplitude are reflected back to the transducer. The microbubble pulses persist because of the nonlinear response it elicits.

ULTRASOUND IMAGE QUALITY AND ARTIFACTS

Image quality

Quality measures of ultrasound images include spatial resolution, contrast resolution, noise, and image uniformity. Ultrasound spatial resolution is composed of three directions: axial, lateral, and elevational. Introduced earlier, the topic of spatial resolution is further discussed in this section. Resolution in the axial direction refers to the ability to delineate two objects lying along the axis of the beam. The pulse length is the most important factor affecting axial resolution. Every ultrasound pulse consists of approximately two wavelengths. Short pulses are generated with damping of the transducer. Axial resolution is equal to one-half of the SPL, which is determined by the frequency of the ultrasound and the damping factor. Depth has no effect on axial resolution. High-frequency transducers are required to achieve good axial resolution. Consider the example of a 2 MHz transducer. The axial resolution will be approximately 1 mm, which is one-half of the pulse length of 2 mm. If a 4 MHz transducer is used, the axial resolution improves to approximately 0.5 mm. However, the trade-off with higher frequency transducers is the poor penetration. Thus, to achieve optimal axial resolution, the distance between the transducer and the region of interest needs to be minimized. Breast ultrasound uses high-frequency transducers (typically 8-10 MHz) to achieve high resolution. Of course, penetration decreases with increasing breast thickness.

Lateral resolution describes the ability to delineate two objects adjacent to one another perpendicular to the axial direction within the image plane. Determinants of resolution in the lateral direction include the width of the ultrasound beam, the depth of the object, and mechanical and electronic focusing. Lateral resolution is improved by using focused transducers, which produce a narrow beam, and by increasing the number of lines per frame. Imaging within the focal zone provides the most optimal lateral resolution. The resolution can be adjusted by moving the focal position. Using multiple focal lengths may improve lateral resolution; however, this leads to a reduced frame rate. Lateral resolution is typically degraded at greater depths from the transducer.

The axial and lateral resolutions are relatively easy to discern because they are both in the plane of the image. Elevational resolution is difficult to perceive and interpret because it is perpendicular to the image, essentially serving as slice thickness. Elevational resolution is directly related to the height of the transducer. An acoustic lens can be used to improve elevational focusing. Similar to lateral resolution, the resolution in the elevational plane is dependent on depth. Elevational resolution is improved by using a 1.5D array, which contains approximately six rows of transducers in the direction of slice thickness. Elevational resolution approximates the lateral resolution.

Contrast resolution is determined by several factors, two of which include acoustic impedance differences and spatial resolution. The recognition of tissue boundaries and internal architecture is possible because of reflections caused by acoustic impedance differences between tissues. Variations in attenuation cause differences in the grayscale appearance. Areas of low attenuation (eg, simple cyst) commonly cause increased signal distally ("increased through transmission" or "posterior enhancement"). Alternatively, areas of high attenuation (eg, gallstone) may cause loss of signal distally ("posterior shadowing"). Several techniques can improve contrast, including the administration of microbubble contrast agents, the use of harmonic imaging, or Doppler imaging. Contrast resolution is also affected by spatial resolution. As mentioned earlier, elevational resolution is equivalent to the slice thickness of an ultrasound image. The slice thickness is wide at deep depths and also in regions close to the transducer array surface. Small objects in one of these two areas will return echoes that are averaged over the volume element, which results in a lower signal and loss of detection. Large objects may achieve improved contrast compared to the background because potential degrading noise components are reduced by averaging over the volume.

A high contrast-to-noise ratio is crucial to detecting subtle anatomy. Contrast depends on signal amplitude generated by tissue attenuation differences. The main generator of noise is from the electronic amplifiers of the system. An amplifier with low noise and high gain specifications is necessary for low-contrast imaging. Noise can be reduced with certain imaging processing techniques, including spatial or temporal averaging, thus increasing contrast-to-noise ratio. This can lead to poor spatial resolution, however, which is a trade-off. Higher electronic signal application is needed in low-power operations to increase the weak echo amplitudes to useful levels. Of course, this will lead to low contrast-to-noise ratios.

Artifacts

As in other imaging modalities, there are numerous artifacts that can degrade the quality of an examination. Understanding the common artifacts that occur in ultrasound imaging is important so that apparent abnormalities are correctly interpreted. An artifact is the false or incorrect display of anatomy, including an object's location, size, or brightness. An ultrasound machine processes images with the assumption that the detected echoes are returning from the main ultrasound beam. However, strong reflectors outside of the main ultrasound beam can create echoes. If detected, the transducer will falsely assume that these echoes originated from the mean beam, which leads to an incorrect display. Artifacts in ultrasound imaging include machine- and operator-related causes, in addition to those occurring from the

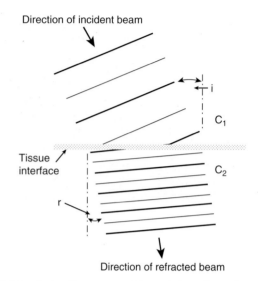

FIG. 7.32 ● **Refraction occurs at boundaries of two tissues with different speeds of sound when an ultrasound beam has nonperpendicular incidence and can lead to misplacement of objects.** Reprinted with permission from Beggs I. *Musculoskeletal Ultrasound.* 1st ed. Philadelphia, PA: Lippincott Williams & Wilkins, A Wolters Kluwer business; 2013.

interaction of ultrasound with tissue. Specific artifacts in ultrasound include refraction, shadowing and enhancement, and reverberation. Although labeled as artifacts, several of these actually improve the specificity and diagnostic confidence depending on their characteristic appearance.

Refraction refers to the change in direction the ultrasound beam takes when passing through a tissue boundary at nonperpendicular angles. For refraction to occur, the two tissues must have different speeds of sound. Refraction leads to spatial distortion, misregistration, or lateral defocusing at the edges of curved structures. The transmitted ultrasound pulse changes direction with nonperpendicular incidence, which leads to misplaced display of the anatomy (Figure 7.32). The amount of anatomic displacement will vary depending on the position of the transducer as well as on the incidence angle with the tissue boundaries.

Acoustic shadowing is an artifact that describes the dark signal displayed beyond an object of high echogenicity. This is classically seen with calcific structures, such as bones, gallstones, and kidney stones. These objects of high echogenicity absorb or attenuate the ultrasound beam, which reduces the intensity of the transmitted beam distally (Figure 7.33). Shadowing can also occur at curved interfaces secondary to reflection of the incident beam. Although shadowing is technically an artifact, it often aids in the diagnosis of echogenic foci.

Acoustic enhancement is essentially the opposite of shadowing. It is characterized as a region of high-intensity distal to an object of low ultrasound attenuation secondary to increased transmission of the sound waves. Classically, this occurs in fluid-filled cavities, including simple cysts, the urinary bladder, and blood vessels (Figure 7.34A). Again, although technically an artifact, the presence (or absence) of posterior enhancement often has crucial clinical implications. It can help differentiate a lesion in the kidney as a simple cyst versus a solid mass (Figure 7.34).

Twinkling (or twinkle) artifact refers to a mixture of alternating colors extending distal to an echogenic object (eg, renal calculus) when using color Doppler imaging (Figure 7.35). Speckle

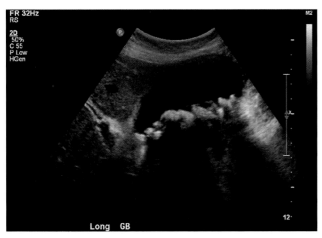

FIG. 7.33 • Multiple dependent gallstones within the gallbladder cause posterior shadowing.

artifact describes a textured appearance, which results from small structures that are in close proximity. Reflectors with rough surfaces will also lead to speckling due to scattering of the ultrasound beam.

Reverberation occurs when ultrasound waves reflect back and forth between two adjacent interfaces before the next pulse is generated. This leads to the transducer falsely interpreting the waves coming from a deeper depth because it took longer for the wave to return. The extent of reverberation is affected by the beam power and sensitivity of the detector. Reverberation commonly occurs between highly reflective interfaces demonstrating a high acoustic impedance mismatch, such as metallic objects, calcified tissues, or an air pocket. The artifact manifests as multiple equally spaced echoes in direct line with the transducer (Figure 7.36).

Comet tail artifact is a type of reverberation artifact, but demonstrating a triangular or conical shape. It occurs when two highly reflective surfaces are in close proximity. Because the generated echoes are closely spaced, the transducer is unable to

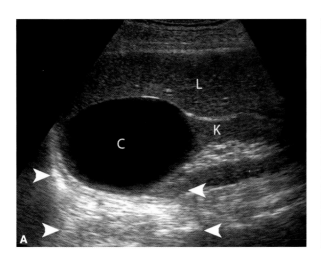

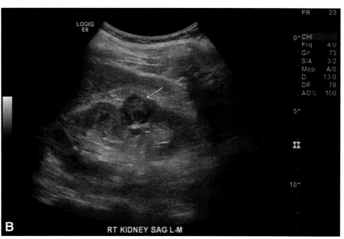

FIG. 7.34 • A. Acoustic enhancement (labeled E) posterior to an anechoic simple renal cyst (C). B. For comparison, a solid renal mass does not show posterior enhancement. Reprinted with permission from Daffner RH, Hartman M. *Clinical Radiology*. 4th ed. Philadelphia, PA: Lippincott Williams & Wilkins, A Wolters Kluwer business; 2013. K, kidney; L, liver.

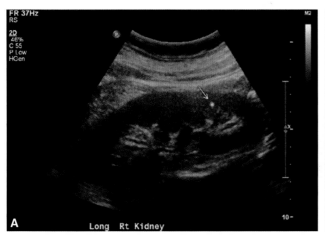

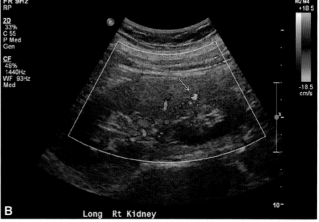

FIG. 7.35 • A renal calculus on conventional grayscale imaging appears a small echogenic focus (A) and demonstrates twinkle artifact when using color Doppler imaging (B).

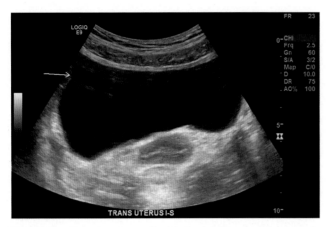

FIG. 7.36 ● Reverberation artifact in the bladder resulting from the skin-transducer interface during the transabdominal portion of a pelvic ultrasound exam.

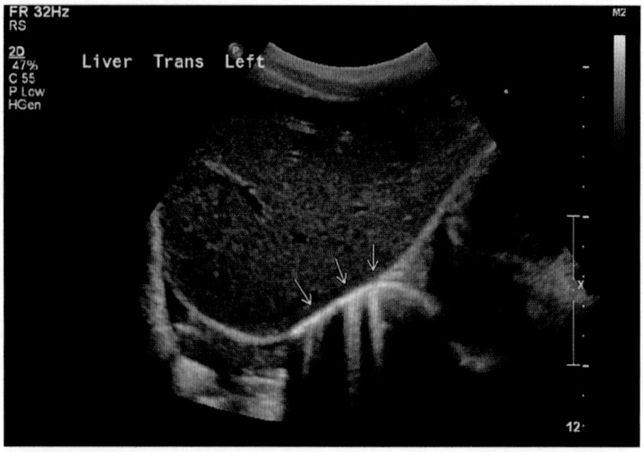

FIG. 7.38 ● Ring-down artifact extending posterior to the right hemidiaphragm.

resolve the individual signals. Furthermore, the delayed echoes may have lower amplitude due to attenuation, which is displayed as decreased echo width. Comet tail artifact occurs with metal objects (eg, surgical clips, needles, and foreign bodies), calcifications (eg, nephrolithiasis), granulomas, and cholesterolosis of the gallbladder wall (Figure 7.37).

Once classified as a variant of the comet tail artifact because of the similarity in appearance, ring-down artifact is now considered a separate entity on account of having different mechanisms. The theory of ring-down artifact is that ultrasound energy transmitted through air bubbles causes resonant vibration within the trapped liquid between the bubbles. This leads to a continuous sound wave, which is transmitted back to the transducer. The result is displayed as a line or series of parallel bands behind the gas collection. Ring-down artifact results from physiologic and normal anatomic effects, such as along the diaphragmatic surface (Figure 7.38), fluid and gas within bowel, or pathologic processes, such as abdominal abscesses and emphysematous cholecystitis.

The mirror image artifact occurs at highly reflective interfaces with large differences in acoustic impedance. Multiple ultrasound refractions and reflections at the interface return to the transducer with a delay. These delays cause the anatomy to be falsely interpreted as deeper along the beam position than their true

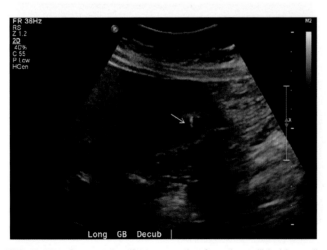

FIG. 7.37 ● Comet tail artifact emanating from the gallbladder wall, representing adenomyomatosis (hyperplastic cholecystosis).

position. One common example involves the liver and diaphragm interface. Echoes generated from a liver mass reflect back to the diaphragm, which produces a very strong echo. The echo then travels back to the mass, thus creating a second echo, which repeats the process of the first echo. These echoes then get reflected back to the transducer from the diaphragm. Ultimately, the second set of echoes from the mass to the transducer creates a mirror image of the mass, which is displayed on the opposite side of the diaphragm. Figure 7.39 demonstrates a clinical example of mirror image artifact.

Beam width artifact relates to the shape of the ultrasound beam as it leaves the transducer. The width of the beam is nearly equal to that of the transducer upon exiting, but narrows as it approaches the focal zone. The ultrasound beam widens distal to this point, potentially to a greater width than the transducer. A highly reflective surface located within the widened beam and outside the margin of the transducer can generate echoes that are detected by the transducer. Classic examples of beam width artifact include imaging of structures that should be anechoic (eg, urinary bladder), but demonstrate intraluminal peripheral echoes. The sonographer can reduce these echoes by moving the transducer and the focal zone closer to the region of interest.

Side lobes and grating globes are low-energy ultrasound beams that are emitted off-axis from the main beam. Side lobes arise from radial expansion and contraction of the piezoelectric crystals (Figure 7.40). The number of side lobes emitted is relatively high during continuous mode operation, in which the transducer has a narrow frequency bandwidth (high Q). The emission of side lobes is reduced in pulse mode operation, in which an ultrasound beam with low Q generates a spectrum of acoustic wavelengths. Side lobe emissions are also reduced with small individual transducer element widths of less than half the wavelength. Grating lobes are beams of low energy emitted much more off-axis than are side lobes. They occur as a result of the noncontinuous transducer surface of the individual elements.

Speed displacement artifacts are caused by variability in the speed of sound of different tissues. These manifest on grayscale imaging as a focal area of discontinuity and displacement of an echo deeper than its actual position. The image processor makes two assumptions in regard to the ultrasound beam. Firstly, it assumes the ultrasound beam propagates with a stable velocity of 1540 m/s. Secondly, it assumes that the round-trip length time of an echo is solely related to the distance it travels. Echoes returning

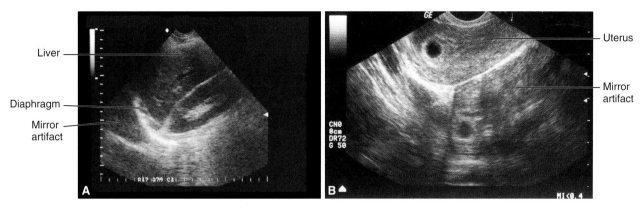

FIG. 7.39 ● **Mirror image artifact may arise between an organ and a strong reflector nearby; multiple echoes result in the display of a mirror image of the organ.** A: liver parenchyma appears on both sides of the diaphragm due to mirror artifacts; B: Identical images of the uterus side by side come from mirror artifacts. Reprinted with permission from Cosby KS, Kendall JL. *Practical Guide to Emergency Ultrasound.* 2nd ed. Philadelphia, PA: Lippincott Williams & Wilkins, A Wolters Kluwer business; 2013.

from tissues with velocities of sound significantly lower than 1540 m/s will appear discontinuous and deep (Figure 7.41).

Sonographers perform quality assurance on the ultrasound equipment in real time during scanning. However, there are certain objective measurements and protocols in place that must be performed on a periodic basis. For instance, phantoms mimicking the acoustic characteristics of a range of tissues are required to test the ultrasound system. The phantoms should have uniform attenuation with a speed of sound representative of soft tissues and also contain embedded echogenic material. General-purpose quality assurance ultrasound phantoms contain multiple modules. The first module contains system resolution targets, vertical and horizontal distance accuracy targets, grayscale targets, dead zone depth, and low-scatter targets. The filling gel within the phantom typically provides high attenuation in the range of 0.5 to 0.7 (dB/cm)/MHz. Low-contrast agents are placed within a scatter matrix to closely replicate background tissue. Axial and lateral

spatial resolution, horizontal and vertical distance measurements, and dead zone depth are tested by placing small, high-contrast reflecting agents at known depths. The second module is composed of small-diameter (2-4 mm), low-contrast, uniformly spaced spheres, which allow for the measurement of elevation resolution variation with depth. The final module contains uniformly distributed scattering material, which tests image uniformity and penetration depth.

One module is typically used to evaluate spatial resolution, contrast resolution, and distance. Axial resolution should be consistent with depth and improve at higher operational frequencies. Lateral resolution is evaluated by assessing the lateral distance of targets as a function of two components, depth and transmit focus. Grayscale objects that have attenuation higher and lower than that of tissue mimicking gel are used to assess contrast resolution. In an optimum system, contrast resolution will improve as transmit power is increased. The accuracy of horizontal and vertical

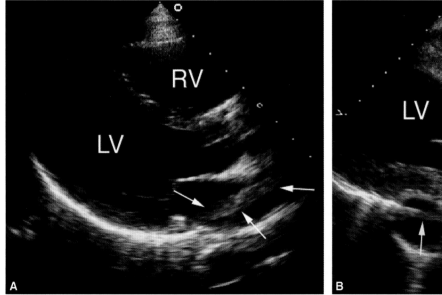
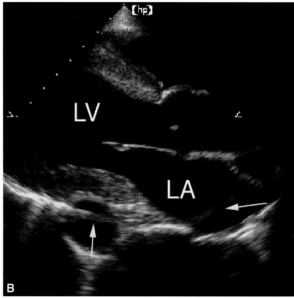

FIG. 7.40 ● **Side lobe emissions can cause anatomy outside of the main beam to be mapped into the main beam.** Two echocardiographic examples of side lobe artifacts are shown here: (A) the mass within the left atrium is actually a side lobe artifact produced by strong echoes from the posterior mitral annulus and the atrioventricular groove; and (B) the linear artifact within the descending aorta is also a side lobe artifact created by echoes from the pericardium. Reprinted with permission from Feigenbaum H, Armstrong WF, Ryan T. *Feigenbaum's Echocardiography.* 6th ed. Philadelphia, PA: Lippincott Williams & Wilkins, A Wolters Kluwer business; 2004.

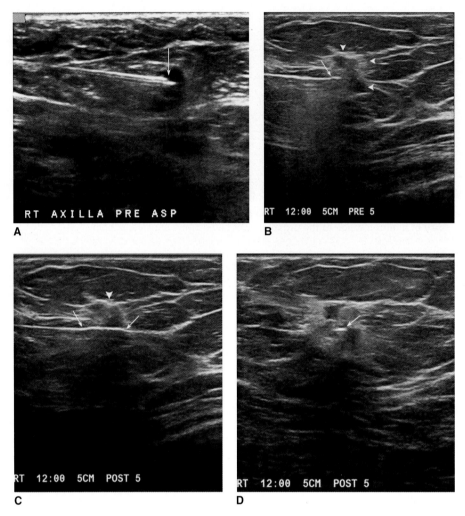

FIG. 7.41 ● **Variation of the speed of ultrasound through different tissues may lead to artifacts, as demonstrated on three of the four images shown here from ultrasound guided breast biopsy.** A: the tip of the needle appears broken (arrow; also known as Bayonet sign) because it is placed in a fluid filled structure. B: the tip of the needle appears bent as it is in the echogenic rim surrounded by a vertically oriented irregular mass (arrowheads). C: a portion of the needle that is through the lesion gives the "bent" appearance. D: this is just an orthogonal view obtained to confirm that the needle is through the center of the mass. Reprinted with permission from Cardenosa G. *Breast Imaging Companion.* 4th ed. Philadelphia, PA: Wolters Kluwer; 2017.

measurements is evaluated using small objects of high contrast. Targets that reside in the axial beam direction (vertical targets) are to have high precision and accuracy. A sphere module is used to assess elevational resolution and partial volume effects. The effects of slice-thickness differences at varying degrees of depth are manifested on the ultrasound image of the spherical targets. Uniformity and penetration depth are measured with a dedicated module. It is expected that an optimally adjusted ultrasound system will display a uniform response up to the penetration depth capabilities of a transducer array. Lower depths of penetration are reached with higher operational frequencies.

Transducers are evaluated during the initial testing of a new ultrasound unit. To determine the maximum depth capability of the transducer, the deepest low-contrast scatterers are identified within a uniform phantom. Multiple parameters dictate how deep the transducer can penetrate, including the type of the transducer and the operating frequency. The depth should be measured and compared with technical standards.

Continuous QC is not only suggested but, effective June 1, 2014, the American College of Radiology (ACR) also began

requiring documentation for ultrasound and breast ultrasound accreditation processes. Per the ACR's website, QC procedures should ideally be performed with the guidance and supervision of a medical physicist. The physicist must be qualified and his or her assistants should be approved in the testing techniques, functions and limitations of the equipment, and the importance of the tests and testing results. If a qualified medical physicist is unable to perform the required procedures, then an appropriately trained individual with experience in ultrasound imaging can be employed with these tasks. Additional required QC measures include acceptance testing and an annual survey. Acceptance testing refers to the initial performance review of new ultrasound equipment before its use in clinical practice. Testing procedures that should be performed every year as part of an annual survey include physical and mechanical inspection, image uniformity and artifact survey, geometric accuracy, ultrasound scanner electronic image display performance, and evaluation of the QC program. Primary interpretation display performance is only required if this is located at the facility where ultrasound examinations are being performed. It is recommended that all ultrasound scanners and transducers being used in routine clinical care be tested quarterly, although the requirement is for at least semiannual testing. Routine QC tests to be done on at least a semiannual basis include physical and mechanical inspection, image uniformity and artifact survey, geometric accuracy, and ultrasound scanner electronic image display performance. In addition, preventative maintenance must be performed by a qualified service engineer routinely, with strict documentation of service records.

An important aspect of quality assurance is the detection of nonfunctioning elements within a transducer probe because these can severely degrade the accuracy of a clinical examination. It has been shown that up to 13% of transducers may contain at least one nonfunctioning or very poorly functioning element. A simple (and cost-effective) method of assessing image uniformity of a transducer is a tool commonly referred to as the "paperclip" test, which was introduced by Goldstein et al.[1] The test was originally designed to directly measure the transmit/receive aperture, an important image acquisition parameter that provides information regarding nonfunctioning elements. Upon its introduction, the test was shown to have several important applications, such as the assessment of the transmit/receive aperture range as image depth varies, evaluation of quality of the equipment in different focusing schemes, and the discovery of nonfunctioning elements of array transducers. The test can be applied to curved array transducers in addition to linear transducers because of the similarities between the two. Phased-array transducers are poorly evaluated with this technique because the reverberation pattern emanating from the paperclip encompasses the entire field of view.

Transducer elements can become nonfunctioning because of several reasons, including poor connections, cable failures, or element damage, all of which can lead to streaking of the image. Disabled elements can be especially problematic in Doppler ultrasound applications, in part because the technical issue may not be readily apparent to the user. Doppler ultrasound techniques are very common in medical practice today and thus it is imperative that measurements be accurate. Relying on these measurements necessitates both accurate acquisition and processing of the flow data. Vachutka et al[2] demonstrated that the overall power of a Doppler system and the detection of maximum and average velocities deteriorate as the number of nonfunctioning elements increases. The presence of three consecutive disabled elements has a relatively small effect on the detection of maximum and average velocities. However, this leads to a clinically significant decrease in the sensitivity and power of the Doppler system, resulting in a degraded examination. Furthermore, if the number of nonfunctioning elements is four or greater, the Doppler measurements typically cannot be regarded as accurate. Different probe types have different sensitivities to element failures. The variability in measured parameters is greatest with convex array probes, whereas linear array probes tend to be more resistant to dead elements, which likely relates to the differences in element arrangements between linear and curvilinear array probes. Color flow Doppler is also significantly affected by nonfunctioning transducer elements. The negative effect primarily involves loss of the total signal amplitude, which can prevent the detection of flow data from small vessels or vessels with slow flow.

Another method of testing Doppler measurements involves the use of a QC phantom, which can evaluate flow and velocity. Phantoms used for this purpose contain tubes embedded with tissue mimicking materials at differing depths. As a fluid mimicking the characteristics of blood is passed through the tubes, pumps calibrated with a known velocity are used to evaluate the accuracy of the Doppler velocity measurements. Parameters that can be tested with this method include the accuracy of the velocity measurements, maximum penetration depth that a flow waveform can be perceived, volume flow, and the alignment of the sample volume with the duplex B-mode image. Sensitivity and alignment of the color flow image with the B-mode grayscale image are evaluated in color flow systems.

ACOUSTIC POWER AND BIOEFFECTS

Acoustic power refers to the production, absorption, and flow of energy. The unit of power is the watt (W), which equals 1 J/s. Intensity is the rate of sound energy flowing through a unit area and is typically expressed as watts or milliwatts per square centimeter (W/cm^2 or mW/cm^2). Power depends strongly on the operational components of the system, which includes PRF, transducer frequency, transmit power, and operation mode. Biologic effects (bioeffects) relate to the heating of tissues from high-intensity ultrasound energy. High-power ultrasound beams can lead to cavitation, which is the generation and collapse of microscopic bubbles. Structures that naturally contain gas, such as the lungs and bowel, are most susceptible to the effects of cavitation. The wavelength of the ultrasound alters the chance of cavitation. Ultrasound with short wavelengths, and thus higher frequencies, do not provide enough time for significant bubble growth. The appearance and extent of cavitation varies widely and ranges from subtle to readily observable to unpredictable and violent. Cavitation may be stable or transient. Stable cavitation, which occurs at relatively low ultrasound intensities, describes persistent pulsation of microbubbles in the tissue. Transient cavitation, which occurs at higher intensities, describes bubbles that expand to a radius at least 2 times their original size before collapsing to a speed approaching that of sound. Transient cavitation is generally considered to be the primary source of chemical and mechanical effects of ultrasound. Each bubble that collapses can reach temperatures of several thousand degrees and pressures greater than 1000 atm instantaneously. Following collapse, the bubbles may disintegrate, dissolve, or rebound. This may lead to the formation of highly reactive radicals, such as hydroxide and hydrogen peroxide, which can chemically damage important biologic materials, including DNA. Ultrasound contrast agents substantially increase the chance of cavitation by its reduction in the intensity threshold.

Cavitation is of particular concern in harmonic imaging because of the high peak pressures used. The risk of tissue heating is increased when using spectral Doppler because the transducer stays in one place. Acoustic intensity levels are maintained below established bioeffect thresholds in clinical diagnostic imaging, keeping in mind the ALARA (as low as reasonably achievable) principle.

Acoustic power and intensity of pulsed ultrasound

The amplitude of the emitted pulse is affected by the transmit power. Stronger echoes are generated from more powerful pulses. High transmit power yields multiple advantages, including an improved signal-to-noise ratio and an increased maximum

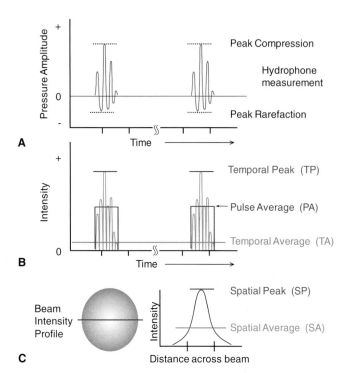

A. A hydrophone measures pressure amplitude variations, which include peak compression and peak rarefaction as a function of time. **B.** Temporal intensity variations have a wide range. Pulse average intensity represents the average intensity over the pulse duration. **C.** Spatial intensity variations are illustrated by the spatial peak and spatial average values measured over the beam profile. Reprinted with permission from Bushberg JT, Seibert JA, Leidholdt EM, Boone JM. *Essential Physics of Medical Imaging*. 3rd ed. Philadelphia, PA: Lippincott Williams & Wilkins, a Wolters Kluwer business; 2012.

penetration depth. However, increased power also leads to increased risks of bioeffects. A hydrophone is a device containing small piezoelectric elements coupled to external conductors and is used to measure the pressure amplitude of an ultrasound beam. The hydrophone generates voltage proportional to the pressure amplitude of the ultrasound beam. This allows for the determination of several parameters, including pulse duration, PRP, and peak compression and rarefaction amplitude (Figure 7.42). Acoustic intensity can be calculated from the measured pressure amplitudes if the acoustic impedance of the tissue medium is known.

Intensity measures of pulsed ultrasound

During pulse mode operation, the intensity of the ultrasound beam at the time the pulse passes through the tissues (instantaneous intensity) is very high. However, the pulse lasts for such a short amount of time (1 μs or less) that the tissues are not greatly affected. During the remainder of the pulse repetition time, the intensity of the beam is negligible. The temporal peak (I_{TP}) is the point at which the ultrasound beam intensity is the highest. The temporal average (I_{TA}) is the average intensity over the PRP in units of time. The pulse average (I_{PA}) is the intensity averaged over the pulse duration. The spatial peak (I_{SP}) is the greatest intensity of the beam spatially. The spatial average (I_{SA}) is the intensity averaged over the beam area (see Figure 7.42). The spatial average-temporal average intensity (I_{SATA}) is obtained by averaging the power within the beam over at least one PRP and dividing by the beam area. Several additional important measures for

pulsed ultrasound intensity can be derived from I_{SATA}. The spatial average-pulse average intensity (I_{SAPA}) is calculated by dividing I_{SATA} by the duty cycle ($I_{SAPA} - I_{SATA}$/duty cycle). The spatial peak-temporal average intensity (I_{SPTA}), which is a useful measure of thermal ultrasound effects, is calculated as follows: $I_{SPTA} = I_{SATA}$ (I_{SP}/I_{SA}). The spatial peak-pulse average intensity (I_{SPPA}), which indicates potential mechanical bioeffects and cavitation, is calculated as follows: $I_{SPPA} = I_{SATA}$ (I_{SP}/I_{SA})/duty cycle. The two most important values are the spatial peak-pulse average intensity (I_{SPPA}) and the spatial peak-temporal average intensity (I_{SPTA}), both of which are required by the United States Food and Drug Administration (FDA) for instrumentation certification. The I_{SPTA} is usually kept under 100 mW/cm^2 for diagnostic ultrasound imaging, although levels above 1000 mW/cm^2 are used for certain Doppler applications. The relative values for acoustic ultrasound intensity output are as follows: $I_{SPPA} > I_{SPTA} > I_{SAPA} > I_{SATA}$.

MI and TI are parameters that estimate the risk of bioeffects. These two indices are displayed on the monitor for the sonographer to view during an ultrasound examination to quantitatively estimate the amount of power being deposited in the patient. These were first required to be displayed in 1993 in the United States. for FDA-approved "Track 3" machines. MI is a value that estimates the probability of cavitation and is proportional to the peak pressure values of the ultrasound beam. As mentioned earlier, cavitation is the generation of microscopic bubbles, which occurs from the extraction of dissolved gases within a tissue medium. The MI is directly proportional to the peak negative (rarefactional) pressure and is inversely proportional to the square root of the ultrasound frequency (in MHz).

$$MI \propto \text{peak negative pressure}$$
$$MI \propto 1/\sqrt{f}$$

In general, if the MI is greater than 0.5, a thorough risk versus benefit analysis should be performed for the scan to proceed.

Tissue heating occurs because of the absorption of ultrasound energy. The amount of heat generated from energy absorption is dependent on several factors, including the intensity of the ultrasound beam, the duration of exposure, and the absorption characteristics of the tissue medium, which takes into account diffusion of heat within the tissues and the rate of heat removal via blood flow. The majority of the total temperature change typically occurs within the first minute of exposure. Stationary ultrasound beams center the beam energy into a smaller volume. The most effective way to mitigate potential thermal injury is to minimize exposure time. The TI refers to the potential tissue temperature rise due to heating effects of ultrasound. The ultrasound system estimates the TI with algorithms, which take into account the acoustic power of the transducer, the ultrasound frequency, and the beam area. TI is a ratio of the acoustic power generated by the transducer over the power needed to raise the temperature of the tissue by 1°C. For example, a TI of 3 indicates a potential tissue temperature rise of 3°C if the transducer is stationary. The TI is associated with the spatial peak-temporal average intensity (I_{SPTA}). More specific TIs are displayed by some scanners for that of soft tissues (TIS), bone (TIB), and cranial bone (TIC). This proves useful because heat can build up relatively quickly at bone-soft tissue interfaces, especially in obstetrics during scanning of late-term pregnancies. The two best markers of heat deposition to the patient during an ultrasound examination are spatial peak-temporal average intensity (I_{SPTA}) and the TI. The amount of heat deposited depends on the average intensity of the ultrasound beam within the focal zone and the absorption coefficient of the tissue medium. Structures with a high absorption coefficient (eg, bone) attenuate more of the ultrasound energy than the adjacent soft tissue, which leads to a large amount of heat deposition. The temperature of tissues typically only rises about 1°C to 2°C in standard diagnostic ultrasound imaging, which is far below what is considered potentially harmful.

Biologic effects are such an important topic that the American Institute of Ultrasound in Medicine (AIUM) has a Bioeffects Committee, which specifically reviews patient safety in ultrasound imaging. The TI has several strengths in the monitoring of potential bioeffects. Firstly, it serves as an indicator to the sonographer of the relative risk of thermal effects on tissues, particularly when changing operating conditions. Secondly, its convenient display on the ultrasound monitor makes it an easily accessible, easily understandable parameter during real-time scanning. Finally, it has generally been accepted by international standards and regulatory bodies as a useful parameter of thermal risk. However, several criticisms and shortcomings of the TI formulations have led to a recent review by the AIUM Output Standards Subcommittee. Specifically, it was believed that the TI did not adequately provide information to determine the full risk posed to the patient. This was suggested because TI did not provide an accurate estimate of the absolute risk of the thermal risk. Additional weaknesses of the previous TI formulations included inconsistencies when using different transmit apertures and the difficulty in implementing ALARA when changing the focusing. The subcommittee addressed multiple proposed changes and ultimately recommended that three key changes be made. The first is to refine the break point distance, which had been previously utilized in TIS formulations to prevent measurements in the ultrasonic near field. The proposed change would allow for measurements to be made in the region of maximum intensity, which previously may have been excluded. The second recommendation is to redefine the source power terms used in TIS formulations, which would eliminate the inconsistencies that occurred when using different sized apertures. The third recommendation is to define "below-surface" TIS and TIB formulations for scanned modes. This would improve the accuracy of the relative risk when multiple scanned modes are operating simultaneously. Ultimately, the AIUM concludes that ultrasound does not cause significant biologic effects unless exposure duration is prolonged.

References

1. Goldstein A, Ranney D, McLeary RD. Linear array test tool. *J Ultrasound Med*. 1989;8:385–397.
2. Vachutka J, Dolezal L, Kollman C, Klein J. The effect of dead elements on the accuracy of Doppler ultrasound measurements. *Ultrason Imaging*. 2014;36(1):18–34.

Suggested Reading

ACR. Ultrasound and breast ultrasound accreditation program requirements. September 2013. https://www.acr.org/Quality-Safety/eNews/Issue-03-September-2013/New-Quality-Control-Requirements. Accessed May 6, 2019.

AIUM. *Performance criteria and measurements for Doppler ultrasound devices*. American Institute of Ultrasound in Medicine. Laurel, Maryland; 2002.

Bigelow T, Church C, Sandstrom K, et al. The thermal index: its strengths, weaknesses, and proposed improvements. *J Ultrasound Med*. 2011;30(5):714–734.

Bushberg JT, Seibert JA, Leidholdt EM, Boone JM. *The Essential Physics of Medical Imaging*. 3rd ed. Philadelphia, PA: Lippincott Williams & Wilkins, a Wolters Kluwer business; 2012.

Caronti A, Caliano G, Carotenuto, et al. Capacitive micromachined ultrasonic transducer (CMUT) arrays for medical imaging. *Microelectron J*. 2005;37:770–777.

Deane C, Lees C. Doppler obstetric ultrasound: a graphical display of temporal changes in safety indices. *Ultrasound Obstet Gynecol*. 2000;15:418–423.

Dillman J, Kappil M, Weadock W, et al. Sonographic twinkling artifact for renal calculus detection: correlation with CT. *Radiology*. 2011;259(3):911–916.

Doody C, Porter H, Duck F, Humphrey VF. In vitro heating of human fetal vertebra by pulsed diagnostic ultrasound. *Ultrasound Med Biol*. 1999;25:1289–1294.

Dudley N, Woolley D. A simple uniformity test for ultrasound phased arrays. *Phys Med*. 2016;32(9):1162–1166.

Feldman M, Katyal S, Blackwood M. US artifacts. *Radiographics*. 2009;29:1179–1189.

Garrido S, Duran J, Melendez A. Ring-down versus comet tail: two artifacts uncovered. *Eur Soc Radiol*. 2013;1–17. doi:10.1594/ecr2013/C-2288.

Huda W. *Review of Radiologic Physics*. 3rd ed. Philadelphia, PA: Lippincott Williams & Wilkins, a Wolters Kluwer business; 2010.

IPEM. Quality assurance of ultrasound imaging systems. New York, United Kingdom: Institute of Physics and Engineering in Medicine; 2010. Report number 102.

Khuri-Yakub B, Oralkan O. Capacitive micromachined ultrasonic transducers for medical imaging and therapy. *J Micromech Microeng*. 2011;21(5):54004–54014.

Kofler JM Jr. Quality assurance of ultrasound imagers: procedures, expectations, and philosophies. *AAPM 43rd Annual Meeting*, Salt Lake City, UT. 2001.

Kupnik M, Ergun A, Huang Y, Khuri-Yakub B. Extended insulation layer structure for CMUTs. *Proc IEEE Ultrason Symp*. 2007;511–514.

Martensson M, Olsson M, Segall B, Fraser AG, Winter R, Brodin LA. High incidence of defective ultrasound transducers in use in routine clinical practice. *Eur J Echocardiogr*. 2009;10:389–394.

Oralkan O, Ergun A, Johnson J, et al. Capacitive micromachined ultrasound transducers: next-generation arrays for acoustic imaging? *IEEE Trans Ultrason Ferroelectr Freq Control*. 2002;49(11):1596–1610.

Thijssen J, Weijers G, de Korte C. Objective performance testing and quality assurance of medical ultrasound equipment. *Ultrasound Med Biol*. 2007;33(3):460–471.

CHAPTER SELF-ASSESSMENT QUESTIONS

1. Which of the following is NOT true regarding spatial resolution of ultrasound images?
   A. Axial resolution worsens with an increase in the number of cycles emitted per pulse by the transducer
   B. Axial resolution worsens with an increase in the frequency of the ultrasound wave
   C. Lateral resolution varies with tissue depth
   D. Lateral resolution at different depths may be kept constant by using multiple transmit/receive focal zones

2. Which of the following leads to lower frame rate of real-time ultrasound images?
   A. Decreased depth of the field of view
   B. Decreased angle of the field of view
   C. Decreased number of lines across the field of view
   D. The use of more transmit/receive focal zones

3. Which of the following increases the maximum blood velocity that can be measured by pulsed Doppler ultrasound and therefore reduces aliasing artifacts?

A. Higher pulse repetition frequency (PRF)

B. Lower frequency of the ultrasound beam

C. Higher frequency of the ultrasound beam

D. Larger angle between the ultrasound beam and the axis of the blood vessel

Answers to Chapter Self-Assessment Questions

1. B   Axial resolution is determined by the spatial pulse length (SPL), which is equal to the product of the number of cycles emitted per pulse by the transducer and the wavelength. Increased frequency of the ultrasound wave leads to decreased wavelength and therefore poorer axial resolution.

2. D   The frame rate is inversely proportional to the time spent acquiring each frame. Decreases in the depth and the angle of the field of view and the number of lines across the field of view all result in shorter acquisition per frame. More focal zones lead to longer acquisition per frame and therefore lower frame rate.

3. C   The maximum blood velocity that can be measured by pulsed Doppler ultrasound follows , where is the speed of ultrasound in tissue, is the frequency of the ultrasound beam, PRF is the pulse repetition frequency, and is the angle between the ultrasound beam and the axis of the blood vessel. Higher frequency of the ultrasound beam actually results in an decrease in the maximum blood velocity that can be accurately measured by pulsed Doppler ultrasound.

Nuclear Medicine: Fundamentals

8

Bruce Mahoney, MD and Vineeth Yeluru, MBBS

LEARNING OBJECTIVES

1. Define the terms *radioactivity*, *radionuclide*, and *radiopharmaceutical*.
2. Explain the structural difference between radioisotopes and stable isotopes.
3. Define the terms *activity*, *radioactive decay*, and *physical half-life*.
4. Name five modes of radioactive decay. For each mode, name the nuclear deficiency of the parent, the common emissions, and an example radionuclide.
5. Describe the function of a radionuclide reactor. State the most common nuclear deficiency of reactor-produced radionuclides and their decay mode. Provide examples of two reactor-produced radionuclides.
6. Describe the function of a cyclotron. State the most common nuclear deficiency of cyclotron-produced radionuclides and their decay mode. Provide examples of two cyclotron-produced radionuclides.
7. Describe the function of a radionuclide generator. Define the terms transient equilibrium and secular equilibrium. Provide examples of two generator-produced radionuclides.
8. Name five mechanisms of radiopharmaceutical localization and provide an example radiopharmaceutical for each.
9. Describe the effects of half-life and gamma photon energy on patient radiation dose.
10. Define the terms *deterministic effect* and *stochastic effect*.
11. Describe a scenario leading to a medical event, and the reporting requirements in a Non-Agreement State.

INTRODUCTION

Nuclear medicine is a medical specialty that employs radioisotopes in the diagnosis and treatment of disease. A *radioisotope* is an unstable atomic species that can undergo nuclear transformation, releasing radiation. The term *radionuclide* refers specifically to the unstable atomic nucleus, although is often used interchangeably with radioisotope. Some of the forms of radiation released can be used for imaging, quantitative measurement, and radiation therapy. A *radiopharmaceutical* is a radioisotope or radiolabeled molecule able to localize within the body. Refer to Chapter 1 for a review of atomic structure and terminology.

Atomic nuclei are composed of protons and neutrons held together by the strong nuclear force. The repulsive force of the positively charged protons must be overcome by the strong force for nuclei to be stable. This stability occurs when there is an ideal ratio of neutrons and protons (the N/Z ratio) (Figure 8.1). This ideal ratio is approximately 1:1 for smaller nuclides, and approaches 1.5:1 for heavy nuclides. Nuclei with too many neutrons fall above the line and are termed proton deficient. Those with too few neutrons, falling below the line, are said to be neutron deficient.

Both proton-deficient and neutron-deficient radionuclides can undergo nuclear transformation to bring their N/Z ratio toward greater stability. *Radioactivity* is the release of particles and photons by radionuclides during these nuclear transformations.

Unlike most other imaging modalities in medicine, nuclear medicine imaging generally focuses on depicting normal physiology and disturbances of function. Gamma rays and X-rays produced during nuclear transformation can be detected for image creation as well as for quantification. The resolutions of planar gamma camera imaging, single-photon emission computed tomography (SPECT) and positron emission tomography (PET) are lower than that of X-ray computed tomography (CT) and magnetic resonance imaging (MRI) by an order of magnitude or more (Figure 8.2). Radiopharmaceuticals localize to tissues or compartments on the basis of various mechanisms (see Section "Mechanisms of Radiopharmaceutical Localization" later), and therefore nuclear imaging does not illustrate the full spectrum of anatomy within a region of interest. This corresponding anatomic information can be provided by combining nuclear imaging data with anatomic imaging data, such as CT. Such *hybrid imaging* allows

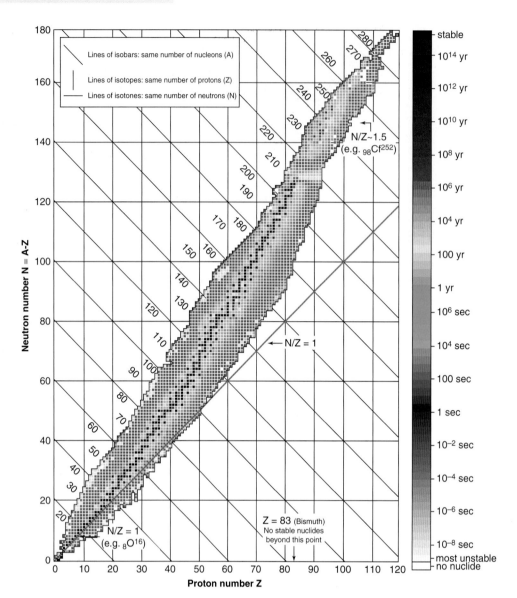

FIG. 8.1 ● **A plot of the nuclides where the number of protons (ie, atomic number or Z) and neutrons of each nuclide is shown on the x- and y-axes, respectively.** The stable nuclides form the so-called line of stability in which the neutron-to-proton ratio is approximately 1 for low Z nuclides and increases to approximately 1.5 for high Z nuclides. Note that all nuclides with $Z > 83$ (bismuth) are radioactive and that, in general, the further the radionuclide is from the line of stability, the more unstable it is and the shorter the half-life it has. Radionuclides to the left of the line of stability are neutron rich and are likely to undergo beta-minus decay, whereas radionuclides to the right of the line of stability are neutron poor and thus often decay by positron emission or electron capture. Extremely unstable radionuclides and those with high Z often decay by alpha particle emission. Reprinted with permission from Bushberg JT, Seibert JA, Leidholdt EM, Boone JM. *Essential Physics of Medical Imaging*. 3rd ed. Philadelphia, PA: Wolters Kluwer Health/Lippincott Williams & Wilkins; 2012.

for increased diagnostic accuracy of nuclear imaging. SPECT/CT, PET/CT, and PET/MRI are powerful hybrid imaging tools.

RADIOACTIVITY

Radioactive material (RAM) contains atoms undergoing radioactive decay. Each individual unstable nucleus has a likelihood of undergoing nuclear transformation in a given span of time that is based on its stability. Each decay event appears to be random

and unaffected by outside events. However, a sample containing a large number of unstable nuclei will appear to emit radiation continuously at a rate that declines steadily. This rate is known as the *activity* of the sample.

The radioactivity of a sample is proportional to the number of unstable nuclei present. Thus, a quantity of RAM may be expressed in terms of its activity A, which refers to the number of nuclear transformations per unit time. The International System of Units (SI) unit of activity is the bequerel (Bq), which is defined

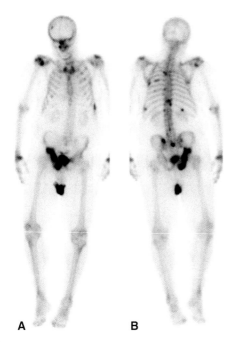

A   **B**

FIG. 8.2 ● (A) Anterior and (B) posterior views from a whole-body **99mTc** methylene diphosphonate (MDP) bone scan in a patient with prostate cancer. Focal areas of increased MDP uptake in the ribs, spine, sacrum, and pelvis are due to metastatic prostate cancer. Uptake in the wrists and right shoulder is related to arthritis. Excreted activity is present in the bladder and there is a small amount of contamination more inferiorly. A focus of uptake in the right skull corresponds with the site of a ventriculoperitoneal shunt.

as an activity of 1 disintegration per second (dps). The curie (Ci), named after radioactivity pioneers Pierre and Marie Curie, is the traditional unit of activity equal to 3.70×10^{10} dps. Thus,

$$1 \text{ Ci} = 3.7 \times 10^{10} \text{ Bq} = 37 \text{ GBq}$$

and

$$1 \text{ mCi} = 37 \text{ MBq}$$

Within the context of nuclear medicine, 1 Curie represents a large amount of radioactivity. The activity of most dosages of radiopharmaceuticals used in clinical nuclear medicine are measured in millicuries or microcuries (megabequerels). Despite the wide adoption of SI, traditional units such as the curie and millicurie are also still used in many countries, including in the United States.

Decay Constant and Physical Half-Life

The activity A of a sample of RAM is proportional to the number of available unstable nuclei in the sample, N. The decay constant λ relates activity with N

$$A = \lambda N$$

Ongoing nuclear disintegrations reduce the number of available unstable nuclei over time, with a corresponding decrease in activity A. A decreases over time as an exponential decay function known as the *fundamental decay equation*:

$$A_t = A_0 e^{-\lambda t}$$

where A_0 is the original activity and A_t is the activity at time t.

The length of time for the number of radioactive atoms (N) and the activity of the sample (A) to decrease by half is a constant known as the *physical half-life* $T_p\frac{1}{2}$. Physical half-life is inversely proportional to the decay constant

$$T_p\frac{1}{2} = 0.693/\lambda$$

λ and $T_p\frac{1}{2}$ are properties unique to each radionuclide.

Physical half-life is an intuitive and useful concept. It is more convenient than applying the fundamental decay equation for calculating or quickly estimating the remaining activity in a sample following the passage of time. With each half-life, the activity of a sample decreases by half. After n half-lives have elapsed, activity A is given by the equation

$$A = A_0/2^n$$

where A_0 is the original activity.
Examples:

1. ^{99m}Tc has a physical half-life of 6.02 hours. Approximately how much of a sample of ^{99m}Tc remains after 24 hours?
   - 24 hours represents almost four half-lives.
   - $A = A_0/2^{(4)} = A_0/16$.
   - Approximately 1/16th of the original activity remains after 24 hours.
2. If 20 mCi of ^{99m}Tc sestamibi is administered to a patient, how much activity remains after 24 hours, assuming no physiologic clearance?
   - 20 mCi/16 = 1.26 mCi
3. As a rule of thumb, a radioactive sample will decay to approximately 1/1000th its original activity after 10 half-lives ($2^{10} = 1024$). How long will it take a sample of ^{99m}Tc to decay to 1/1000th of its original activity?
   - For ^{99m}Tc, 10 half-lives is approximately 60 hours, or 2½ days.
4. At 8 PM on Friday evening, a 100 mCi vial of ^{99m}Tc pertechnetate is spilled on a carpeted surface in the nuclear medicine department, completely soaks in, and cannot be removed. How much activity remains when the first patient shows up at 8 AM Monday morning, 2½ days later? (Figure 8.3).
   - 100 mCi/1000 = 0.1 mCi = 100 µCi

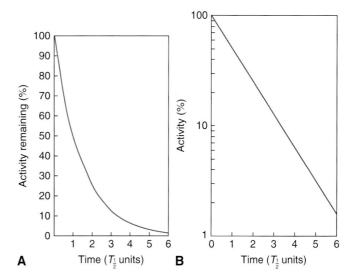

A   **B**

FIG. 8.3 ● **Percentage of initial activity as a function of time.** A. Plot on linear graph. B. Plot on semilogarithmic graph. Reprinted with permission from Bushberg JT, Seibert JA, Leidholdt EM, Boone JM. *Essential Physics of Medical Imaging*. 3rd ed. Philadelphia, PA: Wolters Kluwer Health/Lippincott Williams & Wilkins; 2012.

Table 8.1 **PHYSICAL HALF-LIFE ($T_p\frac{1}{2}$) AND DECAY CONSTANT (λ) FOR RADIONUCLIDES USED IN NUCLEAR MEDICINE**

Radionuclide	$T_p\frac{1}{2}$	λ
Rubidium-82 (^{82}Rb)	75 s	0.0092 s^{-1}
Fluorine-18 (^{18}F)	110 min	0.0063 min^{-1}
Technetium-99m (^{99m}Tc)	6.02 h	0.1151 h^{-1}
Iodine-123 (^{123}I)	13.27 h	0.0522 h^{-1}
Samarium-153 (^{153}Sm)	1.93 d	0.3591 d^{-1}
Yttrium-90 (^{90}Y)	2.69 d	0.2575 d^{-1}
Molybdenum-99 (^{99}Mo)	2.75 d	0.2522 d^{-1}
Indium-111 (^{111}In)	2.81 d	0.2466 d^{-1}
Thallium-201 (^{201}Tl)	3.04 d	0.2281 d^{-1}
Gallium-67 (^{67}Ga)	3.26 d	0.2126 d^{-1}
Xenon-133 (^{133}Xe)	5.24 d	0.1323 d^{-1}
Iodine-131 (^{131}I)	8.02 d	0.0864 d^{-1}
Phosphorus-32 (^{32}P)	14.26 d	0.0486 d^{-1}
Strontium-82 (^{82}Sr)	25.60 d	0.0271 d^{-1}
Chromium-51 (^{51}Cr)	27.70 d	0.0250 d^{-1}
Strontium-89 (^{89}Sr)	50.53 d	0.0137 d^{-1}
Iodine-125 (^{125}I)	59.41 d	0.0117 d^{-1}
Cobalt-57 (^{57}Co)	271.79 d	0.0025 d^{-1}

Reprinted with permission from Bushberg JT, Seibert JA, Leidholdt EM, Boone JM. *Essential Physics of Medical Imaging*. 3rd ed. Philadelphia, PA: Wolters Kluwer Health/Lippincott Williams & Wilkins; 2012.

The half-lives of most radionuclides used for clinical nuclear imaging are measured in hours. Rubidium-82 (Rb-82), used in myocardial perfusion PET imaging, has a relatively short half-life of 1 minute 15 seconds. To perform PET imaging with Rb-82, it is necessary to have an on-site strontium-82/rubidium-82 (Sr-82/Rb-82) generator. In contrast, fluorine-18 (F-18) has a half-life of nearly 2 hours, allowing for a central facility to produce doses and distribute them regionally. Reusable sources for determining gamma camera image uniformity employ Cobalt-57, which has a half-life of approximately 9 months (Table 8.1).

Modes of Decay

Unstable isotopes undergo radioactive decay by one or more of several mechanisms. The parent nuclide undergoes decay, producing one or more daughter species, which may be stable and/or radioactive (Table 8.2).

Isotopes which are proton deficient seek to increase their atomic number for greater stability. One example is phosphorus-32 (P-32). The stable isotope of phosphorus is phosphorus-31 (P-31), with 15 protons and 16 neutrons. Radioisotope P-32 has a higher atomic weight because of having an extra neutron compared with P-31 (high N/Z). This extra neutron results in its instability.

β^- decay

In beta-minus decay (β^- decay, negatron decay, beta emission), the nucleus emits a beta particle β^-, which is an electron, as well as an antineutrino $\bar{v}$, allowing a proton-deficient radioisotope to reduce its N/Z ratio.

$$^A_ZX \to {}^A_{Z+1}Y + \beta^- + \bar{v} + \text{energy}$$

The antineutrino is a very small uncharged particle that goes undetected by clinical nuclear imaging apparatus and has no significant effect on the patient. The effect of β^- decay is the conversion of a neutron to a proton, producing an element with increased atomic number Z and with no change in atomic mass number A (an isobaric transition). The emitted beta particle has a spectrum of energies up to a maximum energy. Many nuclear fission products are proton deficient and undergo β^- decay (Figure 8.4).

Beta particles demonstrate limited penetration of soft tissues and detector materials compared with gamma rays, and are not effectively detected by clinical nuclear medicine camera systems. Pure beta emitters are therefore not used for diagnostic imaging. However, some isotopes, including phosphorus-32 and yttrium-90 are employed as therapeutic agents in clinical nuclear medicine. Their in vivo distribution following radioisotope therapy can be demonstrated by imaging the bremsstrahlung radiation they generate (Figure 8.5).

Decay schemes illustrate radioactive decay graphically. The horizontal axis represents atomic number, and the vertical axis represents energy. The higher energy parent appears at the top of the diagram, and the lower energy daughter(s) appear to the left or right. For beta emitters such as P-32, the daughter has $Z + 1$ compared with the parent, and thus lies to the right (Figure 8.6).

Table 8.2 **RADIOACTIVE DECAY MODES FOR UNSTABLE NUCLEI CONTAINING PROTONS (Z), NEUTRONS (N), AND MASS NUMBER (A)**

Decay Mode	Daughter Nucleus Value			Comments
	Mass Number	Atomic Number	Neutron Number	
Isomeric transition	A	Z	N	Metastable if half-life is long
Beta minus (β^-)	A	$Z + 1$	$N - 1$	Nucleus emits electrons
Beta plus (β^+)	A	$Z - 1$	$N + 1$	Nucleus emits positrons
Electron capture	A	$Z - 1$	$N + 1$	Atoms emit characteristic X-rays[a]
Alpha decay	$A - 4$	$Z - 2$	$N - 2$	Occurs with heavy nuclei ($Z > 82$)

[a]When inner shell vacancies are filled.
Reprinted with permission from Huda W. *Review of Radiologic Physics*. 4th ed. Philadelphia, PA: Wolters Kluwer; 2016.

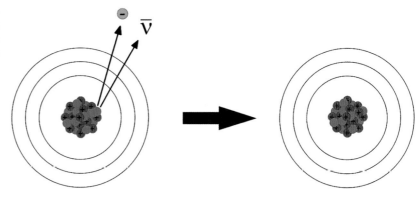

FIG. 8.4 ● **Beta decay.** A proton-deficient radionuclide emits a beta particle (−) and an antineutrino ($\bar{\nu}$). The result is a daughter nuclide with an increase in atomic number and no change in atomic mass number.

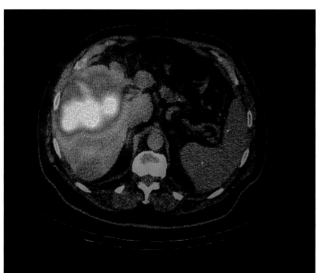

FIG. 8.5 ● Bremsstrahlung single-photon emission computed tomography/computed tomography following selective internal radiation therapy with Y-90 microspheres demonstrates the expected distribution of the microspheres within the liver, and no significant extrahepatic activity.

PHOSPHORUS-32
Beta-Minus Decay
$T_{1/2}$ = 14.3 days

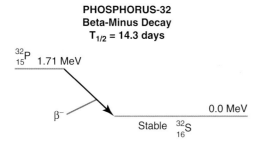

Decay Data Table

Radiation	Mean Number per Disintegration	Mean Energy per Particle (MeV)
Beta Minus	1.000	0.6948

FIG. 8.6 ● **Principal decay scheme of phosphorus-32.** Reprinted with permission from Bushberg JT, Seibert JA, Leidholdt EM, Boone JM. *Essential Physics of Medical Imaging.* 3rd ed. Philadelphia, PA: Wolters Kluwer Health/Lippincott Williams & Wilkins; 2012.

(β⁻, γ) emission

Following beta emission, the daughter nuclide may temporarily exist in one or more excited states, subsequently giving one or more gamma rays to reach the stable state.

$$^{A}_{Z}X \rightarrow ^{A}_{Z+1}Y^{\star} + \beta^{-} + \bar{\nu} + \text{energy}$$

$$^{A}_{Z+1}Y^{\star} \rightarrow ^{A}_{Z+1}Y + \gamma$$

The total energy of the beta particle, neutrino, and gamma ray is equal to the transition energy for the reaction. There may be many different possible combinations of energies given off during beta decay of a radioisotope (Figure 8.7).

The gamma ray from (β⁻, γ) emission may be imaged by nuclear medicine gamma cameras. For example, this may be useful to demonstrate treated lesions following therapy with (β⁻, γ) emitter I-131 for thyroid cancer (Figure 8.8). However, owing to the radiation dose imparted by the beta particle, (β⁻, γ) emitters are not routinely used for clinical nuclear imaging.

β⁻ decay (positron emission)

Neutron-deficient isotopes may undergo *positron emission* (beta-plus decay). For example, positron emitter carbon-11 (^{11}C) has a lower atomic mass than does the common, stable isotope, carbon-12 (^{12}C). This difference is due to the presence of six neutrons on the ^{12}C nucleus, but only five neutrons in the ^{11}C nucleus. This neutron deficiency is responsible for the instability of ^{11}C.

In positron emission, a proton is effectively converted to a neutron, positron β⁺, and neutrino ν, with concomitant decrease in atomic number Z and no change in atomic mass number A (an isobaric transition).

$$^{A}_{Z}X \rightarrow ^{A}_{Z-1}Y + \beta^{+} + \nu + \text{energy}$$

The positron is the antiparticle of the electron. It has unit positive charge, a mass identical to that of the electron, and a variable amount of kinetic energy. The positron travels some distance from the site of its generation as it loses kinetic energy, and the distance is generally greater for more energetic positrons. The emitted positron eventually loses sufficient kinetic energy that it is able to interact with an electron, with which it is mutually attracted. Both particles convert all of their rest mass to energy, which is released in the form of two 511 keV photons emitted approximately 180° apart. (By the law of conservation of momentum, the photon pair will conserve the momentum of the positron-electron pair, and therefore the two photons' paths will be slightly <180° apart if the positron is not completely at rest at the beginning of the interaction.) This event is known as *annihilation* (see Figure 8.9).

The 1.022 MeV energy released in annihilation is the minimum transition energy necessary for positron emission to occur.

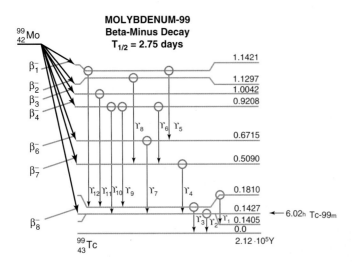

MOLYBDENUM-99
Beta-Minus Decay
$T_{1/2}$ = 2.75 days

FIG. 8.7 ● **Principal decay scheme of Mo-99.** The many possible radiation decay products are listed on the accompanying decay data table.

Decay Data Table

Radiation		Mean Number per Disintegration	Mean Energy per Particle (MeV)	Radiation		Mean Number per Disintegration	Mean Energy per Particle (MeV)
Beta Minus	1	0.0010	0.0658	Gamma	4	0.0119	0.3664
Beta Minus	3	0.0014	0.1112	Gamma	5	0.0001	0.4706
Beta Minus	4	0.1640	0.1331	Gamma	6	0.0002	0.4115
Beta Minus	6	0.0004	0.2541	Gamma	7	0.0006	0.5288
Beta Minus	7	0.0114	0.2897	Gamma	8	0.0002	0.6207
Beta Minus	8	0.8220	0.4428	Gamma	9	0.1367	0.7397
Gamma	1	0.0105	0.0406	K Int Con Elect		0.0002	0.7186
K Int Con Elect		0.0428	0.0195	Gamma	10	0.0426	0.7779
L Int Con Elect		0.0053	0.0377	K Int Con Elect		0.0000	0.7571
M Int Con Elect		0.0017	0.0401	Gamma	11	0.0013	0.8230
Gamma	2	0.0452	0.1405	Gamma	12	0.0010	0.9608
K Int Con Elect		0.0058	0.1194	K Alpha-1 X-Ray		0.0253	0.0183
L Int Con Elect		0.0007	0.1377	K Alpha-2 X-Ray		0.0127	0.0182
Gamma	3	0.0600	0.1811	K Beta-1 X-Ray		0.0060	0.0206
K Int Con Elect		0.0085	0.1600	KLL Auger Elect		0.0087	0.0154
L Int Con Elect		0.0012	0.1782	KLX Auger Elect		0.0032	0.0178
M Int Con Elect		0.0004	0.1806	LMM Auger Elect		0.0615	0.0019
				MXY Auger Elect		0.1403	0.0004

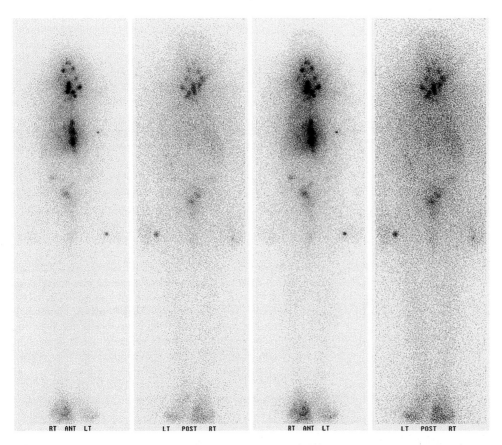

FIG. 8.8 ● **I-131 posttherapy images.** Anterior and posterior whole-body images obtained 5 days following therapy for thyroid cancer with I-131 demonstrate uptake within cervical, mediastinal, and upper abdominal lymph nodes, pelvic bones, and a left-sided rib, consistent with metastatic disease. Activity within the liver, bowel, nose, and mouth is physiologic. Diffuse activity on the skin of the feet is due to perspiration.

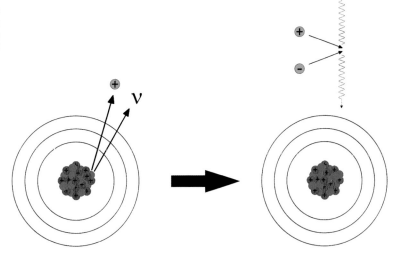

FIG. 8.9 ● **Positron emission.** A neutron-deficient radio-nuclide emits a positron (+) and a neutrino (ν), resulting in a daughter nuclide with a decrease in atomic number and no change in atomic mass number. When the positron loses energy, it interacts with an electron to form two 511 MeV photons directed approximately 180° apart.

Below this threshold, positron emission does not take place, but the neutron-deficient isotope may undergo electron capture, discussed later. Above the threshold, electron capture may compete with positron emission. This threshold is also reflected in the minimum mass difference between the parent and daughter atoms required for positron emission. Like the antineutrino seen in β^- decay, the neutrino does not significantly interact with the patient or the clinical nuclear imaging system (Figure 8.10).

Positron emitters used in clinical applications are usually cyclotron produced or generator produced. These radioisotopes, such as fluorine-18, nitrogen-13, rubidium-82, carbon-11, and gallium-68, are widely employed in PET (Table 8.3).

Electron Capture

Electron capture provides a second mechanism for the neutron-deficient radioisotope to increase stability (Figure 8.11). An orbital electron, usually from the K or L shell, combines with a proton in the nucleus. This results in conversion of a proton to a neutron and liberation of a neutrino ν, producing a daughter with decreased atomic number Z and unchanged atomic mass number A (an isobaric transition).

$$^A_Z X + e- \rightarrow\ ^A_{Z-1} Y + v + \text{energy}$$

Energy may be released as gamma rays from the nucleus, or as characteristic X-rays and Auger electrons from filling the vacancy left by the captured orbital electron.

Electron capture is the decay mode for neutron-deficient radioisotopes below the 1.022 MeV threshold. Isotopes with transition energies above this threshold may undergo electron capture, positron emission, or both (see Figure 8.10). Heavier elements, which have orbital electrons closer to the nucleus, tend to favor electron capture, and lighter elements favor positron emission. As with positron emitters, neutron-deficient radioisotopes undergoing electron capture are frequently cyclotron produced. Example isotopes used in clinical practice include gallium-67, indium-111, iodine-123, thallium-201, and cobalt-57.

Isomeric Transition

Isomeric transition occurs in nuclides undergoing transition from a *metastable* state to a stable state. Following nuclear transformations, nuclei may temporarily exist in excited states, releasing gamma rays as they decay to their stable form. This phenomenon has been demonstrated in the case of (β^-, γ) emission mentioned earlier (see Figure 8.7). When this initial excited state decays with a relatively long half-life, it is termed a *metastable* state, denoted by "m." The decay involves liberation of energy from the nucleus,

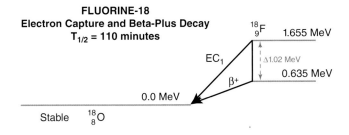

FLUORINE-18
Electron Capture and Beta-Plus Decay
$T_{1/2}$ = 110 minutes

$^{18}_{9}$F 1.655 MeV

EC₁

Δ1.02 MeV

0.635 MeV

β+

0.0 MeV

Stable $^{18}_{8}$O

Decay Data Table

Radiation	Mean Number per Disintegration	Mean Energy Particle (MeV)
Beta Plus	0.9700	0.2496
Annih. Radiation	1.9400	0.5110

FIG. 8.10 ● **Principal decay scheme of fluorine-18.** Reprinted with permission from Bushberg JT, Seibert JA, Leidholdt EM, Boone JM. *Essential Physics of Medical Imaging.* 3rd ed. Philadelphia, PA: Wolters Kluwer Health/Lippincott Williams & Wilkins; 2012.

Table 8.3 **FDA-APPROVED PET RADIOPHARMACEUTICALS**
Carbon-11 choline
Fluorine-18 florbetaben (Neuraceq)
Fluorine-18 florbetapir (Amyvid)
Fluorine-18 fludeoxyglucose (FDG)
Fluorine-18 fluciclovine (Axumin)
Fluorine-18 flutemetamol (Vizamyl)
Fluorine-18 sodium fluoride
Gallium-68 dotatate (Netspot)
Nitrogen-13 ammonia
Rubidium-82 chloride (Cardiogen-82)
Abbreviations: FDA, U.S. Food and Drug Administration; FDG, fluorodeoxyglucose; PET, positron emission tomography.

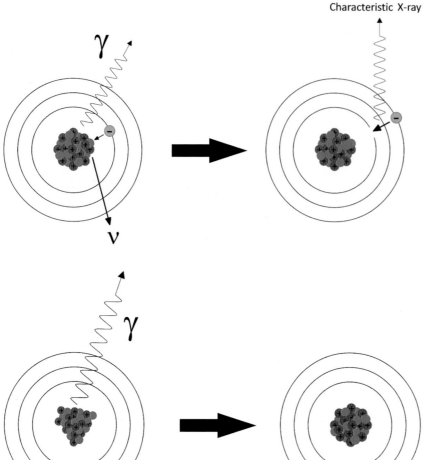

Characteristic X-ray

FIG. 8.11 ● **Electron capture.** A neutron-deficient radionuclide incorporates an inner shell electron into the nucleus with emission of a neutrino (ν) and a gamma ray. The vacancy may be filled by an outer shell electron and will result in characteristic X-rays or Auger electrons. The daughter nuclide has a decreased atomic number and an unchanged atomic mass number.

FIG. 8.12 ● **Isomeric transition.** The excited nucleus emits energy in the form of a gamma ray without gain or loss of particles and without change in atomic number or atomic mass number. Isomeric transition may compete with internal conversion (not pictured).

and does not involve the gain or loss of particles as in other decay modes discussed (Figure 8.12).

$$^{Am}_{Z}X \rightarrow ^{A}_{Z}X + \text{energy}$$

As there is no change in Z or A, the transition is isomeric, that is, isotonic and isobaric. The energy may be released in the form of one or more gamma rays, or may be absorbed by an inner shell electron which is subsequently ejected as an *internal conversion* electron. Filling of the resulting vacancy results in characteristic X-rays or Auger electrons. Technetium-99m, the most widely used radionuclide, decays by isomeric transition (Figure 8.13).

Alpha Decay

Alpha decay involves loss of an alpha particle and energy. The alpha particle is composed of two protons and two neutrons and is identical with a helium-4 nucleus. Alpha decay provides a mechanism for heavy nuclides to reduce their size. It results in a daughter element with decreased atomic number Z and atomic mass number A (Figures 8.14 and 8.15).

$$^{A}_{Z}X \rightarrow ^{A-4}_{Z-2}Y + ^{4}_{2}He^{2+} + \text{energy}$$

Alpha particles are the heaviest form of radiation as well as the least penetrating, failing to pass beyond the dead cells of the epidermis. However, they can induce significant damage when internalized within the body. Alpha emitters are not useful for nuclear imaging. However, intravenous administration of alpha

TECHNETIUM 99m
Isomeric Transition
T$_{1/2}$ = 6.02 hrs.

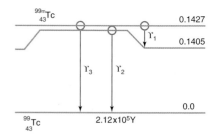

Decay Data Table

Radiation		Mean Number per Disintegration	Mean Energy per Particle (MeV)
Gamma	1	0.0000	0.0021
M Int Con Elect		0.8620	0.0018
N Int Con Elect		0.1300	0.0022
Gamma	2	0.8910	0.1405
K Int Con Elect		0.0892	0.1194
L Int Con Elect		0.0109	0.1375
M Int Con Elect		0.0020	0.1377
Gamma	3	0.0003	0.1426
K Int Con Elect		0.0088	0.1215
L Int Con Elect		0.0035	0.1398
M Int Con Elect		0.0011	0.1422
K Alpha-1 X-Ray		0.0441	0.0183
K Alpha-2 X-Ray		0.0221	0.0182
K Beta-1 X-Ray		0.0105	0.0206
KLL Auger Elect		0.0152	0.0154
KLX Auger Elect		0.0055	0.0178
LMM Auger Elect		0.1093	0.0019
MXY Auger Elect		1.2359	0.0004

FIG. 8.13 ● ^{99m}Tc decay scheme and decay data table.

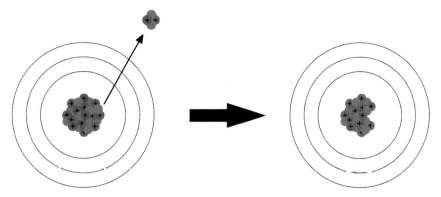

FIG. 8.14 • **Alpha decay.** The parent nucleus emits an alpha particle, which is composed of two protons and two neutrons, with corresponding decrease in atomic number and atomic mass number.

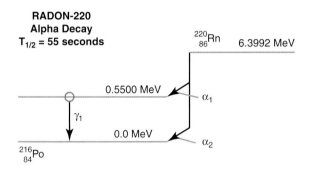

RADON-220
Alpha Decay
$T_{1/2}$ = 55 seconds

$^{220}_{86}$Rn   6.3992 MeV

0.5500 MeV α_1

γ_1

0.0 MeV α_2

$^{216}_{84}$Po

Decay Data Table

Radiation		Mean Number per Disintegration	Mean Energy per Particle (MeV)
Alpha	1	0.0007	5.7470
Recoil Atom		0.0007	0.1064
Alpha	2	0.9993	6.2870
Recoil Atom		0.9993	0.1164
Gamma	1	0.0006	0.5500

FIG. 8.15 • **Principal decay scheme of radon-220.** Reprinted with permission from Bushberg JT, Seibert JA, Leidholdt EM, Boone JM. *Essential Physics of Medical Imaging.* 3rd ed. Philadelphia, PA: Wolters Kluwer Health/Lippincott Williams & Wilkins; 2012.

emitter radium-223 dichloride has found therapeutic application in treating skeletal metastases of castration-resistant prostate cancer (Tables 8.4 and 8.5).

RADIOISOTOPE PRODUCTION

Radionuclides commonly used in radiopharmaceuticals are artificially produced in nuclear reactors, cyclotrons, and generators. In general, they are created by bombarding stable nuclides with protons or neutrons to produce unstable nuclides with desirable properties, or, in some cases, they may be decay products of nuclear fission. Although naturally occurring radionuclides played important roles in nuclear medicine historically, they are not used in modern applications.

Nuclear reactors produce energy and nuclear materials by nuclear fission, usually employing uranium-235 (U-235). When U-235 absorbs a neutron, the resulting U-236 quickly decays to two of many possible fission fragments as well as to a variable number of neutrons. These neutrons can trigger further U-235 fission, leading to a chain reaction. If, on average, one of the neutrons produced by fission is absorbed to produce a subsequent fission reaction, the reaction is said to be *critical* and will proceed at a constant rate. If fewer than one neutron is absorbed on average, the reaction is termed *subcritical*, and if more than one neutron is absorbed, the reaction is said to be *supercritical*. The rate of a supercritical reaction will increase exponentially and can quickly escalate to a runaway reaction (Figure 8.16).

A runaway chain reaction can produce an explosion, as seen in atomic weapons. However, the nuclear fuel used in nuclear reactors is structured in such a way as to be incapable of explosion, although it is subject to overheating and *meltdown*. Modern nuclear reactors are designed with features to help to prevent runaway reactions and meltdown.

Nuclear reactors are found in varied applications, including nuclear power plants, nuclear propulsion systems for ships and submarines, and radionuclide reactors for radionuclide production and research. Many of the reactors in these various applications share common features. Within a nuclear reactor, the reaction takes place in the reactor core. Inside the core is the U-235 nuclear fuel, present in the form of fuel rods, interposed between control rods, and surrounded by a moderator, such as water. The control rods are composed of a material, such as boron or cadmium, which effectively absorbs neutrons. By withdrawing

Table 8.4 KEY CHARACTERISTICS OF COMMON GAMMA-EMITTING RADIONUCLIDES

Nuclide	Photons (keV)	Production Mode	Decay Mode	Half-Life ($T_{1/2}$)
^{67}Ga	93, 185, 300	Cyclotron	EC	78 h
^{99m}Tc	140	Generator	IT	6 h
^{111}In	173, 247	Cyclotron	EC	68 h
^{123}I	159	Cyclotron	EC	13 h
^{131}I	364	Fission product	β	8 d

Abbreviations: β, beta decay; EC, electron capture; IT, isomeric transition.
Reprinted with permission from Huda W. *Review of Radiologic Physics.* 4th ed. Philadelphia, PA: Wolters Kluwer; 2016.

Table 8.5 **SUMMARY OF RADIONUCLIDE DECAY**

Type of Decay	Primary Radiation Emitted	Other Radiation Emitted	Nuclear Transformation	Change In		Nuclear Condition Before Transformation
				Z		A
Alpha		λ-rays C X-rays AE, ICE		−2	−4	Z > 83
Beta minus	β^{-1}	λ-rays C X-rays AE, ICE		+1	0	N/Z too large
Beta plus	β^{+1}	γ-rays C X-rays AE, ICE, v		−1	0	N/Z too small
Electron capture	C X-rays	λ-rays AE, ICE, v		−1	0	N/Z too small
Isomeric transition	λ-rays	C X-rays AE, ICE		0	0	Excited or metastable nucleus

Abbreviations: AE, Auger e^{-1}; ICE, internal conversion e^{-1}; C X-rays, characteristic X-rays; *v*, neutrino.
Reprinted with permission from Bushberg JT, Seibert JA, Leidholdt EM, Boone JM. *Essential Physics of Medical Imaging*. 3rd ed. Philadelphia, PA: Wolters Kluwer Health/Lippincott Williams & Wilkins; 2012.

and advancing the control rods, the operator can cover the fuel rods or expose them to neutron bombardment by one another. In this way, one can adjust the rate at which neutrons are available for reaction, and thus control the reaction rate. The moderator serves to slow the neutrons. Following fission, the produced neutrons are too energetic to be efficiently absorbed for subsequent fission reactions. By slowing the neutrons, the moderator increases the reaction rate. These slowed neutrons are known as *thermal neutrons*, because they have kinetic energies similar to their surroundings. In the case of water as a moderator, as the reaction rate increases, the water temperature rises, reducing the water density. Decreased density results in a decrease in the moderator effect of the water, and therefore a slowing of the reaction. This negative feedback loop serves as a safety feature to help prevent a runaway reaction.

The water surrounding the fuel rods serves not only as a moderator but also as a coolant. This coolant water usually transfers its heat to a separate water system, from which it isolated, by way of a heat exchanger. In nuclear power reactors, this secondary coolant water is used to drive turbines which power generators for production of electricity. Radionuclide reactors release this heat to the environment.

Heavy elements, such as U-235, tend to have a significantly higher N/Z ratio than do lighter elements (see Figure 8.1). Likewise, the daughter species of nuclear fission, known as fission fragments, tend to be proton deficient. They frequently undergo one or more subsequent decay events, usually beta emission, producing additional proton-deficient species. Several of these fission products are used in clinical nuclear medicine. Because the parent and various fission products represent different elements, fission

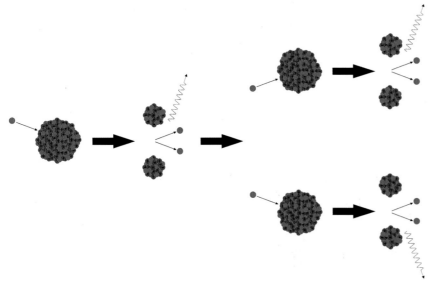

FIG. 8.16 ● **Fissile nuclides such as U-235 can absorb a neutron and subsequently decay to form fission fragments as well as gamma emissions and a variable number of neutrons, a process known as a nuclear fission.** Emitted neutrons can be absorbed by nearby nuclei, triggering further nuclear fission and sustaining the reaction. If enough emitted neutrons are absorbed, a chain reaction will occur.

products of interest often have the advantage of being readily isolated on the basis of chemical properties. The resultant material is said to be carrier free, that is, free from contaminating stable isotopes of the same element. Because they are proton deficient, fission products typically decay by beta emission. Examples used in clinical nuclear medicine include iodine-131, xenon-133, and molybdenum-99.

A second mechanism by which reactors may produce radio-isotopes is by *neutron activation*. Stable target material is placed within the reactor and bombarded with neutrons. Absorption of neutrons is accompanied by emission of gamma rays, protons, or alpha particles. Such reactions are termed (n, γ), (n, p), and (n, α), respectively. The (n, γ) reaction is the most common mechanism of neutron activation used in radionuclide production. Because (n, γ) neutron activation results in no change in atomic number, the radionuclide products are generally not carrier free. They exist in small quantities admixed with their stable isotope, yielding low specific activity. An exception is iodine-125 (I-125), which is produced from xenon-124 (Xe-124) by the (n, γ) reaction, yielding Xe-125. Xe-125 subsequently undergoes positron emission or electron capture, producing I-125. Other example radionuclides used in clinical nuclear medicine produced by the (n, γ) reaction are phosphorus-32 and chromium-51. Most products of neutron activation decay by beta emission.

A cyclotron is a type of charged-particle accelerator used in the production of medical radioisotopes. A high-energy beam of charged particles, most commonly protons (p, H^+), deuterons (d, $^2H^+$), or negatively charged hydrogen ions (H^-), bombards a target of suitable material. The target absorbs positively charged particles from the beam, undergoing nuclear reactions. In the case of H^-, the orbital electrons are removed before the beam impacting the target. The energy of the beam must be sufficiently high to overcome the repulsive forces between the positively charged particles and the target nuclei.

Two common particle-target reactions in the production of medical radionuclides are the (p, n) and (d, n) reactions. In the (p, n) reaction, a proton is absorbed and a neutron is emitted, resulting in a product with equal atomic mass number and increased atomic number compared with the parent (target). An example is ^{18}F, commonly used in PET imaging:

$$^{18}O(p, n)\ ^{18}F$$

In the (d, n) reaction, a deuteron is absorbed and a neutron is emitted, producing a daughter with increased atomic mass number and increased atomic number. ^{57}Co is produced from the common, stable isotope of iron in this way:

$$^{56}Fe(d, n)\ ^{57}Co$$

In each case, the daughter is a different element from the parent and therefore carrier free.

The cyclotron consists of a circular vacuum chamber containing two semicircular, D-shaped electrodes ("dees") within a magnetic field, separated by a gap (Figure 8.17). The dees are connected with an oscillator that produces alternating voltage between the dees. A source situated in the center of the circle, between the dees, releases charged particles, which are attracted to

FIG. 8.17 ● Schematic view of a cyclotron. Two "dees" (A, B) are separated by a small gap. Reprinted with permission from Bushberg JT, Seibert JA, Leidholdt EM, Boone JM. *Essential Physics of Medical Imaging.* 3rd ed. Philadelphia, PA: Wolters Kluwer Health/Lippincott Williams & Wilkins; 2012.

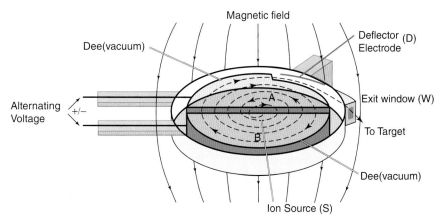

Top and bottom magnet removed

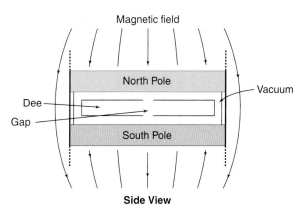

Side View

the oppositely charged dee. The magnetic field causes the particle to travel toward the dee in a circular path. As the particle travels around the dee and approaches the gap, the potential of the dees reverses, and the particle is accelerated toward the opposite dee. With subsequent alternating accelerations, the speed of the particle increases and it traces a spiral path outward. As it approaches the outer margin of the dees, the particle is diverted to impact the target, producing the nuclear reaction. Positively charged particles, such as protons, deuterons, and alpha particles, are diverted by an electrostatic deflector positioned at the periphery of the chamber. Most of the particles in the beam impact the target, but some impact the walls of the cyclotron, producing radioactive species within the structure. In the case of negatively charged H^- particles, stripping foil made from carbon is placed along the outer margin of the chamber, in the path of the beam. The two electrons are stripped away from H^-, leaving a positively charged hydrogen nucleus, H^+. The magnetic field deflects the subsequent beam of bare protons because of the reversal of charge, causing it to impact the target. Negative-ion cyclotrons have the advantage that nearly all the particles impact the target, producing little radioactivity of the structure.

Cyclotron-produced radionuclides are generally neutron deficient and decay by positron emission or electron capture. Examples include indium-111, gallium-67, iodine-123, and cobalt-57, as well as PET agents fluorine-18, nitrogen-13, oxygen-15, and carbon-11.

When a desired radionuclide is the decay product of a relatively long-lived parent radioisotope, a *radionuclide generator* may be employed for ongoing production of the daughter from the parent. The most common radionuclide generator used in clinical nuclear medicine is the molybdenum-99/technetium-99m (Mo-99/^{99m}Tc) generator.

In the Mo-99/^{99m}Tc generator, aluminum molybdenate is adsorbed onto a porous column of alumina resin immersed in saline. Mo-99 molybdenate decays to ^{99m}Tc pertechnetate, which is less tightly bound to the column. ^{99m}Tc can be efficiently removed by flushing with saline, a process known as *elution* (or "milking" the generator, which is sometimes colloquially referred to as the "cow"). Elution is typically performed by connecting a vacuum vial, which draws eluant from a saline reservoir within the generator across the column and into the vial (Figure 8.18). Elution of the generator with saline produces sodium pertechnetate solution.

As parent Mo-99 in the generator decays, activity of ^{99m}Tc increases over time until it is either removed from the generator by elution, or until the daughter ^{99m}Tc reaches a state of maximum activity. At this state, known as *transient equilibrium*, the rate of decay of ^{99m}Tc equals its production, and its activity decreases with the decay of the parent Mo-99 (Figure 8.19). Transient equilibrium is observed in cases in which the parent half-life is approximately 10 times the half-life of the daughter. At transient equilibrium, the daughter activity may exceed that of the parent. However, in the case of the Mo-99/^{99m}Tc generator, the activity of ^{99m}Tc is slightly less than that of Mo-99, because a portion of the Mo-99 decays directly to Tc-99. The Mo-99/^{99m}Tc generator reaches transient equilibrium in approximately 23 hours (depending upon elution efficiency), making daily elution practical and efficient. If the generator is eluted sooner, before reaching transient equilibrium, the yield of ^{99m}Tc will be lower (approximately half of the maximum activity at 6 hours). However, more frequent elution will yield more total activity in a day (Figure 8.20).

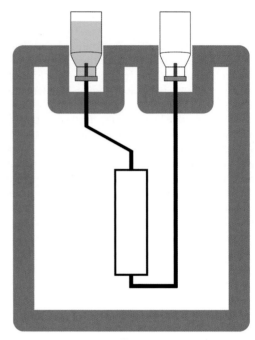

FIG. 8.18 ● **Molybdenum-99/^{99m}Tc generator.** The column (center) is composed of porous alumina resin onto which Mo-99 is adsorbed. Mo-99 decays to ^{99m}Tc, which is less tightly bound. As saline is drawn from a vial (upper left) through the column and into a vacuum vial (upper right), it removes ^{99m}Tc into the eluate. The apparatus is self-contained and housed in lead for shielding (gray).

Generator systems in which the half-life of the parent is greater than that of the daughter by 100 times or more, such as the strontium-82/rubidium-82 (Sr-82/Rb-82) generator, reach a state known as *secular equilibrium*. As with transient equilibrium, the apparent half-life of the daughter will equal that of the parent. However, in secular equilibrium, if the daughter is the only decay product, its activity will equal that of the parent at equilibrium (Figure 8.21).

Generator eluate may be tested for radionuclide and chemical purity. For the Mo-99/^{99m}Tc generator, any Mo-99 in the eluate is a radionuclidic impurity. Alumina present in the eluate is a chemical impurity. Quality control testing for radionuclide and chemical impurities is discussed later.

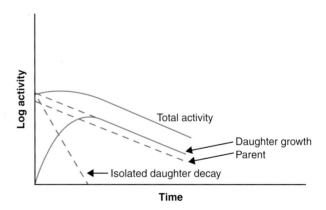

FIG. 8.19 ● **Transient equilibrium.** The concentration of the daughter rises to a maximum, after which it declines along with the decay of the parent.

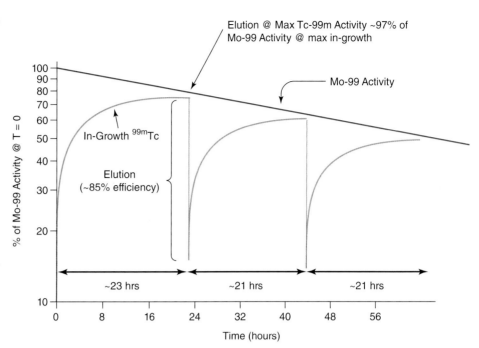

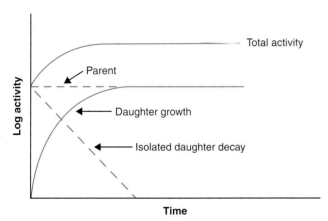

RADIOPHARMACEUTICALS

Radiopharmaceuticals are radioactive ions, molecules, or particles with the ability to localize to cells, tissues, or compartments of the body for diagnostic imaging or for delivery of therapeutic radiation. Most radiopharmaceuticals consist of a radioisotope bound to a pharmaceutical, such as a ligand or particle, which provides localization functionality. For example, ^{18}F fluorodeoxyglucose (FDG) consists of positron emitter F-18 linked with glucose. The glucose ligand causes FDG to localize within cells actively concentrating glucose, and F-18 undergoes beta-plus decay, allowing for PET imaging (see Section "Mechanisms of Radiopharmaceutical Localization" later). Radiopharmaceuticals used in the imaging of physiologic or pathologic processes are known as *radiotracers.* Most modern radiotracers are produced from ^{99m}Tc using simple commercially available kits.

Some radiopharmaceuticals may be administered in an elemental or ionic form, without a separate functional ligand, with localization inherent in the chemistry of the radioisotope or the delivery system. Examples include I-123 sodium iodide used in thyroid imaging, ^{99m}Tc pertechnetate used in Meckel's diverticulum imaging, Xe-133 used for dynamic lung ventilation imaging, and I-131 sodium iodide used for therapy of hyperthyroidism and thyroid cancer. Such radioisotopes are chemically identical with their stable forms, and their chemical behavior is not significantly different. For example, I-123, used in thyroid imaging, has the same orbital electron structure as the common stable form of iodine, I-127. It differs only in atomic weight, which has a negligible effect on its chemical and physiologic behavior. I-123 is taken up in the thyroid gland by the sodium-iodide symporter (NIS), and participates in the same chemical reactions as I-127, permitting imaging and functional evaluation of iodine metabolism.

Most *therapeutic radiopharmaceuticals* utilize beta emitters such as Y-90, Lu-177, or I-131. Beta-emitting radiopharmaceuticals localize to areas of pathology and deposit beta particles, which induce cellular damage and cell death. However, alpha emitter Ra-223 is FDA approved for treating skeletal metastases of castration-resistant prostate cancer. The heavier alpha particle is capable of providing greater cell damage with less tissue penetration compared with traditional beta-emitting agents, reducing damage to surrounding normal tissues. Additional therapeutic applications of alpha emitters are an active area of research.

The nuclear decay properties of a diagnostic or therapeutic radionuclide are not significantly affected by its chemical environment. For example, the decay of ^{99m}Tc proceeds identically whether in the form of ^{99m}Tc pertechnetate or bound to sestamibi.

The theranostic approach in nuclear medicine combines imaging and therapy. The term *theranostic* (or theragnostic) is a portmanteau of "therapy" and "diagnostic." Within the context of nuclear medicine, it refers to a pair of functionally similar radiopharmaceuticals: a diagnostic agent able to depict sites of disease, usually malignancy, with high specificity, and a therapeutic agent able to target those sites of disease by a similar mechanism of localization. Advantages of the theranostic pair over conventional imaging modalities include (1) verification that the tumor lesions avidly concentrate the radiopharmaceutical before therapeutic administration, (2) the ability to map the entire biodistribution of the radiopharmaceutical and thus identify nontarget sites of dose delivery before therapy, and (3) functional assessment of response to therapy.

The first theranostic application in nuclear medicine was likely the diagnosis and treatment of diseases of the thyroid gland with radioisotopes of iodine. These techniques remain in wide use today. The thyroid gland and most thyroid cancers concentrate iodine. In patients with hyperthyroidism, administration of gamma emitter iodine-123 (I-123) permits functional imaging of the gland to confirm the etiology of hyperthyroidism, as well as quantitative assessment of radioiodine uptake to assess disease activity and to plan the therapeutic dosage. Iodine-131 (I-131) is a beta, gamma emitter that is useful for treatment of many cases of hyperthyroidism. Following administration, I-131 will concentrate within the gland, killing thyroid cells and slowing the function of the overactive gland. In patients with thyroid cancer, I-123 imaging and quantitation is useful for estimating the amount of remnant thyroid tissue following total thyroidectomy, and can demonstrate sites of metastatic disease. Therapy with I-131 will kill suspected or known sites of thyroid cancer, and will ablate the remnant normal thyroid tissue, which facilitates laboratory and imaging follow-up and decreases the risk of development of subsequent thyroid cancer.

The theranostic agent dotatate is a more recent example. It is a peptide analog of the hormone somatostatin that localizes to neuroendocrine tumors (NETs). It binds to somatostatin receptors on the cell membranes of both normal and tumor cells. Most NETs express somatostatin receptors. Ga-68 dotatate PET imaging demonstrates NETs expressing somatostatin receptors, and beta emitter Lu-177 dotatate delivers targeted therapy.

Mechanisms of radiopharmaceutical localization

Most imaging radiopharmaceuticals provide functional information by one or more of various mechanisms (Table 8.6). Active transport involves the energy-dependent concentration of the radiopharmaceutical into the cell against a concentration gradient. I-123 and I-131 are concentrated in thyroid follicular cells by the NIS, a transmembrane glycoprotein. Sodium ions crossing the cell membrane flowing down their concentration gradient provide the energy for iodide ions traveling up their concentration gradient into the follicular cell, a mechanism known as *cotransport*. In contrast, FDG and glucose are transported into cells by glucose transporters (GLUTs) *down* their concentration gradients by facilitated diffusion. The intracellular concentration of FDG is kept low by hexokinases, which phosphorylate FDG and glucose. Glucose-6-phosphate then enters the metabolic pathways, while FDG-6-phosphate does not, accumulating within the cell (Figure 8.22). In cisternography, In-111 diethylenetriaminepentaacetic acid (DTPA) is introduced by lumbar puncture, with subsequent diffusion through the cerebrospinal fluid.

When introduced into the bloodstream, particles larger than about 10 μm will lodge within arterioles and capillaries, a process known as *capillary blockade*. This allows for imaging of a perfused area of tissue as well as assessing the integrity of the capillary bed. For example, ^{99m}Tc macroaggregated albumin (MAA) can depict the perfusion defects within the lung created by pulmonary emboli, and also be used to quantify vascular shunting (Figure 8.23). The introduction of much smaller particles, such as ^{99m}Tc sulfur colloid, into the bloodstream results in *phagocytosis* by cells of the mononuclear phagocyte system in the liver, spleen, and bone marrow.

Radiopharmaceuticals may localize to tumors and other tissues by receptor binding. In-111 pentetreotide and Ga-68 dotatate are ligands for somatostatin receptors in NETs and other sites in the body. Y-90 ibritumomab tiuxetan localizes by antibody-antigen *binding* and is used in the treatment of non-Hodgkin's lymphoma. It is a radiolabeled monoclonal antibody that binds the surface glycoprotein CD20 on normal and malignant B cells.

Radionuclide ventriculography uses compartment localization of ^{99m}Tc-labeled red blood cells within the blood pool for imaging and quantification of ventricular anatomy and function. On the other hand, compartment leakage of ^{99m}Tc-labeled red blood cells can depict lower gastrointestinal bleeding (Figure 8.24).

Radiolabeled autologous white blood cells, when administered intravenously, migrate to areas of infection by chemotaxis. In the radionuclide bone scan, ^{99m}Tc methylene diphosphonate (MDP, medronate) is incorporated into areas of osteogenic activity by chemisorption (see Figure 8.2).

Many nuclear medicine and PET imaging studies are examples of *molecular imaging*. *Molecular imaging* is the depiction and

---

Table 8.6 MECHANISMS OF RADIOPHARMACEUTICAL LOCALIZATION

Mechanism	Example(s)
Active transport	I-123, I-131
Facilitated diffusion	F-18 FDG
Diffusion	In-111 DTPA in CSF
Capillary blockade	^{99m}Tc MAA
Phagocytosis	^{99m}Tc sulfur colloid
Receptor binding	In-111 pentetreotide, Ga-68 dotatate
Antibody-antigen binding	Y-90 ibritumomab tiuxetan
Compartment localization	^{99m}Tc RBC in MUGA
Compartment leakage	^{99m}Tc-labeled red blood cells in gastrointestinal bleeding
Chemotaxis	In-111-labeled white blood cells
Chemisorption	^{99m}Tc MDP in bone scan

Abbreviations: CSF, cerebrospinal fluid; DTPA, diethylenetriaminepentaacetic acid; FDG, fluorodeoxyglucose; MAA, macroaggregated albumin; MDP, methylene diphosphonate; MUGA, multigated acquisition; RBC, red blood cell.

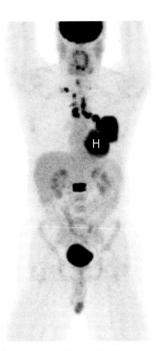

FIG. 8.22 ● **Maximum intensity projection image from a fluoro-deoxyglucose (FDG) positron emission tomography/computed tomography scan of a patient with lung cancer.** A mass is present within the left lung adjacent to the heart (H). There is FDG-avid left hilar, mediastinal, and right supraclavicular lymphadenopathy as well as a metastatic lesion within the L2 vertebral body. Intense activity is also present within the brain and bladder. Glucose transporters facilitate FDG diffusion into cells.

Radionuclide and radiopharmaceutical characteristics

An ideal radiopharmaceutical for clinical nuclear imaging would be readily available and deliver maximum diagnostic information with minimal negative effects and cost. Several features of a radiopharmaceutical and its radionuclide determine its suitability for clinical use. Low radiation dose limits the exposure of the patient, radiation workers, and the public. It is dependent in part on the photon energy and half-life of the radionuclide. Ideally, an agent used for imaging would not emit particle radiation, which may greatly increase the dose to the patient and which generally does not contribute to imaging. Rather, it would emit only photons of sufficient energy to penetrate the patient and clothing to reach camera, but not so high that it penetrates the collimators or detectors.

Gamma cameras are optimized to detect 140 keV photons. Having a high proportion of emissions near 140 keV and minimal other photon or particle emissions reduces dose. Gamma emissions of lower energy are more readily deposited in the patient's body, reducing diagnostic information and increasing patient dose, and those of higher energy are detected with low efficiency by the gamma camera.

Dose is also minimized when the half-life of the imaging agent is no longer than necessary to deliver sufficient photon flux for the imaging examination. For example, positron emitter F-18 has a half-life of approximately 2 hours, providing a convenient time window for PET imaging while decaying away rapidly. In contrast, single-photon agents gallium-67, thallium-201, and indium-111 all have half-lives of approximately 3 days. Although these relatively long half-lives permit multiday imaging, which may be useful for certain applications, in most situations they result in needless irradiation of the patient for days after the imaging examination. These agents have largely been replaced by ^{99m}Tc-based radiopharmaceuticals or PET agents for most applications.

The ability of a radiopharmaceutical to localize in a tissue or structure of interest, with minimal activity in surrounding tissues, is known as its *target-to-background ratio*. Having a high target-to-background ratio contributes to image contrast and is a major factor in lesion detectability. In many cases, such as bone imaging with ^{99m}Tc methylene diphosphonate and tumor imaging

quantitation of biologic processes in living subjects using tracers that function at the cellular or molecular level. In addition to gamma imaging and PET, molecular imaging encompasses other techniques such as MRI and optical imaging.

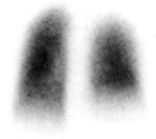

A

FIG. 8.23 ● **Capillary blockade.** Ventilation/perfusion (V/Q) lung scan and preselective internal radiation therapy (pre-SIRT) scans. A, Normal V/Q lung scan, anterior and posterior views. Patient with shortness of breath and chest pain has been referred for evaluation for possible pulmonary embolism. There is uniform activity throughout both lungs, reflecting the distribution of peripherally intravenously injected ^{99m}Tc macroaggregated albumin (MAA) particles embolized to the lungs. B, V/Q lung scan, pulmonary embolism. There are multiple perfusion defects, including large areas involving the left lung apex, the right mid lung, and the posterior left lung base. C, Normal pre-SIRT study, anterior and posterior whole-body views. Patient with planned selective internal radiation therapy (SIRT) procedure treatment of hepatic malignancy is evaluated for possible intrahepatic shunting as a safety measure before the SIRT procedure. ^{99m}Tc MAA injected via catheter within the hepatic artery has embolized within the hepatic vascular bed, with minimal activity shunted to the lungs. D, Abnormal pre-SIRT study. The presence of lung activity reflects intrahepatic shunting. ^{99m}Tc MAA particles bypass the hepatic vascular bed, returning to the systemic venous circulation, right heart, and pulmonary vascular bed. Shunted activity calculated at 18%.

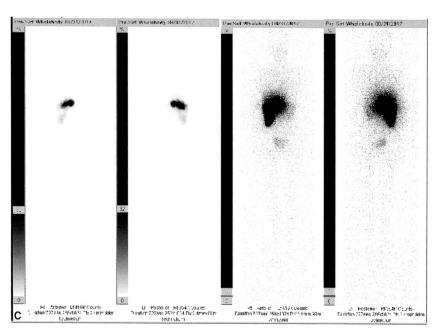

B

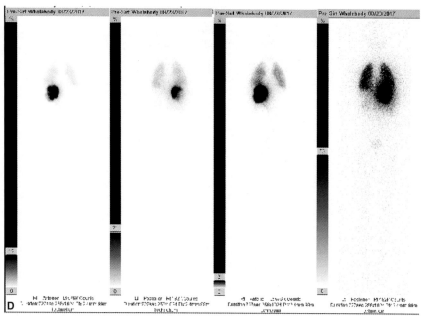

FIG. 8.23 ● (*continued*)

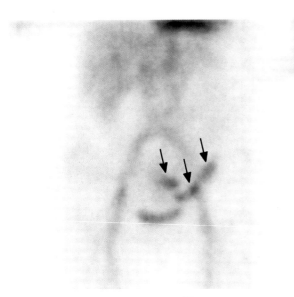

FIG. 8.24 • **Anterior view from a ^{99m}Tc-labeled red blood cell study for lower gastrointestinal bleeding.** Activity is largely confined to the blood pool, with visualization of the larger vessels of the abdomen, pelvis, and thighs, as well as partial visualization of the heart at the top of the image. Curvilinear activity in the pelvis (arrows) indicates bleeding into the sigmoid colon. Activity is present in the bladder because of urinary excretion of a small amount of untagged ^{99m}Tc pertechnetate.

with F-18 fluorodeoxyglucose, choosing an appropriate delay between radiopharmaceutical administration and imaging can allow for a high degree of radiopharmaceutical uptake and background clearance while preserving sufficient activity for imaging.

The *specific activity* of a radionuclide refers to its activity relative to the quantity present. It varies inversely with the half-life. For a given radiopharmaceutical, specific activity can be affected by several factors. Radiopharmaceuticals with high specific activity can yield sufficient photon flux for imaging and quantitation techniques, while ensuring that no significant pharmacologic effect is produced by the administered dosage and minimizing potential toxicity.

Radiopharmaceuticals should be nontoxic and apyrogenic in the quantities typically administered, and should have a high degree of purity. Ensuring high radionuclidic purity, or a low concentration of undesired radionuclides, reduces unnecessary radiation dose. Radionuclidic impurities can also interfere with imaging. Having a high proportion of radionuclide in the desired radiopharmaceutical form, known as high radiochemical purity, maximizes the target-to-background ratio and helps reduce unnecessary radiation.

The wide use of ^{99m}Tc as a radionuclide for single-photon nuclear imaging is, in part, related to these factors. ^{99m}Tc emits gamma rays of 140 keV, which are optimal for gamma camera imaging. Its 6-hour half-life is well suited to many nuclear imaging examinations, and it is sufficiently long to permit distribution of doses from a centralized nuclear pharmacy. Mo-99/^{99m}Tc generators are readily available and economic, and they produce ^{99m}Tc pertechnetate with high specific activity and radionuclidic purity.

Radionuclide and radiopharmaceutical quality control

The presence of contaminant Mo-99 in eluate from a Mo-99/^{99m}Tc generator is known as "molybdenum breakthrough" and is a *radionuclidic impurity*. Molybdenum breakthrough is tested in a dose calibrator. The sample is placed in a lead shield sufficient

to block the 140 keV photons from ^{99m}Tc, permitting detection of the higher energy gamma emissions from Mo-99 contaminant and quantification of small amounts within a sample.

Mo-99 emits a beta particle and high-energy gamma rays. The presence of significant Mo-99 in a sample of a ^{99m}Tc-based radiopharmaceutical exposes the patient to unnecessary radiation. The maximum concentration of Mo-99 contamination allowed by the US Pharmacopeia (USP) and the US Nuclear Regulatory Commission (NRC) is 15 µCi Mo-99/1 mCi ^{99m}Tc. Other examples of radionuclidic impurity include I-124 in samples of I-123 and Tl-202 in samples of Tl-201.

Radiochemical purity refers to the degree to which an isotope is present in the desired radiopharmaceutical form. It is tested by paper chromatography using filter paper or thin-layer chromatography using a plastic plate coated with silica gel. In both cases, a drop of the sample to be tested is placed near the end of the paper or plate (the stationary phase), the end of which is placed in a solvent (the mobile phase). As the solvent advances along the stationary phase (paper or plate) by capillary action, the radiopharmaceutical and impurities advance at differing rates depending on their solubility and become separated on the stationary phase. The relative amounts of radiopharmaceutical and impurities can be quantified by cutting the stationary phase and testing the activity of the separated components. Free ^{99m}Tc pertechnetate and hydrolyzed reduced ^{99m}Tc in a sample of ^{99m}Tc MDP are examples of radiochemical impurities (Figure 8.25).

Alumina breakthrough in generator eluate is a *chemical impurity* detected by commercially available chemical test kits. Its maximum permissible concentration set by the USP is 10 µg alumina/mL eluate.

RADIATION DOSES FROM RADIONUCLIDES

Radiation capable of removing electrons from atoms and molecules is known as *ionizing radiation*. Gamma rays, X-rays, and particle radiation released in nuclear reactions are all ionizing forms of radiation. Radiation can directly damage target molecules or can produce fast electrons or free radicals that go on to produce damage. Ionizing radiation can damage many cellular structures; however, of greatest concern is damage to DNA. DNA damage can result in cell death or dysregulation and malignancy, and DNA errors in germ cells can be passed down to future generations. In most human cells, DNA repair mechanisms can repair the strand breaks and other damage induced by ionization. However, incomplete or incorrect repair can result in DNA mutations.

Sufficiently widespread cell damage can cause clinically evident tissue or organ dysfunction. The resulting signs and symptoms are known as *deterministic effects* or tissue effects. Examples of deterministic effects include skin erythema and epilation (hair loss), cataracts, decreased sperm count, and death. Each of these effects generally occurs at a threshold radiation dose, is not observed below the threshold, and may be more severe with increasing dose. Deterministic effects are invariably seen when radiation doses are sufficiently high.

The induction of cancer or birth defects are examples of *stochastic effects* of radiation. Stochastic effects are random events, and the likelihood of such an event occurring increases with increasing radiation dose. However, if the effect occurs, its severity is independent of radiation dose. The most widely applied model of the risk of stochastic effects of radiation exposure is the *linear no-threshold* hypothesis, in which the risk increases in a linear

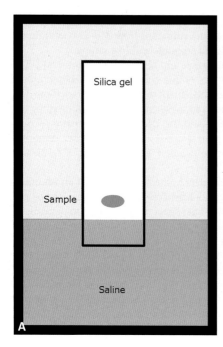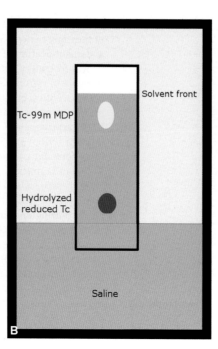

FIG. 8.25 ● Thin-layer chromatography. A, The sample is placed on the plate above the level of the mobile phase (in this case, saline). B, As the mobile phase migrates up the plate, the radiopharmaceutical and the impurities advance at different rates because of differences in solubility. They become separated on the plate and can be isolated by cutting the plate. Measuring the activity of the plate fragments can be used to quantify the amounts of impurities.

manner with increasing dose, and the risk is increased for even very low doses of radiation. The linear no-threshold hypothesis is not universally accepted and is considered a conservative approach to radiation dose risk estimation. A consequence of its no-threshold approach is the principle that there is no level of radiation safe from stochastic effects.

Deterministic effects are generally not seen at the radiation doses typically received in diagnostic nuclear medicine, in which stochastic effects are the main concern. In radionuclide therapy, on the other hand, both stochastic and deterministic effects may be seen.

Measures of Patient Radiation Dose

There are several measures of radiation and radiation dose that are worth defining and contrasting: activity, dose, dosage, absorbed dose, dose equivalent, and effective dose.

Activity (A) means radioactivity. It describes the *rate of nuclear decay*, and is discussed at the beginning of this chapter. SI unit = bequerel (Bq), traditional unit = curie (Ci). It is typically measured in megabequerels (MBq), gigabequerels (GBq), microcuries (μCi), and millicuries (mCi).

Dose refers to a quantity of radiation a patient receives from a radiopharmaceutical administration or another source. It is a nonspecific term, although it usually refers to absorbed dose, which is discussed later.

Dosage is the quantity of a radiopharmaceutical prescribed or administered to an individual patient, expressed as its activity. The term is also used to refer to a specific sample of radiopharmaceutical prescribed or administered to an individual patient.

Absorbed dose (D) refers to the radiation dose to tissue (or other material). Absorbed dose equals the amount of *energy deposited per gram of tissue*. SI unit = gray (Gy), traditional unit = rad (acronym of *radiation absorbed dose*). It is typically measured in milligray (mGy).

$$1 \text{ Gy} = 1 \text{ J of energy deposited per gram of tissue}$$
$$= 100 \text{ rads}$$
$$1 \text{ rad} = 100 \text{ ergs of energy deposited per gram of tissue}$$
$$= 10^{-2} \text{ Gy}$$
$$= 1 \text{ cGy}$$

Equivalent dose (H) is a measure of radiation *dose to an organ, taking into account the type of radiation involved*. It equals the absorbed dose to an organ or tissue multiplied by the radiation weighting factor. The *radiation weighting factor W_R* accounts for differences in biologic effect for different types of radiation. For example, $W_R = 1$ for photons and beta particles, 2 for protons, and 4 for alpha particles. SI unit = sievert (Sv), traditional unit = rem (acronym of *roentgen equivalent man*). It is typically measured in millisieverts (mSv) or millirem (mrem).

Note that for X-rays and gamma rays:

$$W_R = 1$$

and so equivalent dose (in mSv) = Absorbed dose (in mGy)

Effective dose is the *whole-body dose, accounting for the radiation sensitivity of each organ*. It reflects the *stochastic risk* of a radiation dose. It is calculated as the sum, for all specified tissues and organs of the body, of the equivalent dose for each organ times its tissue weighting factor. The *tissue weighting factor W_T* expresses the relative risk of stochastic effects for a given organ or tissue. SI unit = sievert Sv, traditional unit = rem (acronym of *roentgen equivalent man*). It is typically measured in millisieverts (mSv) or millirem (mrem).

Effective doses are useful for radiation protection. However, they are not valid for estimating the risk of malignancy or other stochastic effects for individual patients. They do not take into account patient size and other factors that significantly impact the individual patient's dose.

In addition to the effective dose, the radiation dose from a nuclear medicine procedure may be expressed in terms of organ doses. Important organ doses in nuclear medicine include the doses to the target organ and the critical organ. The *target organ* is the organ of interest in a diagnostic study or the target of radionuclide therapy. The organ most susceptible to radiation from a given radiopharmaceutical is known as the *critical organ*. The critical organ is not necessarily the target organ, and its dose frequently limits the activity administered (Table 8.7).

REGULATORY CONSIDERATIONS IN CLINICAL NUCLEAR MEDICINE

The NRC regulates the use of by-product material for medical use in the United States according to Title 10 Part 35 of the Code of Federal Regulations (10 CFR 35). This by-product material includes both unsealed sources of radioactivity as well as sealed sources, such as brachytherapy seeds. However, most states have entered an agreement with the NRC to regulate by-product material within their borders. These *agreement states* enact and enforce regulations that must be equally or more restrictive compared with NRC regulations. These regulations specify many aspects of the handling and use of radioisotopes relevant to the practice of nuclear medicine, including the following:

- Recordkeeping
- Research with human subjects
- Licensure
- Written directives
- Training and supervision of radiation workers
- Training of radiation safety officers (RSOs) and associate RSOs
- Training for authorized medical physicists and nuclear pharmacists
- Training of authorized users (AUs)
- Calibration of radiation measuring instruments
- Determination of dose

Table 8.7 **EFFECTIVE DOSES FOR ADULTS FROM VARIOUS NUCLEAR MEDICINE EXAMINATIONS**

Examination	Effective Dose (mSv)	Administered Activity (MBq)	Effective Dose (mSv/MBq)[a]
Brain (^{99m}Tc-HMPAO-exametazime)	6.9	740	0.0093
Brain (^{99m}Tc-ECD-Neurolite)	5.7	740	0.0077
Brain (^{18}F-FDG)	14.1	740	0.019
Thyroid scan (sodium iodine-123)	1.9	25	0.075 (15% uptake)
Thyroid scan (^{99m}Tc-pertechnetate)	4.8	370	0.013
Parathyroid scan (^{99m}Tc-sestamibi)	6.7	740	0.009
Cardiac stress-rest test (thallium-201 chloride)	40.7	185	0.22
Cardiac rest-stress test (^{99m}Tc-sestamibi 1-d protocol)	9.4	1100	0.0085 (0.0079 stress, 0.0090 rest)
Cardiac rest-stress test (^{99m}Tc-sestamibi 2-d protocol)	12.8	1500	0.0085 (0.0079 stress, 0.0090 rest)
Cardiac rest-stress test (Tc-tetrofosmin)	11.4	1500	0.0076
Cardiac ventriculography (^{99m}Tc-labeled red blood cells)	7.8	1110	0.007
Cardiac (^{18}F-FDG)	14.1	740	0.019
Lung perfusion (^{99m}Tc-MAA)	2.0	185	0.011
Lung ventilation (xenon-133)	0.5	740	0.00074
Lung ventilation (^{99m}Tc-DTPA)	0.2	1300 (40 actually inhaled)	0.0049
Liver-spleen (^{99m}Tc-sulfur colloid)	2.1	222	0.0094
Biliary tract (^{99m}Tc-disofenin)	3.1	185	0.017
Gastrointestinal bleeding (^{99m}Tc-labeled red blood cells)	7.8	1110	0.007
Gastrointestinal emptying (^{99m}Tc-labeled solids)	0.4	14.8	0.024
Renal (^{99m}Tc-DTPA)	1.8	370	0.0049
Renal (^{99m}Tc-MAG3)	2.6	370	0.007
Renal (^{99m}Tc-DMSA)	3.3	370	0.0088
Renal (^{99m}Tc-glucoheptonate)	2.0	370	0.0054
Bone (^{99m}Tc-MDP)	6.3	1110	0.0057
Gallium-67 citrate	15	150	0.100
Pentreotide (^{111}In)	12	222	0.054
White blood cells (^{99m}Tc)	8.1	740	0.011
White blood cells (^{111}In)	6.7	18.5	0.360
Tumor (^{11}F-FDG)	14.1	740	0.019

[a]Recommended ranges vary, although most laboratories tend to use the upper end of suggested ranges.

Abbreviations: DMSA, dimercaptosuccinic acid; DTPA, diethylenetriaminepentaacetic acid; ECD, ethyl cysteinate dimer; FDG, fluorodeoxyglucose; HMPAO, hexamethylpropyleneamine oxime; MAA, macroaggregated albumin; MAG3, mercaptoacetyltriglycine; MDP, methylene diphosphonate. Reprinted from Mettler FA Jr, Huda W, Yoshizumi TT, Mahesh M. Effective doses in radiology and diagnostic nuclear medicine: a catalog. *Radiology*. 2008;248:254–263. Copyright © 2008 Radiological Society of North America. With permission.

- Radionuclidic purity of administered radiopharmaceuticals
- Area surveys
- Release criteria for individuals containing by-product material
- Storage and disposal of by-product material

The NRC or state agency issues licenses for the use of RAM to hospitals and other organizations. Individual users of RAM must be designated AUs or supervised users. An AU is a physician who has completed training in the medical use of RAM specified in 10 CFR 35. A supervised user, such as a nuclear medicine technologist, works under the supervision of an AU.

Each licensee must designate an RSO. The RSO is a physicist, physician, or other professional who meets requirements for education, training, and experience and who is responsible for implementing the radiation safety program.

The administration of therapeutic radiopharmaceuticals or I-131 in amounts greater than 1.11 MBq (30 μCi) requires completion of a written directive. This document records details of the administration including the patient's name, the radiopharmaceutical, its activity, and route of administration. The written directive must be signed by the AU before administration).

Medical Events

Significant deviation of administered activity from the prescribed activity or other errors in administration that result in significant patient exposure or functional harm are defined as *medical events* by the NRC and state agencies. The regulations specify criteria for significant deviation of administered dosage, types and levels of patient exposure, and functional harm. Medical events must be reported to the NRC or state agency initially by phone, with a subsequent written report of the event. The licensee is also responsible for notifying the referring provider, and in many cases the patient, of the event.

Medical event criteria are defined in 10 CFR 35 for unsealed sources, discussed later, as well as sealed sources, which are not discussed here. Any event involving by-product material that is due to patient action is only considered a medical event if it results in "unintended permanent functional damage to an organ or a physiological system." However, if patient action is not the cause of the event, there are three scenarios in nuclear medicine that may result in a medical event.

Scenario 1

One or both of the following has occurred:

- The total dose delivered differs from the prescribed dose by 20% or more.
- The total dosage delivered differs from the prescribed dosage by 20% or more or falls outside the prescribed dosage range.

And the dose differs from (1) the prescribed dose or (2) the dose that would have resulted from the prescribed dosage by at least one of the following:

- More than 0.05 Sv (5 rem) effective dose equivalent
- 0.5 Sv (50 rem) to an organ or tissue
- 0.5 Sv (50 rem) shallow dose equivalent to the skin

Scenario 2

One or more of the following has occurred:

- Administration of a wrong radioactive drug

- Administration of a radioactive drug by the wrong route of administration
- Administration of a dose or dosage to the wrong individual

And the dose exceeds at least one of the following:

- 0.05 Sv (5 rem) effective dose equivalent
- 0.5 Sv (50 rem) to an organ or tissue
- 0.5 Sv (50 rem) shallow dose equivalent to the skin

Scenario 3

For an administration that was given in accordance with a written directive, a dose that exceeds the expected dose to at least one of these sites:

- The skin
- An organ or tissue other than the treatment site

By both of the following:

- At least 0.5 Sv (50 rem)
- At least 50% of the expected dose to that site from the procedure

NOTIFICATION OF A MEDICAL EVENT

Upon discovering a medical event, the licensee must notify the referring physician of the event within 24 hours of the event, or as soon as possible thereafter. The licensee is also required to notify the patient or their responsible party within 24 hours, unless the referring physician agrees to inform the patient, or if informing the patient would be harmful. Any delays in notification should not delay medical care related to the incident or other care for the patient. The licensee must notify the NRC by telephone no later than the next calendar day after discovering the medical event.

Within 15 days of the event, the licensee must submit a written report of the event to the NRC. The report must include the following information:

- Licensee's name
- Name of the prescribing physician
- Brief description of the event
- Why the event occurred
- The effect, if any, on the individual(s) who received the administration
- What actions, if any, have been taken or are planned to prevent recurrence
- Certification that the licensee notified the individual (or the individual's responsible relative or guardian), and if not, why not

The patient's name or other identifying information must not be present in the report.

In addition, within 15 days of the event, the licensee must submit a copy of the written report of the event to the referring physician, annotated with the patient's name and social security number or other identification number.

Agreement states may have different requirements, and the licensee under such a state license must notify the appropriate state board rather than the NRC.

See Chapter 10 for a further discussion of regulatory agencies relevant to nuclear medicine.

CHAPTER SELF-ASSESSMENT QUESTIONS

1. A patient undergoing FDG PET/CT scanning is concerned about possible side effects of radiation from the scan. Which of the following effects could be seen as a result of radiation from this scan?

   A. Skin erythema (redness)
   B. Epilation (hair loss)
   C. Nausea
   D. Cancer induction

2. Which of the following measures is intended to correlate with stochastic risk?

   A. Activity
   B. Absorbed dose
   C. Effective dose
   D. Equivalent dose

3. Which of the following is true for most cyclotron-produced radionuclides used in nuclear medicine?

   A. They are proton deficient and undergo beta-plus decay.
   B. They are neutron deficient and undergo beta-plus decay.
   C. They are neutron deficient and undergo beta-minus decay.
   D. They are neutron deficient and undergo alpha decay.

4. What would be the result of eluting a Mo-99/^{99m}Tc generator every 8 hours, compared with once per day?

   A. Higher activity of ^{99m}Tc pertechnetate for each elution
   B. Lower activity of ^{99m}Tc pertechnetate for each elution, but higher total activity yield for the day
   C. Generator life decreased by two-thirds
   D. Decrease in the half-life of Mo-99 by two-thirds

Answers to Chapter Self-Assessment Questions

1. D   Cancer induction. By the linear no-threshold model, there is no radiation dose free from stochastic effects such as the (low) risk of cancer induction. The doses received in diagnostic studies such as FDG PET/CT are ordinarily below the thresholds for deterministic effects (tissue reactions) such as erythema, epilation, and sterility.

2. C   Effective dose. The stochastic risk of a radiation exposure is, in part, related to the amount and types of radiation involved, the distribution in the organs of the body, and the radiation sensitivity of organs. These factors are reflected in the effective dose. Effective dose can be a useful gauge of risk for the purposes of radiation protection; however, it is important to note that it is not useful for determining risk for individual patients.

3. B   They are neutron deficient and undergo beta-plus decay. Medical cyclotrons bombard stable target material with protons, producing neutron-deficient radioisotopes that decay by beta-plus decay (positron emission) or electron capture. Most radionuclides used in PET imaging are cyclotron produced.

4. B   Lower activity of ^{99m}Tc pertechnetate for each elution, but higher total activity yield for the day. Figure 8.21 shows that at 8 hours, ^{99m}Tc has regenerated to more than half the activity that would be obtained at 24 hours. The sum of the activities for the three 8-hour elutions will be greater than that of a single elution obtained at 24 hours.

Nuclear Medicine: Radiation Detection and Nuclear Imaging

Jennifer L. Scheler, MD, and Nabeel Porbandarwala, MD

LEARNING OBJECTIVES

1. List the components of a gas-filled detector.
2. Describe each region of the voltage response curve.
3. Describe the operation of a dose calibrator.
4. List the differences between an ion survey meter and a Geiger-Mueller (GM) survey meter.
5. Describe the relationship between gamma photon energy and the scintillation event.
6. List the function of the following components of a scintillation detector: crystal, photomultiplier tube (PMT), and pulse height analyzer.
7. Describe energy spectra and energy resolution.
8. Describe the principles of nuclear counting statistics and their application to counting measurements.
9. List detector quality control (QC) tests and their frequencies.
10. Describe the components of a scintillation camera.
11. Describe the role of collimators in imaging of gamma photons by scintigraphy and single photon emission computed tomography (SPECT).
12. Explain the importance of attenuation correction in SPECT and positron emission tomography (PET) and how it is typically performed.
13. Describe the principle of annihilation coincidence detection (ACD) in PET imaging.
14. Explain the difference between 2D and 3D modes of PET scans.

RADIATION DETECTION

Detecting and measuring radiation is essential to diagnostic imaging and nonimaging applications. Radiation detectors rely on the interaction of radiation with matter. As radiation interacts with the atoms or molecules of a material, energy is transferred to it, resulting in *ionization* and *excitation*.

Ionization occurs when the transferred energy is great enough to remove an orbital electron from an atom or molecule, producing an ion pair—a negatively charged electron (anion) and a positively charged atom or molecule (cation). Excitation is the transfer of energy to a *bound* electron in atoms or molecules, including crystals, which are often used in detectors.

Radiation detectors can be grouped into the following categories: gas-filled detectors, scintillation detectors, and semiconductor detectors.

Gas-filled detectors

Basics

A rudimentary model includes a gas-filled chamber and an electric circuit. As radiation passes through the gas, molecules in the gas are ionized, forming ion pairs. When high voltage is applied between two areas of the chamber, the positive ions are attracted to the negative side of the detector (*cathode*), and the free electrons travel to the positive side (*anode*). Often, the cathode is the wall or coating of the chamber and the anode is the wire in the chamber. Electrons move through the circuit to the cathode and reunite with the cations, generating a current. This small current is measured and displayed as a signal. With more radiation, there is greater current. Common gas-filled detectors include ionization chambers, proportional chambers, and GM counters (Figure 9.1).

The type of gas within the chamber determines the needed energy for ionization. Typically, 20 to 45 electron volts (eV) is required to form an ion pair. The number of electrons measured depends on several factors, such as the radiation being measured, energy of the radiation, geometric configuration of the detector, and gas composition and volume within the chamber, as well as the pressure and temperature of the gas. The most important determinant, however, is the applied voltage between the anode and cathode.

Voltage response curve

The voltage response curve for a gas-filled detector illustrates the relationship between the applied voltage and the amount of

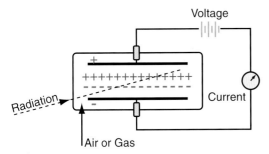

FIG. 9.1 ● **The schematic of a gas-filled radiation detector.** Reprinted with permission from Chandra R, Rahmim A. *Nuclear Medicine Physics: The Basics.* 8th ed. Philadelphia, PA: Wolters Kluwer; 2017.

electrical charge collected, or signal, after a single photon or particle interaction. The shape of the curve is best understood by examining each of its six regions in detail.

- *Recombination region*: If the applied voltage is low, then the electrons move so slowly that they can recombine with ionized gas molecules. With increasing voltage, more ions are gathered and fewer reunite, resulting in increasing current. No usable detectors operate in this range.
- *Ionization (saturation) region*: Most ion pairs are collected and further voltage increase does not result in increased current. There is a wide range over which the response is relatively flat, and the size of the signal is proportional to the rate at which photons or particles are interacting with the detector. Dose calibrator and ionization survey meter operate in this range.
- *Proportional region*: At higher voltages, the electrons are accelerated to such a degree that they produce further ionization, known as *gas multiplication*, resulting in amplified current. As applied voltage is increased, amplification increases. Proportional detectors operate in this region.

- *Limited proportionality region*: In this region, the positive ions formed from radiation interaction with the gas molecules slowly drift to the cathode and the electrons are attracted to the cloud of positive ions as well as to the anode. Gas amplification decreases and there is no longer a linear relationship with increasing voltage, limiting radiation detection.
- *GM region*: Gas multiplication extends the length of the anode and further current amplification cannot occur. The amount of electrical charge collected from each radiation interaction is the same, independent of the amount of energy collected at the detector.
- *Continuous discharge region*: At voltages greater than the GM region, gas-filled detectors continuously discharge and cannot be utilized (Figure 9.2).

Current mode and pulse mode operation

Electrons formed in the gas-filled chamber travel to the anode. The number of electrons at the anode correlates to the amount of radioactivity or strength of the radiation field. Most detectors generate an electrical signal after each photon or particle interaction. Signal modification by electronic circuitry includes amplification, processing, or data storage. **Pulse mode** and **current mode** are two main ways a signal is processed.

In **pulse mode**, a signal from each photon or particle interaction is processed individually. Each interaction must be separated by a sufficient time interval to render a separate signal electrical pulse, termed the *dead time* of a detector system. If an interaction occurs during this dead time, its signal is lost. At higher interaction rates, the percentage of interactions lost from dead-time effects is greater. Dead time varies depending on the detector system. Pulse mode detectors require a lower rate of radiation interactions than do current mode detectors. Geiger counter, semiconductor detectors, and scintillation detectors operate in pulse mode.

FIG. 9.2 ● **A typical voltage response curve for a gas-filled detector.** Note the six different regions. Reprinted with permission from Bushberg JT, Seibert JA, Leidholdt EM, Boone JM. *Essential Physics of Medical Imaging.* 3rd ed. Philadelphia, PA: Wolters Kluwer Health/Lippincott Williams & Wilkins; 2012.

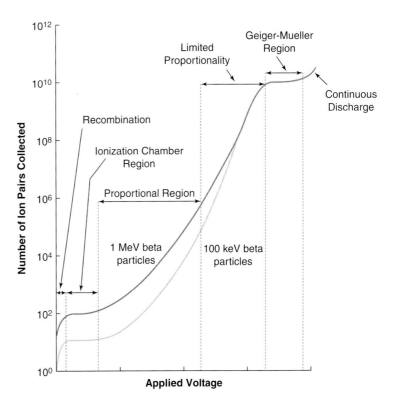

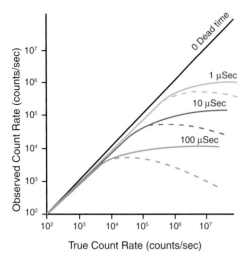

FIG. 9.3 ● **The observed count rate as a function of the true count rate for detectors with different dead times.** Note the differences between nonparalyzable (solid lines) and paralyzable detector (dashed lines) in their behaviors. Reprinted with permission from Chandra R, Rahmim A. *Nuclear Medicine Physics: The Basics*. 8th ed. Philadelphia, PA: Wolters Kluwer; 2017.

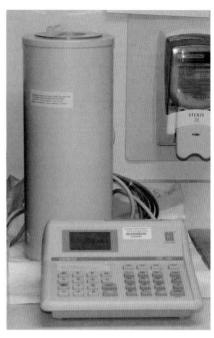

FIG. 9.4 ● **The photograph of a dose calibrator, a gas-filled ionization chamber used to measure radioactivity.** Reprinted with permission from Kanne JP. *Quality and Safety in Medical Imaging: The Essentials*. Philadelphia, PA: Wolters Kluwer; 2016.

Detectors operated in pulse mode can be further divided into **paralyzable** and **nonparalyzable** systems. In a **paralyzable** system, an interaction occurring in the dead time will extend the dead time. At very high interaction rates, the dead time will lengthen infinitely, and a paralyzable system will not detect subsequent interactions after the first interaction, falsely lowering the count rate. In a **nonparalyzable** system, an interaction occurring during the dead time is not recorded but does not extend the dead time.

In practice, dead time ranges from about 2 μs in a scintillation detector, to about 5 μs in a gamma camera, to about 50 to 100 μs in a Geiger counter. One should be aware that the true count may vary from the detector records, particularly at high count rates (Figure 9.3).

In **current mode**, the signals from separate interactions are averaged together, forming a net current signal. Detectors operating in current mode utilize a power supply that constantly keeps the anode and cathode charged to full capacity. As electrons produced from radiation-induced ionization neutralize some of the charge at the capacitor, electrons flow from the power supply to restore charge. This electron flow is the measured current, which is based on time-averaged numbered ionizations per second. These detectors, like dose calibrators and ionization survey meters, encounter high interaction rates and operate in the ionization range of the voltage response curve. They often operate in current mode to avoid dead-time losses. At low levels of radiation, current mode detectors are susceptible to statistical variations.

Dose calibrators

Dose calibrators assay activities of patient radiopharmaceutical doses. Federal and state regulations require that doses of X- and gamma ray–emitting radiopharmaceuticals be measured before patient administration. It is calibrated in units of Curies (Ci) and/or becquerels (Bq) (Figure 9.4).

The majority of dose calibrators are sealed-well-type ionization chambers containing pressurized argon gas ($Z = 18$) to increase sensitivity. These detectors operate in the ionization range of the voltage response curve, so all primary electrons from ionization in the gas chamber travel to the anode without gas amplification. Current mode operation allows for steady state to be achieved within a couple of seconds, and the voltage supply is approximately 150 V.

The surrounding cylindrical lead shielding reduces exposure to the operator and minimizes contamination from nearby external radioactive sources. There is gamma-ray backscatter from the lead into the ionization chamber, causing increased ionization events and, therefore, increased current. Because the calibrator is calibrated with shielding present, the detector's readings are valid only with shield in place. The calibrator does not directly measure activity and cannot discriminate between different radioisotopes. Instead, it measures the intensity of the emitted radiation by the radiopharmaceutical dose. The manufacturer determines calibration factors relating the magnitude of the signal from the detector to the activity for specific radioisotopes. This calibration curve is developed using a series of long-lived radioisotope standards from the National Institute of Standards and Testing (NIST). From this curve, conversion factors for the short-lived radioisotopes used in clinical practice are determined and programmed into the instrument. The technologist selects the radioisotope being measured, the appropriate conversion factor is applied, and the instrument displays the measured activity. Importantly, if the wrong isotope is selected, the measurement will be inaccurate. Dose calibrators are accurate down to about 20 μCi. If measurement is desired below this limit, a sodium iodide scintillation detector should be utilized.

Dose calibrators have an electronic means of zeroing the background when the well is empty. This process should be performed at least once per day and ideally throughout the day. The chamber contains a removable liner to protect it from potential contamination. Liners and ladles can be cleaned if contamination is suspected.

Pure beta-emitting radionuclides usually cannot be measured directly in a dose calibrator because the particle cannot penetrate the liner and wall of the chamber to interact with the pressurized gas. Nevertheless, most calibrators can estimate the dose using a programmed correction table on the basis of the Bremsstrahlung emissions of the radioisotope.

Ionization survey meters

Also called ion chambers or exposure rate meters, ionization survey meters typically measure exposure rates in radiation fields. They are battery powered (50-500 V) gas-filled detectors that function in the ionization region of the voltage response curve and are operated in current mode. Various gases can be used in the ionization chamber. However, most ionization survey meters utilize air in the chamber, and the material of the chamber walls has an effective atomic number comparable to air. In this way, the generated current is proportional to the *exposure rate* (exposure is the amount of electrical charge produced per mass of air). Primarily, these portable survey meters are used for radiation protection purposes and can detect exposure rates over a large range.

In very high radiation fields, there can be signal loss from the recombination of ions in the chamber before they contribute to the generated current. To minimize this loss, these detectors are modified to have a small gas volume, low gas density, or a high applied voltage. They have a thin entrance window made of a low atomic number material, like mylar or mica, that has a sliding or removable cover. If gamma-emitting radiation is to be detected, then the cover is left in place, thereby excluding particles like beta or alpha particles. If particles or low-energy gamma photons are to be measured, then the cover is removed (Figure 9.5).

Ionization survey meters and GM survey meters/Geiger counters often have overlapping uses; however, there are notable distinctions between these types of instruments. Ionization survey meters function best with higher radiation fields and are accurate to a lower limit of 1 mR/h. They are ideally suited for monitoring patients receiving therapeutic doses of radiopharmaceuticals or radioactive implants, but are not effective for radioactive contamination surveys. Because they have a fairly constant response over a wide range of gamma energies, they are useful for measuring radiation fields containing multiple radioisotopes.

Proportional counters

In contrast to ion chambers, proportional counters operate in the *proportional range* of the voltage response curve and rely on gas multiplication. These chambers are designed to optimize gas multiplication using gases with low electron affinity, like xenon and argon. The primary advantage of proportional counters over ion chambers is that the electrical signal generated by a single radiation event is much greater. Because of their low efficiency for higher X-rays and gamma rays used in medical imaging, they are usually restricted to research applications measuring nonpenetrating radiations, like alpha and beta particles.

GM survey meters/Geiger counters

GM counters are gas-filled detectors designed for maximum gas multiplication effect and function in the GM region of the voltage response curve. They need minimal additional signal amplification and are primarily used as survey meters for radiation protection purposes because they can detect minimal amounts of gamma contamination.

GM counters are operated in pulse mode, and the units of measurement can be displayed as counts per minute (cpm), exposure units of mR/h, or both. Calibration for exposure units is performed using a fixed gamma-ray source. In this way, the reading will vary with source strength at energy. If the measured radiation field contains gamma photons of differing energies, the conversion to mR/h is not accurate for all of the gamma rays and displayed readings are only approximations. They also cannot discriminate between radiation events of different energies based on pulse size, because all pulses are the same size. Therefore, GM counters should not be used as precise dose-rate meters. Rather, they are better suited in a qualitative or semiquantitative manner to detect small amounts of gamma photons (Figure 9.6).

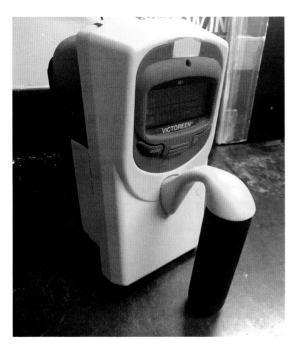

FIG. 9.5 ● The photograph of an ionization chamber–based survey meter.

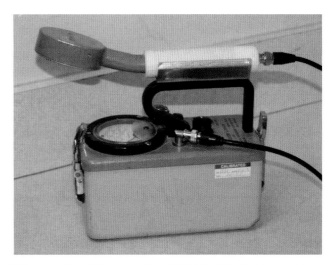

FIG. 9.6 ● **The photograph of a Geiger-Mueller survey meter.** The detector in the photo, in the pancake shape, is attached to handle and connected to the electrometer; the dial reads in counts per minute (cpm) or milliroentgens per hour (mR/h). Reprinted with permission from Kanne JP. *Quality and Safety in Medical Imaging: The Essentials*. Philadelphia, PA: Wolters Kluwer; 2016.

GM survey meters can be battery operated using direct current or can be powered from a wall outlet, converting alternating current to direct current internally. Often, the gas in the ion chamber is argon or helium. These meters are usually portable and are relatively sturdy. Some have audible alarms, allowing the operator to "hear" the radiation detection. They have a logarithmic scale permitting detection over a wide range, and the detector can be pancake or tube shaped depending on its use.

As with ionization survey meters, GM counters have a thin entrance window to allow radiation particles to enter, protected by a screen or cover. The cover must be removed if particles are to be detected in addition to gamma photons. These windows are easily damaged, so the survey meter should be handled with care. Otherwise, the ion chamber gas may escape, and the instrument may become useless.

GM counters have long dead times and are infrequently used when accurate measurements are needed at count rates greater than a few hundred counts per second. Portable GM survey meters can become paralyzed in very high radiation fields, rendering a zero reading. Instead, ionization chamber survey meters should be employed in high gamma-ray or high X-ray fields.

Quality control

Radiation detection systems are subject to a variety of malfunctions, resulting in their performance deterioration either acutely or gradually. For this reason, a nuclear medicine department must rigorously adhere to a QC program. A QC program also includes documentation of these practices and organized record keeping in chronologic order.

Often, QC tests are not performed with short-lived radioisotopes used clinically. Instead, long-lived surrogate radioisotope standards are employed. These standards must be traceable to the NIST to ensure the accuracy of its calibrated activity. Frequently, standards can be used for months to years because they are long-lived. Reference standards must be tested annually for radioactivity leakage (wipe tested), and a current list of these sources must be maintained. These long-lived sources remain radioactive even after they are no longer useful as a standard. They must be returned to their manufacturer or be disposed of as radioactive waste through an authorized third party.

Common Long-Lived Radioisotopes Used in Instrument QC

Refer to Table 9.1 for a list of commonly used radioisotopes.

QC for Ionization Survey Meters and GM Survey Meters

Generally, QC tests for survey meters include daily battery check with a readout displaying whether the supply voltage is within acceptable range. Background exposure or counting rate should be checked daily in a nonradioactive area to ensure the instrument is not contaminated. These meters should be assessed daily for constancy of response by measuring the exposure rate or counting rate of a reference source. Readings from day to day should be similar, to within about 10%. Accuracy testing of the survey meter is performed at installation, yearly and after service/repair by a commercial calibration facility or the institutional radiation safety office.

QC for Dose Calibrators

Dose calibrator *constancy* must be tested daily using an NIST-traceable reference source, like ^{57}Co, ^{133}Ba, ^{68}Ge, or ^{137}Cs. Daily activity readings should fall within $\pm10\%$ agreement.

Quarterly assessment of activity *linearity* can be performed using the decay method or the shield method. Decay method utilizes an independently calibrated ^{99m}Tc source that is assayed at 12-hour time points over 3 days. The measured activities are plotted on a semilogarithmic graph with time in the *x*-axis. For each time point, the difference between the measured activity and the best-fit straight line at that point should be less than 10%. The shield method uses a set of commercially available lead sleeves of varying thickness that simulate decay via attenuation. Before use, these sleeves must be calibrated by comparing with the decay method.

Accuracy is checked annually using a reference standard traceable to the NIST. It requires three separate measurements of the source, which are averaged and compared to the known activity. This procedure is repeated with two or three sources of differing gamma energies. The reading must be within $\pm5\%$ of the reference activity to be accurate.

Geometry testing occurs at installation and after repair or adjustment and is performed by the manufacturer. A small volume of the radiopharmaceutical, such as ^{99m}Tc pertechnetate, is placed

---

Table 9.1 COMMONLY USED LONG-LIVED RADIOISOTOPES AND THEIR QC

Radioisotope	Half-Life	Energy of Principal X-ray or Gamma Ray (keV)	QC Application
^{57}Co	272 d	122 (86%)	• Well counter constancy and accuracy • Dose calibrator constancy and accuracy • Gamma camera uniformity
^{68}Ge	287 d	511 (178%)	• Well counter constancy and accuracy • Dose calibrator constancy and accuracy • Positron emission tomography scanner response
^{133}Ba	10.7 y	356 (62%)	• Well counter constancy and accuracy • Dose calibrator constancy and accuracy
^{137}Cs	30 y	662 (86%)	• Well counter constancy and accuracy • Dose calibrator constancy and accuracy

Abbreviation: QC, quality control.

in a vial or syringe and its activity is measured after each dilution. If the volume affects the measurements by more than ±10%, a correction factor must be established.

Molybdenum-99 Concentration Testing

With ^{99}Mo/^{99m}Tc generator elution, there is a potential for ^{99}Mo contamination in the eluate. If the eluate is administered to a patient, the patient will receive increased radiation dose (^{99}Mo emits high-energy beta particles and has a half-life of 66 hours). Furthermore, the image quality can be compromised by the high-energy ^{99}Mo gamma photons. The limit at time of administration is 0.15 µCi of ^{99}Mo per 1 mCi of ^{99m}Tc. The first elution of the generator must be assayed for ^{99}Mo concentration.

The concentration of ^{99}Mo is usually measured with a dose calibrator using a lead container provided by the manufacturer. The walls of the container will prevent 140 keV gamma photons from ^{99m}Tc but are insufficient to block the higher gamma photons from ^{99}Mo (740 and 778 keV).

^{82}Sr and ^{85}Sr Concentration Testing

PET myocardial perfusion imaging can be performed using ^{82}Rb chloride, which is acquired from an ^{82}Sr/^{82}Rb generator. With generator elution, ^{82}Sr or ^{85}Sr contamination can occur in the eluate. The limit at the time of administration is 0.02 kBq of ^{82}Sr or 0.2 kBq of ^{85}Sr per 1 MBq ^{82}Rb. A dose calibrator is used to measure the contaminants, following the manufacturer instructions in the package insert.

Recommended QC Tests for Gas-Filled Detectors

Refer to Table 9.2 for the recommended QC tests for gas-filled detectors

Scintillation detectors

Scintillation detectors are an essential category of radiation detectors used in nuclear medicine. They have important advantages over gas-filled detectors. Most are solid materials, like crystals, allowing for many more interactions with gamma photons compared to gas-filled detectors. They also provide the means to measure the energy of the radiation interaction, distinguishing energies from different radioisotopes, which is not possible with gas-filled detectors. Scintillation detectors are used in both imaging and nonimaging applications in nuclear medicine, including thyroid probes, well counters, gamma cameras, and PET cameras.

Basics

A *scintillator* is any material that emits a visible or ultraviolet (UV) photon when an excited electron in the material returns to its ground state. Most scintillation detectors use PMTs to convert visible or UV light to an electrical signal, which is then amplified.

Ionizing radiation interacts with a scintillator to excite electrons to a higher energy level. As these electrons return to their lower energy state, visible or UV light is emitted. There can be more than one manner of light emission, each having its own decay constant. *Luminescence* is defined as the emission of light after excitation. *Fluorescence* is the prompt emission of light after excitation, and *phosphorescence* (afterglow) is the delayed emission of light.

Current mode operation of the scintillation detector does not allow for the separation of the signal from fluorescence from the phosphorescence caused by prior radiation interactions. However, with pulse mode operation, the effect of phosphorescence on the signal is minimized. Circuitry is able to distinguish the prompt rise and fall of the fluorescent emission signal from the gradual decline of the phosphorescent emission signal from previous interactions.

Desired characteristics of scintillator materials include the following:

- High conversion efficiency, or the fraction of deposited energy converted to visible or UV radiation
- Short decay times of excited states, resulting in prompt fluorescent emission
- Transparency to its own emissions, minimizing radiation reabsorption
- Frequency spectrum of the emitted visible or UV radiation comparable to the spectral sensitivity of the light receptor (PMT)
- Large mass attenuation coefficient (µ), high atomic number, and high density, for good X-ray and gamma-ray detection efficiency
- Durability, moisture resistance, and inexpensiveness

For all scintillators, the amount of light or UV emission after a radiation interaction increases with the amount of energy deposited by the interaction. For this reason, scintillators can be operated in pulse mode as spectrometers. The energy resolution, or the capability to discriminate between photons or particles of differing energies, is mostly dependent on the conversion efficiency; the higher the conversion efficiency, the greater the energy resolution.

Table 9.2 COMMONLY USED GAS-FILLED DETECTORS AND THEIR QUALITY CONTROL

Instrument	Test	Recommended Frequency
Dose calibrator	• Constancy • Activity linearity • Accuracy • Geometry	• Daily • Quarterly • Annually • At installation and after repair
Ionization survey meter Geiger-Mueller survey meter	• Battery functionality • Contamination • Constancy • Accuracy/calibration	• Daily • Daily • Daily • Installation, annually, and post repair

All of these tests should be performed if a device has been serviced.

Organic scintillators

A variety of materials can be used as scintillators. In organic scintillators, the scintillation is an inherent property of the molecular structure. However, organic scintillators are not utilized in medical imaging, because their low atomic numbers and densities make them inefficient for X-ray and gamma-ray detection.

Inorganic scintillators/crystals

In contrast to organic scintillators, inorganic crystals are often used in medical imaging and nonimaging applications. Their scintillation is a property of their crystalline structure, not the individual elements. These materials have high atomic numbers and densities, superior for X-ray and gamma-ray detection. These crystals are grown with impurity elements to cause disturbances in the crystal matrix. These "activation centers" allow for electron excitation, affect the frequency or color of the light emission, modify promptness of fluorescence, and minimize reabsorption in the crystal.

Most nuclear medicine applications use sodium iodide activated with thallium, NaI(Tl). The crystal is coupled with PMTs and operated in pulse mode in scintillation cameras, thyroid probes, and gamma well counters (Figure 9.7).

NaI(Tl) crystal has a high density ($\rho = 3.67$ g/cm^3) and high atomic number (iodine, $Z = 53$), allowing for good photoelectric absorption. It has a high efficiency for detecting X-rays and gamma rays in the 70 to 250 keV range, which includes most medical radiopharmaceuticals. It has high conversion efficiency with about 13% of the energy deposited at the crystal converted

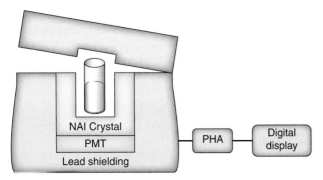

FIG. 9.7 ● **A gamma well counter with the use of a sodium iodide (NaI) crystal.** The scintillator is connected to a photomultiplier tube (PMT), for signal amplification, and a pulse height analyzer (PHA), for spectrum analysis. Reprinted with permission from Brant WE, Helms CA. *Fundamentals of Diagnostic Radiology.* 3rd ed. Philadelphia, PA: Lippincott Williams & Wilkins; 2007.

to light, rendering superior energy resolution. Its fast light emission allows for pulse mode operation at high interaction rates (>100 000/second). It is transparent to its own scintillation emissions with minimal reabsorption, even in large crystals. Crystals can be grown as large plates, useful in imaging equipment.

Its main disadvantages include its susceptibility to mechanical and thermal stresses and its tendency to absorb moisture. At higher gamma energies, the primary interaction is Compton scatter and detection efficiency decreases.

For the detection of the 511 keV emissions from positron emitters, denser scintillators are required. Early PET detectors included bismuth germinate ($Bi_4Ge_3O_{12}$, or "BGO") crystals. Lutetium oxyorthosilicate (Lu_2SiO_4O, or "LSO"), lutetium yttrium oxyorthosilicate ($Lu_xY_{2-x}SiO_4O$, or "LYSO"), and gadolinium oxyorthosilicate (Gd_2SiO_4O, or "GSO"), all activated with cerium, are used in newer PET/CT scanners. These materials have high densities and high atomic numbers, but they have even greater conversion efficiencies and faster light emission compared to BGO.

Photomultiplier tubes

PMTs serve two purposes—conversion of light or UV emission into electrical signal and signal amplification. Thyroid probe and well counters each have one PMT, whereas gamma cameras have many PMTs, permitting both energy and position determination (Figure 9.8).

As depicted in Figure 9.8, a PMT is an evacuated glass tube containing a photocathode, a series of 10 to 12 electrodes (dynodes), and an anode. The photocathode is the front surface of the entrance window of the PMT coated with a photoemissive material that ejects electrons (photoelectrons) when struck by light photons, usually metal alloys with extra electrons, like bialkali antimonide compounds (K_2CsSb and Na_2CsSb). Conversion efficiency is about 1 to 3 photoelectrons per 10 light photons. The focusing grid is an electrical field that directs the emitted photoelectrons to the first dynode. It is critical that the vacuum of the PMT is maintained so that no electrons are lost via gas molecule interactions. PMTs are also shielded from magnetic fields so that electron trajectory is not altered.

The first dynode is a curved metal plate a short distance from the photocathode, and it is coated with a material having high secondary emission properties. The dynode is maintained at a positive voltage (+100 to 200 V) relative to the photocathode, attracting the photoelectrons to it. The accelerated photoelectron strikes the dynode, ejecting about five secondary electrons from it. Each dynode is maintained at successively higher voltages (+100 V increments), resulting in greater electron multiplication.

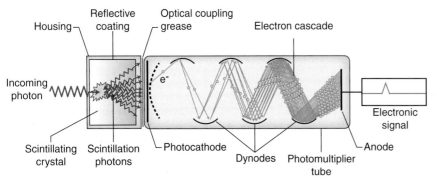

FIG. 9.8 ● **Diagram of a photomultiplier tube (PMT) coupled with a scintillator crystal for gamma photon detection.** PMT receives the scintillation photons from the crystal, converts them to electrons, and sends the electrons through a number of dynodes for amplification. A much larger number of electrons PMT at its anode and gets measured as the produced signal. Reprinted with permission from Klein J, Vinson EN, Brant WE, Helms CA. *Brant and Helms' Fundamentals of Diagnostic Radiology.* 5th ed. Philadelphia, PA: Wolters Kluwer Health; 2018.

The total amplification of the PMT is equal to the product of the individual multiplication at each dynode. For example, if a PMT has 10 dynodes and the multiplication at each step is 5, then the total amplification is

$$5^{10}, \text{ or approximately } 10\ 000\ 000.$$

In this manner, a large electrical current is produced despite a relatively weak light emission. Amplification can be modified by changing the applied voltage to the PMT. PMTs require a high voltage supply, which must remain stable given the sensitivity of the electron multiplication factor to dynode voltage changes.

Between the back of the crystal and the PMT, there is usually a light pipe consisting of quartz or lucite, reflecting back any wide-angled scintillation photons toward the PMT photocathode. Optical coupling grease minimizes scintillation photon loss by preventing reflections at component interfaces. If the grease degrades, fewer scintillation photons will reach the PMT.

Preamplifier and amplifier

The preamplifier is directly attached to the PMT to lessen signal distortion, and augments the output signal. The amplifier further increases the signal as well as shapes the pulse for the pulse height analyzer (PHA).

Pulse height analyzer

The PHA determines the height of the pulse generated by the PMT, which is proportional to the energy absorbed in the crystal from gamma photon interaction. However, with each step in this conversion process, gamma photon to light photon to electrons, there is inefficiency and energy loss. For this reason, the pulse height, or measured output, is not exactly proportional to the incidental gamma ray, and instead is a distribution of pulse heights around the true gamma ray energy. Such broadening of energy peaks in the measured spectra poses challenges for discrimination between gamma photons of similar energies (Figure 9.9).

There are two types of PHAs: the single-channel analyzer (SCA) and the multichannel analyzer (MCA).

SCA Systems

Signal pulses from the PMT are routed to the preamplifier and then the amplifier, which augment the signal. The pulses then travel to the SCA. The operator can set a lower voltage level (LL) and an upper voltage level (UL). If a signal pulse is above the UL or is below the LL, the SCA does not accept the pulse. If the pulse falls within the set voltage levels, the SCA produces a single logic pulse of a fixed amplitude and duration. These output pulses can drive counters, rate meters, and other circuits. SCA extracts the gamma-ray energy information from the voltage signal and, based on that energy, accepts or rejects that pulse. The SCA output is a series of binary logic pulses (yes/no or 1/0) that can be counted but contain no additional information about the gamma photons they represent.

MCA Systems

The major disadvantage of an SCA system is the rejection of gamma interactions that do not fall between the LL and UL voltage levels. In contrast, the MCA depicts all energy interactions on an energy graph, or *pulse height spectrum*. The number of

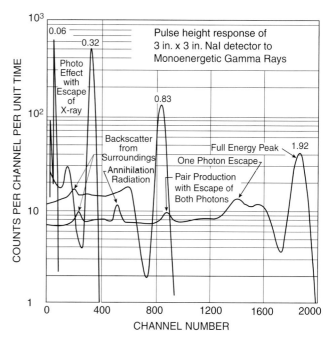

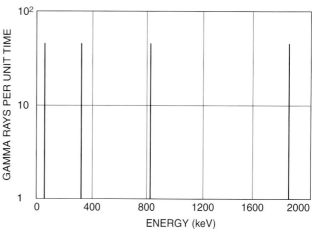

FIG. 9.9 ● **Peak broadening demonstrated by pulse height distributions when measuring monoenergetic gamma-ray sources of 0.06, 0.32, 0.83, and 1.92 MeV with a 3 × 3 inch² NaI(Tl) detector.** From Heath RL. *Scintillation Spectrometry, Gamma-Ray Spectrum Catalogue.* 2nd ed. USAEC Report IDO-16880-1. Springfield, VA: National Technical Information Service; 1964.

detected events, or counts, is graphed against the amplitude of those events, or gamma energy (Figure 9.10).

The MCA system has an analog-to-digital converter (ADC), which measures and sorts the incoming pulses by their amplitudes. Typically, the pulse amplitude range is 0 to 10 V, sorted by the ADC into separate bins, or channels. For example, a 1000-channel analyzer would divide the 0 to 10 V amplitude range into a 1000 channels, each 0.01 V wide (10/1000). Channel 1 would correspond to 0 to 0.01 V, channel 2 would correspond to 0.01 to 0.02 V, channel 3 would correspond to 0.02 to 0.03 V, etc. The ADC would assign a signal pulse to a specific channel number, converting an analog pulse into a digital value. The MCA memory counts and stores the number of pulses within each channel. The pulse height spectrum can then be displayed as counts per channel versus the channel number, or energy.

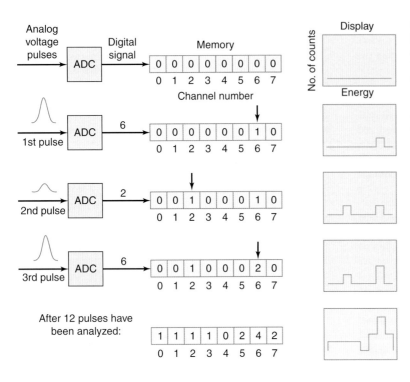

FIG. 9.10 ● Illustration of how a multichannel analyzer works. After an analog signal is digitized by the analog-to-digital converter (ADC), the resulting digital signal can be sorted into one of several bins (8 bins in this example) depending on the amplitude of the signal; with many analog pulses processed in such a way, an energy spectrum can be formed, revealing the energy distribution of the measured signals. Reprinted with permission from Bushberg JT, Seibert JA, Leidholdt EM, Boone JM. Radiation detection and management. In: *The Essentials Physics of Medical Imaging.* Philadelphia, PA: Wolters Kluwer Health/Lippincott Williams & Wilkins; 2012.

Energy spectra

The generated spectrum from the MCA has several identifiable peaks. The right-most peak in the spectrum is the *photopeak*. It corresponds to the gamma rays that have undergone photoelectric conversion in the scintillation crystal. Peaks to the left of the photopeak represent photons that did not deposit their full energy on the crystal, many of which have undergone Compton scatter effects (Figure 9.11).

The photopeak (*A*) is the total absorption of the 140 keV photons by the crystal. The iodine escape peak (*B*) is due to the 140 keV photons interacting with the iodine in the crystal and causing iodine K-shell X-rays (28-33 keV) to escape. Photopeak (*C*) is due to the absorption of K-shell X-rays from the lead shielding. Lower energies represent Compton scattering with the scattered photons escaping the crystal.

An energy window can be set, centered on the photopeak, to exclude the other energy peaks. The window is specified as a percentage of the photopeak energy. A narrow window (2%-5%) would be used for calibration and a wider window (15%-20%) for imaging and other clinical applications.

Energy resolution

Energy resolution describes the detector's ability to discriminate photons of closely spaced energies. The width of the photopeak is a measure of the energy resolution. Because of statistical fluctuations in the detection process, the peak has a spread around

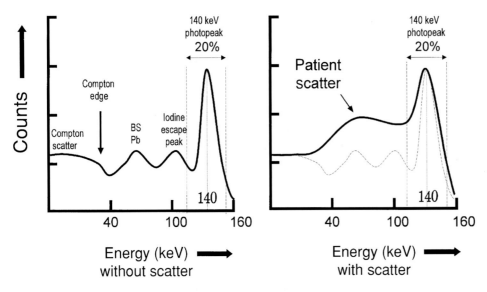

FIG. 9.11 ● The pulse height spectra of ^{99m}Tc, with and without patient scatter. Note that, in addition to the 140 keV photopeak, there are other portions of the measured spectrum caused by Compton scatter, backscatter (BS), iodine escape peak, patient scatter, and others. Reprinted with permission from Brant WE, Helms CA. *Fundamentals of Diagnostic Radiology.* 3rd ed. Philadelphia, PA: Lippincott Williams & Wilkins; 2007.

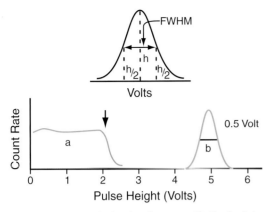

FIG. 9.12 ● **Energy resolution is often quantitatively determined by the measurement of full width at half maximum (FWHM), as is demonstrated at the top of the figure, where *h* is the height of the measured photopeak.** Reprinted with permission from Chandra R, Rahmim A. *Nuclear Medicine Physics: The Basics.* 8th ed. Philadelphia, PA: Wolters Kluwer; 2017.

a mean value. The spread is the full width at half maximum (FWHM) of the photopeak (Figure 9.12).

$$\text{Energy resolution} = \frac{\text{FWHM}}{\text{Pulse amplitude of the photopeak}} \times 100\%$$

The energy resolution can be tracked to assess detector performance over time.

Count-rate effects

If two photon or particle interactions occur within a very brief interval, the detector may produce a single-signal pulse with amplitude equal to their sum. This event is termed *pulse pileup*. Pileups between photopeaks and lower energy events lead to widening of the photopeak. Operating a pulse height spectrometer at a high count rate leads to pulse pileup, distortion of the spectrum, increased dead-time effects, and loss of counts (Figure 9.13).

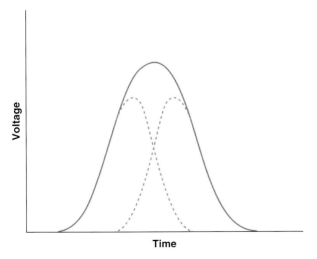

FIG. 9.13 ● **The pulse pileup effect.** When two individual events close to each other in time are detected, the detector, because of its limited response time, may detect a single pulse (solid line) as the sum of the signals from the two actual pulses (dashed lines). Reprinted with permission from Bushberg JT, Seibert JA, Leidholdt EM, Boone JM. *Essential Physics of Medical Imaging.* 3rd ed. Philadelphia, PA: Wolters Kluwer Health/Lippincott Williams & Wilkins; 2012.

Scintillation detector applications

Most scintillation detectors fall within two categories: probe configuration and well configuration. Probe-type detectors are used to measure radioactivity from a specific organ, like the thyroid. Well-type detectors are utilized to measure radioactivity in samples.

Sodium Iodide Thyroid Probe

Thyroid probe is used to measure the uptake of ^{123}I or ^{131}I by the thyroid in patients and to monitor for ^{131}I activity in technologists who handle these radiopharmaceuticals. The probe comprises a cylindrical NaI(Tl) crystal coupled to a PMT, which is connected to a preamplifier. The probe has surrounding lead shielding with a lead collimator and is connected to a high voltage power supply and either an SCA or MCA system (Figure 9.14).

Uptake measurements can be performed using a one- or two-capsule method. A neck phantom (lucite cylinder with a central cavity for the radioiodine capsule) is needed.

In the two-capsule method, the two capsules should have similar activities. Each capsule is placed in the neck phantom and counted separately. The patient then swallows the capsule, and the other capsule remains "the standard." The patient's neck is counted at 4 to 6 hours and then at 24 hours after swallowing. Each time the patient's neck is counted, a thigh count is obtained for the same length of time to approximate nonthyroid neck uptake, and a background count is acquired. For each measurement, the distance of the probe to the source should remain the same. Every time the patient's neck is counted; the second capsule should be placed in the neck phantom and measured.

$$\text{Uptake} = \frac{\text{Thyroid counts} - \text{Thigh counts}}{\text{Standard counts in phantom} - \text{Background counts}}$$

$$\times \frac{\text{Initial counts of standard capsule in phantom}}{\text{Intial counts of patient's capsule in phantom}}$$

In the single-capsule method, the capsule is counted in the neck phantom and is then swallowed by the patient. The patient's neck and thigh are counted at 4 to 6 hours and then 24 hours post swallowing. A background count is also obtained. The time of capsule administration and neck counts are recorded.

$$\text{Uptake} = \frac{\text{Thyroid counts} - \text{Thigh counts}}{\text{Counts of capsule in phantom} - \text{Background counts}} \times e^{0.693t/T_{1/2}}$$

In the given equation, $T_{1/2}$ is the physical half-life of the radionuclide, and t is the time between the count of the capsule in the phantom and the neck count. The one-capsule method is cheaper and relies on fewer measurements, but it is more prone to technologist error, dead-time effects, and instrument instability.

Sodium Iodide Well Counter

NaI(Tl) well counter has clinical applications such as Schilling tests (vitamin B_{12} absorption) and plasma or red blood cell volume measurements. In addition, it is used for wipe surveys to assess for radioactive contamination. It is a single-cylindrical NaI(Tl) crystal with a hole at one end for sample insertion, typically standard-sized test tubes (Figure 9.15).

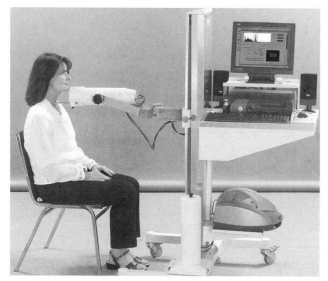

FIG. 9.14 ● Thyroid uptake probe system. A radiation-detecting probe is placed with its open aperture exposed to the patient's thyroid gland region. Radioactive counts from the neck, mainly from the thyroid gland, can be counted with the total counts recorded into a computer system with a printer or interface to a radiology picture archiving and communication system /information system. Counts of the proper energy window are recorded. This type of device is typically used to perform radionuclide thyroid uptake studies. Reprinted with permission from Braverman LE, Cooper D. *Werner & Ingbar's the Thyroid.* 10th ed. Philadelphia, PA: Wolters Kluwer Health/Lippincott Williams & Wilkins; 2012.

Its design allows for high efficiency, detecting activities less than 1 nCi. The crystal is coupled to a PMT, which is connected to a preamplifier, a high voltage power supply, and, usually, an MCA system. Most systems have a thick lead shielding to reduce background counting levels. If needed, an automatic well counter can handle a large number of samples, such as wipe tests.

Sample position and volume can have a significant effect on detection efficiency. In vitro tests often require a reference sample

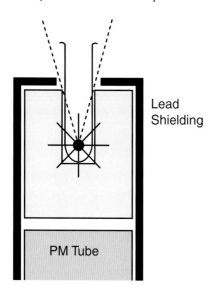

FIG. 9.15 ● The diagram of a NaI(Tl) well counter. Its geometric efficiency is close to 95%, because only a small fraction of the radiation goes undetected (emitting within the angular range indicated by the two dotted lines). PM, photomultiplier. Reprinted with permission from Chandra R, Rahmim A. *Nuclear Medicine Physics: The Basics.* 8th ed. Philadelphia, PA: Wolters Kluwer; 2017.

to compare to the patient sample. It is critical that samples have the same type of vials and volumes. The high efficiency of the well counter can lead to significant dead-time count losses. Sample activity must be small to avoid a falsely low count rate. Typically, well counters should not be operated at count rates above 5000 counts per second.

QC for Scintillation Detectors

Both the thyroid probe and well counter require daily energy calibrations. Daily constancy measurement is made using a long half-life source, like ^{137}Cs. The counts per minute for the standard should be about the same day to day, falling within ±10%. A daily background check also detects any external source of radiation or contamination of the detector.

Energy resolution should be assessed annually, graphing spectra for commonly measured radioisotopes, such as ^{123}I or ^{131}I for the thyroid probe and ^{57}Co, ^{125}I, and ^{51}Cr for the well counter. With an MCA, the FWHM is easily determined in conjunction with daily calibration. Measured energy resolution should be less than 10% using ^{137}Cs as a reference standard. Quarterly, a chi-square test should be performed to measure statistical variability of the detector. The instrument's efficiency factor should be determined annually. The efficiency factor correlates the measured count rate to the absolute activity of a reference (Table 9.3).

Dosimeters

Inorganic scintillators that trap electrons at excited states instead of prompt light emission are useful for storing information regarding radiation exposure, like personnel dosimeter badges. The material within thermoluminescent dosimeters (TLDs) is heated, and the emitted light is converted to an electrical signal by a PMT. The amount of light emitted increases with the amount of energy absorbed by the material and can be used to estimate dose received. LiF is a widely used TLD material. Its effective atomic number is similar to that of tissue, so the amount of light emission is nearly proportional to tissue dose over a range of X-ray and gamma-ray energies. There are also dosimeter badges based on optically stimulated luminescence.

Semiconductor detectors

Basics

Semiconductors are crystalline materials with electrical conductivities less than those of metals but greater than those of crystalline insulators. In crystalline materials, electrons exist in energy bands separated by large energy gaps. In metals, the least bound electrons exist in the conduction band and are freely mobile, contributing to high electrical conductivity. In a semiconductor or insulator, the valence electrons exist in a filled valence band and are immobile, held by covalent bonds, while the conduction band is empty (Figure 9.16).

Table 9.3 **COMMONLY PERFORMED QUALITY CONTROL FOR DOSE CALIBRATORS**	
Test	*Recommended Frequency*
Calibration (peaking)	Daily
Constancy/sensitivity	Daily
Energy resolution	Quarterly/annually
Chi-square test	Monthly/annually
Detector efficiency	Annually

FIG. 9.16 ● The diagram of energy band structures of (A) insulator, semiconductor (B), and conductor (C).

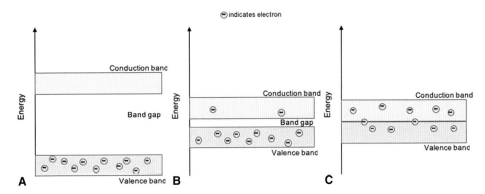

Compared to insulators, semiconductors have a much smaller energy gap separating the valence and conduction bands. With ionizing radiation, the electron is raised to the conduction band and becomes mobile. This excitation creates a "hole" or vacancy in the valence band. Holes are considered a net positive charge of the same magnitude as an electron. When another valence electron fills the hole, a new hole is created. These holes act as mobile, positive charges in the valence band. These hole-electron pairs in a semiconductor are analogous to ion pairs in gas-filled ionization chambers.

Given semiconductor materials' significantly higher densities and atomic numbers relative to gases, they have greater efficiency for detecting X-rays and gamma rays. For example, for every 3 to 5 eV of radiation energy absorbed, a single ionization is produced in a semiconductor. In contrast, for every 34 eV of radiation

absorbed, a single ionization is produced in air. Compared with gas, a semiconductor is more efficient at radiation absorption and produces a higher electrical signal. Unfortunately, the generated signal current can be hidden by the larger applied voltage current. To reduce this effect, the semiconductor crystal is "doped" with trace impurities.

An impurity element with more valence electrons than the semiconductor element is considered an *n-type* material and has mobile electrons in the valence band. An impurity element with fewer valence electrons compared with the semiconductor is a *p-type* material and has mobile holes in the valence band (Figure 9.17).

Semiconductor diode has an n-type region adjacent to a p-type region. With *forward bias*, external voltage is applied with the positive polarity on the p-side of the n-p junction and negative polarity on the n-side. This results in charge carriers flowing

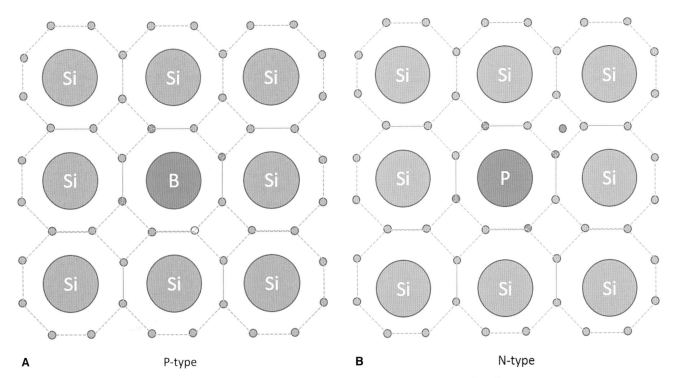

FIG. 9.17 ● **The diagram of p-type (A) and n-type (B) semiconductor materials.** P-type semiconductors are created by doping an intrinsic semiconductor with an electron-receptor element; the dopant in the illustration (A) for p-type silicon is Boron (B). In p-type semiconductors, holes are the majority carriers and electrons are minority carriers. *N-type* semiconductors are created by doping an intrinsic semiconductor with an electron-donor element during manufacture; the dopant in the illustration (B) for n-type silicon is phosphorus (P). In *n-type* semiconductors, electrons are the majority carriers and holes are the minority carriers.

to the junction, and a large current is produced. With *reverse bias*, external voltage is applied with negative polarity on the p-side and positive polarity on the n-side. This results in charge carriers flowing away from the junction, creating a depletion zone and essentially no current.

Reverse bias semiconductor diodes can detect light or UV radiation or an ionization event. The photons or ionization can excite the lower state electrons in the depletion zone to conduction bands, resulting in electron-hole pairs. With applied voltage, these conduction band electrons flow to the n-side and the holes "move" to the p-side, creating a pulse of current (Figure 9.18).

Semiconductor detectors are semiconductor diodes that detect ionizing radiation. The size of the electrical signal produced is proportional to the amount of radiation absorbed; therefore, these detectors can be used to generate energy spectra, similar to scintillation detectors.

Both silicon and germanium are commonly used semiconductor materials, and germanium semiconductor detectors have greater energy resolution than traditional NaI(Tl) scintillators. Unlike scintillation detectors, electrons in semiconductor detectors do not undergo the multiple mass-energy conversions. The energy needed to create a hole-electron pair in a semiconductor is only 3 to 5 eV compared to 30 eV to create a scintillation photon in sodium iodide. In this way, there are many more information carriers per radiation event, resulting in superior energy resolution.

Unfortunately, many semiconductor detectors are susceptible to heat and must be cooled with liquid nitrogen. They also are expensive and produced in small sizes. More recently, though, cadmium zinc telluride has been used in some imaging systems. It has a higher atomic number than does germanium and can be operated at room temperature.

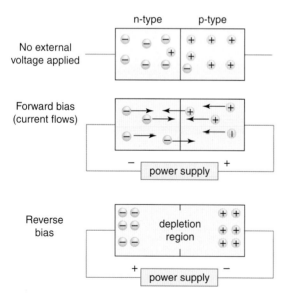

FIG. 9.18 ● The illustration of the electrical behaviors of a semiconductor diode, created by attaching n-type and p-type materials together. With no external voltage applied, there are few migrations of charge carriers (electrons and holes). With forward bias, charge carriers are swept into the junction, and a current begins to flow. With negative bias, charge carriers are moved away from the junction, and a depletion region with no charge carriers is formed, which could potentially serve as a solid-state ion chamber. Reprinted with permission from Bushberg JT, Seibert JA, Leidholdt EM, Boone JM. *Essential Physics of Medical Imaging.* 3rd ed. Philadelphia, PA: Wolters Kluwer Health/Lippincott Williams & Wilkins; 2012.

Detection efficiency

Detection efficiency is the efficiency with which a detector converts emissions from a radiation source to useful signals. It is defined as

$$\text{Efficiency} = \frac{\text{Number of detected events}}{\text{Number of emitted events}}$$

Many factors affect efficiency, including geometric efficiency, intrinsic efficiency of the detector, energy window, and absorption and scatter. The detection efficiency (*D*) is a product of these factors:

$$D = g \times \varepsilon \times f \times F$$

- *g* = geometric efficiency of the detector
- *ε* = intrinsic efficiency of the detector
- *f* = fraction of the output signals that falls within the PHA window
- *F* = factor for absorption and scatter within the source or between the source and detector

Geometric efficiency (*g*) is generally expressed as the fraction or percentage of the total emissions that intersect with the detector in a given source-detector geometry.

$$g \approx A/4\pi r^2$$

- *A* = detector surface area
- *r* = distance of detector from point source

This equation becomes inaccurate as the source is brought close to the detector.

Intrinsic efficiency (*ε*) is derived from the energy of the photons as well as the atomic number, density, and thickness of the detector. It is expressed in the following equation:

$$\varepsilon = 1 - e^{-\mu x} = 1 - e^{-(\mu/\rho)\rho x}$$

- *μ* = linear coefficient of the detector material
- *ρ* = density of the detector material
- *μ/ρ* = mass attenuation coefficient of the detector material
- *x* = thickness of the detector

Intrinsic efficiency increases as detector thickness, material density, and mass attenuation coefficient increase. Mass attenuation coefficient increases with increasing atomic number (*Z*) of the material and decreases with increasing photon energy.

The fraction of detected gamma photons that produce output signals within the PHA is denoted by *f*. If the PHA window size is decreased, the measured count rate in counts per minute will become smaller, even though the radioactivity is unchanged. As the window width decreases, efficiency decreases.

Fortunately, actual detector efficiency is needed in only select situations: performing wipe surveys for contamination, checking packages for contamination, and performing thyroid bioassays.

In these cases, an *efficiency factor* can be determined using a long-lived reference standard that has a known activity and emits a gamma photon similar to the radioisotope of interest. Using a reference source with similar gamma energy, the intrinsic efficiency of the detector remains about the same. The standard is placed into or in front of the detector in same geometric orientation as will be used with the sample. The settings are kept the same as will be used for the sample. Importantly, the efficiency factor is valid only for measurements made under the same parameters. The efficiency factor should be determined annually.

Nuclear counting statistics

Accurate measurement of a radiation source or event is subject to several factors. Although imaging systems are also affected by these variables, counting measurements are more susceptible because there is no resulting image.

All measurements are subject to error. *Blunder, systematic error*, and *random error* are three types of errors that can occur with measurements. An example of a blunder would be using the incorrect instrument setting and is usually easily rectified. As expected, systematic error happens when measured results differ from the correct values by a fixed amount. For instance, measuring a volume with a misshapen vial could produce a systemic error. Systemic errors may be difficult to recognize. Using measurement standards, such as radionuclide standards, which contain a known quantity of radioactivity, are often part of the quality assurance program to test a variety of instruments. Random error is variation in result from one measurement to the next. It is due to many sources, such as the randomness of radioactive decay, the limitations of the radiation detector itself, whether or not a gamma photon interacts with the camera crystal, etc. *Counting statistics* is a method to account for random error in measurements.

Definitions

Accuracy and Precision

If a measured value is near the correct value, it is considered *accurate*. If measurements are reproducible, they are considered *precise*. Precision does not indicate accuracy. If measured values differ from the correct values in a systematic manner (systematic error), they are *biased*.

Mean and Median

The *mean* (*M*) or average of a set of measurements is defined by the following formula:

$$M = \frac{x_1 + x_2 + \cdots + x_N}{N}$$

• N = total number of measurements

To obtain the median, measurements are arranged in order of magnitude. The *median* is the middle measurement if the total number of measurements is odd, and it is the average of the two middle-most numbers if the total number of measurements is even. Compared to the mean, the median is less affected by outliers.

Variance and Standard Deviation

Both variance and standard deviation describe the dispersion, or spread, of a set of measured values around the mean. Variance (σ^2) is defined as follows:

$$\sigma^2 = \frac{(x_1 - M)^2 + (x_2 - M)^2 + \cdots + (x_N - M)^2}{N - 1}$$

• M = sample mean
• N = total number of measurements

Standard deviation (σ) is the square root of the variance (σ^2). *Fractional standard deviation*, also termed the fractional error or coefficient of variation, is the standard deviation divided by the mean (*M*).

Probability distribution functions

Binary Processes

A trial is an event that can have more than one outcome. A binary process is a trial that has two outcomes, one of which is termed a success and the other a failure. A coin toss is an example of a binary process. Whether or not a gamma photon is detected by a radiation detector is considered a binary process. A measurement consists of counting the number of "successes" for a given number of trials. Performing 10 coin tosses and counting the number of heads (successes) is a measurement. Likewise, using a detector to record the number of radiation events from a source is considered a measurement.

A probability distribution function describes the likelihood of obtaining each outcome from a measurement. Three probability distribution functions used in binary processes include binomial, Poisson, and Gaussian. The binomial function describes exactly the probability of each outcome, $P(x)$, from a measured binary process.

$$P(x) = \frac{N!}{x!(N-x)!} \times p^x (1-p)^{N-x}$$

• N = total number of trials in a measurement
• p = probability of success in a single trial
• x = number of successes

$N!$, or factorial notation, represents the following product: $N! = N \times (N-1) \times (N-2) \times \cdots \times 1$. For example, $3! = 3 \times 2 \times 1 = 6$. When x or N is very large, this equation becomes difficult to use. Instead, a Poisson or Gaussian distribution can be applied (Figure 9.19).

Because radioactive decay follows the Poisson statistical model, a single measurement can be utilized to predict the probability distribution that would be obtained from many thousand measurements of the sample. Furthermore, the width of the probability distribution (its standard deviation, σ) can be estimated as the square root of that single measurement, or x.

$$\sigma \approx \sqrt{x}$$

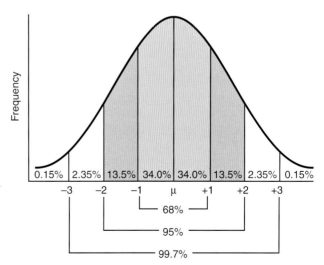

Area under the curve

FIG. 9.19 ● **The normal (Gaussian) distribution.** Reprinted with permission from Fadem B. *High-Yield Behavioral Science.* 4th ed. Baltimore, MD: Wolters Kluwer Health/Lippincott Williams & Wilkins; 2013:126.

Moreover, if there are an infinite number of measurements, the probability distribution curve will have a Gaussian shape and the distribution width will be fixed relative to the standard deviation. Therefore:

- Of all possible measurements, 68.3% is within ± 1 standard deviation of the mean of the sample, M (the peak of the curve).
- Of all possible measurements, 95.4% is within ± 2 standard deviations of M.
- Of all possible measurements, 99.7% is within ± 3 standard deviations of M.

Because the single measurement gives an estimation of the probability distribution curve and its width, it permits an estimation of the mean, M, or peak of the curve. The single measurement, x, directly relates to M in the following ways:

- M of the sample has a 68.3% probability of being within ± 1 standard deviation of x, or $\sqrt{x}$
- M of the sample has a 95.4% probability of being within ± 2 standard deviations of x, or $2\sqrt{x}$
- M of the sample has a 99.7% probability of being within ± 3 standard deviations of x, or $3\sqrt{x}$

These points can be restated in terms of *confidence intervals,* meaning that we are 68.3% confident that M of the sample is within ± 1 standard deviation of our single measurement x, 95.4% confident that M is within ± 2 standard deviations of x, and 99.7% confident that M is within ± 3 standard deviations of x.

Referring back to the equation, $\sigma \approx \sqrt{x}$, where x is the single measurement. The fractional standard deviation, also termed *fractional error* or *coefficient of variation*, can be rewritten as

$$\text{Fractional error} = \sigma/x = \sqrt{x}/x = 1/\sqrt{x}$$

Fractional error permits the comparison of standard deviations for measurements with different x values. Many counting measurements, such as in vitro sample counting, the fractional error should be less than 1%.

$$\text{Fractional error} = 1/\sqrt{x} = 0.01 \text{ or } 1\%$$

Therefore, $x = 10\,000$ counts

The fractional error decreases with increasing number of counts, as demonstrated in Table 9.4.

Propagation of error

Most of the preceding discussion has focused on determining the random error of a single measurement. However, many nuclear medicine applications rely on several counting measurements to calculate a final result.

Table 9.4 FRACTIONAL ERROR FOR DIFFERENT COUNTS

Counts	Fractional Error (%)
100	10
1000	3.16
10 000	1
100 000	0.316

Sums and Differences

For sums or differences of multiple individual measurements, the standard deviations of the individual measurements must be included in the standard deviation for the sum or subtraction, using the following equation.

$$\sigma = \sqrt{\sigma_1^2 + \sigma_2^2}$$

- σ_1 = standard deviation for measurement 1
- σ_2 = standard deviation for measurement 2

Therefore, a significant measurement not only alters the value of the calculated sum or difference but it also changes the statistical certainty of that measurement. Likewise, if one of the measurements is small, then there will be minimal effect on the combined standard deviation. In practice, correcting for background radiation is a commonly encountered situation. Background refers to detected counts not from the measured source. It is determined by taking a measurement without a source present. Contributors of background radiation include cosmic rays, radionuclides in the materials of the surrounding walls, nearby radioactive sources, and electronic noise within the detector itself.

For example, a measurement of a radioactive sample is 2000 counts and a background measurement is 1500 counts.

$$\text{Net counts} = 2000 - 1500 = 500 \text{ counts}$$

$$\sigma_{(\text{sample + background})} = \sqrt{2000} = 44.7 \text{ counts}$$

$$\text{Fractional error} = 44.7/2000 = 2.2\%$$

For the background counts, standard deviation is calculated as follows:

$$\sigma_{\text{background}} = \sqrt{1500} = 38.7 \text{ counts}$$

$$\text{Fractional error} = 38.7/1500 = 2.6\%$$

Therefore, the standard deviation of the sample count corrected for background can be determined by applying the following formula:

$$\sigma = \sqrt{\sigma_1^2 + \sigma_2^2}$$

$$\sigma_{\text{sample}} = \sqrt{44.7^2 + 38.7^2} = 59.1 \text{ counts}$$

$$\text{Fractional error} = 59.1/500 = 11.8\%$$

Importantly, the resulting uncertainty of the difference is far greater than the fractional errors for the individual counts despite their similar values. High background counts are disadvantageous because they increase the uncertainty of the net sample counts.

Multiplication or Division

Sometimes a number containing random error must be multiplied or divided by a number without random error. A common example would be the determination of count rate. For instance, a 5-minute count of a radioactive sample is 1000 counts.

$$\text{Count rate} = 1000 \text{ counts/5 minutes} = 200 \text{ cpm}$$

$$\text{Standard deviation}, \sigma = \sqrt{1000} = 31.6 \text{ counts}$$

$$\text{Fractional error} = 31.6/1000 = 0.0316 = 3.16\%$$

Table 9.5 PROPAGATION OF ERROR FOR COMMON OPERATIONS

Description	Operation	Standard Deviation
Multiplication of a number with random error (x) by a number without random error (c)	$c\,x$	$c\,\sigma$
Division of a number with random error (x) by a number without random error (c)	x/c	σ/c
Addition of two measurements containing random error (x_1, x_2)	$x_1 + x_2$	$\sqrt{(\sigma_1^2 + \sigma_2^2)}$
Subtraction of two measurements containing random error (x_1, x_2)	$x_1 - x_2$	$\sqrt{(\sigma_1^2 + \sigma_2^2)}$

Standard deviation of the count rate = σ/time = 31.6 counts/5 minutes = 6.32 cpm

$$\text{Fractional error for the count rate} = 6.32/200$$
$$\text{cpm} = 0.0316 = 3.16\%$$

Notably, the fractional error is unaffected when a number is multiplied or divided by a number without random error.

Propagation of error equations are summarized in Table 9.5.

Statistical testing

Statistics can aid in QC. The performance of a detector over time can be assessed using a Levey-Jennings plot. Several measurements of a specific QC parameter are determined. The mean and standard deviation of the data set are plotted on a graph with time as the x-axis. If the values follow Poisson statistics, 95% of the plotted values should fall between the standard deviation lines. In this way, trends can be more easily recognized (Figure 9.20).

Chi-square test (χ^2) is a method for determining whether random variations in a series of measurements fall within a Poisson distribution. This test is useful if error is suspected from faulty instrumentation or some other source. The following steps are employed:

1. Obtain a set of counting measurements (a minimum of 20)
2. Calculate the mean (M): $M = (x_1 + x_2 + \ldots + x_N)/N$
   - N = total number of measurements
   - x = individual measurement

1. Apply the following equation: $\chi^2 = (N - 1)\,\sigma^2/M$
   - σ = standard deviation

1. Refer to a χ^2 table or graph and locate the value corresponding to the number of measurements, N, on the horizontal axis
2. Compare the calculated χ^2 to the most closely corresponding P-value curve on the graph (Figure 9.21)

P is the probability that random variations observed in a set of measurements from a Poisson distribution would equal or exceed the computed χ^2. $1 - P$ is the probability that smaller variations would be observed. $P = 0.5$ or 50% is ideal. It indicates that the calculated χ^2 is in the middle of the spread for a Poisson distribution. A low P (<0.01) indicates that the data set has greater variability than expected by Poisson statistics alone. A high P (>0.99) implies less variability than expected. Typically, $0.05 < P < 0.95$ is considered satisfactory. If the P falls outside this range, then the detector is faulty.

NUCLEAR IMAGING: SCINTIGRAPHY
Scintillation camera

Nuclear medicine imaging encompasses the development of images from the distribution of radionuclides in tissues. Imaging equipment for nuclear medicine is designed to image gamma and X-ray-emitting radionuclides using collimators, which permit only photons of particular trajectories to be detected. Collimators, typically made of lead, block more than 99% of emitted photons. Images generated without the implementation of collimators are essentially nondiagnostic.

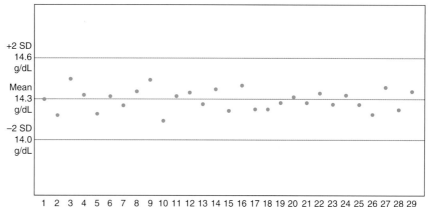

FIG. 9.20 ● **The Levey-Jennings plot.** The data for a hemoglobin assay is used here as example. Normal values are expected to fall within the two standard deviations of the mean value. Reprinted with permission from Turgeon ML. *Clinical Hematology.* 6th ed. Philadelphia, PA: Wolters Kluwer; 2017.

+2 SD
14.6
g/dL

Mean
14.3
g/dL

−2 SD
14.0
g/dL

1 2 3 4 5 6 7 8 9 10 11 12 13 14 15 16 17 18 19 20 21 22 23 24 25 26 27 28 29

Month of February

Hemoglobin assay
Normal control lot No. 12C
Stat lab – Spec. 20

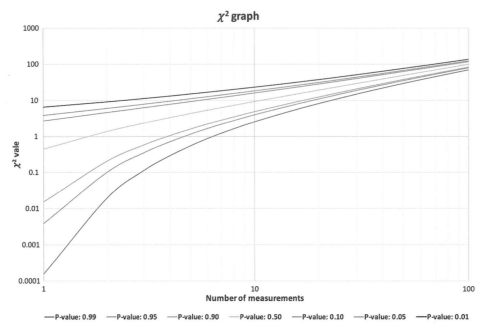

FIG. 9.21 ● χ^2 graph.

Anger scintillation camera

Detector and Electronics

Virtually all clinical nuclear imaging equipment employ solid inorganic scintillators as detectors because of the superior quality of detection. The most common imaging device used is the Anger gamma scintillation camera. Because of the superior efficiency of the Anger camera compared to the rectilinear scanner, it is the predominating device in nuclear imaging. The primary advantage of the scintillation camera is its ability to acquire data over a large area of the patient simultaneously. In comparison, the rectilinear scanner utilizes a moving radiation detector to sample the photons in a small region of the patient at a time. Thus, Anger cameras allow for more rapid acquisitions and for dynamic imaging studies that demonstrate redistribution of the radionuclides (Figure 9.22).

The scintillation camera head comprises a rectangular-shaped sodium iodide thallium crystal combined with a number of PMTs. A collimator is placed on the camera head between the patient and the scintillation camera. A preamplifier connects to the photomultiplier output in most camera designs (Figure 9.23).

The collimator consists of lead walls called septa, which absorb a majority of the photons that are not directed or oriented toward the holes leading to the scintillation camera. Photons passing through the holes in the collimator are absorbed in the sodium iodide crystal. As a result, visible light and ultraviolet radiation

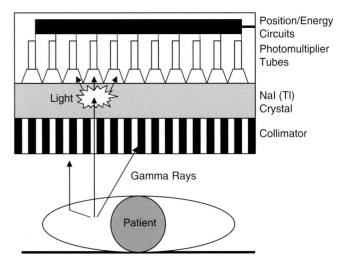

FIG. 9.22 ● **A dual-head gamma camera.** Reprinted with permission from Braverman LE, Cooper D. *Werner & Ingbar's the Thyroid.* 10th ed. Philadelphia, PA: Wolters Kluwer Health/Lippincott Williams & Wilkins; 2012.

FIG. 9.23 ● **Schematic representation of an Anger scintillation camera.** Reprinted with permission from Griffin BP, Kapadia SR, Rimmerman CM. *Cleveland Clinic Cardiology Board Review.* 2nd ed. Philadelphia, PA: Wolters Kluwer Health/Lippincott Williams & Wilkins; 2012.

are emitted and converted into electrical signals that are then amplified by the photomultiplier tubes. The preamplifiers further enhance the electrical signals. The amount of X- or gamma-ray photon interactions in the sodium iodide crystal is directly proportional to the electrical pulse signal amplitude generated by each PMT.

The image generated from the process of photons interacting with the gamma camera crystals is a 2D projection from the 3D emission of the distribution of the radionuclide in the patient. The photons emitted from the patient closest to the PMTs result in higher electrical signals versus the photons emitted further away. The relative amplitudes of the electrical impulses resulting from the photon interactions contain adequate data to distinguish the location of the interaction in the plane of that crystal.

Scintillation cameras are also designed with ADCs, which convert analog signals to digital signals in a process called digitization. Digitization involves sampling and quantization.

ADCs are used for the signal from the preamplifier. The digitized signals are then sent to the additional digital circuitry for signal processing and image generation. One of these additional circuits is a position circuit, which receives signals from the individual preamps after each interaction in the gamma camera crystals. By determining the center point of the signal, an X-coordinate position and a Y-coordinate position localize the interaction in the plane of the crystal. Next, a summing circuit computes all the incoming preamp signals to produce an energy (Z) signal proportional in amplitude to all the energy received by the gamma camera crystal. Correction circuits calculate and adjust position-dependent systematic errors in interaction position localization and energy assignment. The correction circuits enhance the spatial linearity and uniformity of the images generated. The corrected energy signal is analyzed by an energy discrimination circuit. If the interaction in the gamma camera crystal is within a preset range, the interaction is recorded as a count (Figure 9.24).

Scintillation cameras can register up to four discrete energy ranges for imaging radionuclides, such as indium-111 and gallium-67, which emit photons of more than one energy. Once energy discrimination is complete, the X- and Y-position signals are analyzed by a computer and a digital projection image is generated.

Collimators

The use of collimators on gamma cameras allows X- or gamma-ray photons approaching the camera from certain directions to interact with crystal while absorbing a majority of the other incoming photons. Collimators comprise high-density materials, such as lead. The parallel-hole collimator is the most commonly employed collimator and comprises multiple parallel holes. Modern collimators contain holes in a hexagonal configuration. The lead walls between the holes are called septa.

Collimators with thicker septa are designed for various radionuclides that emit higher energy photons. By decreasing the size of the collimator holes or increasing the length of the collimator, the spatial resolution of the collimator improves, but at the expense of the sensitivity of the collimator. The spatial resolution also decreases when the patient distance to the collimator increases. However, the field of view (FOV) of a parallel-hole collimator does not change when the distance to the patient is changed. As such, modern scintillation cameras are equipped with a selection of parallel-hole collimators ranging from low-energy, high-sensitivity to ultrahigh-energy for various imaging purposes.

With the pinhole collimator, the images generated are reverse-oriented magnified views of the selected body part. The pinhole collimator consists of a small opening at the apex of a lead-lined cone. The further the imaging area is from the pinhole collimator, the less magnification applied upon development of the image. Furthermore, if the pinhole is equidistant from the body part and the crystal of the camera, then no magnification will result.

Another type of collimator is the converging collimator, which comprises multiple holes coming to a focal point in front of the camera. In contrast to the pinhole collimator, the converging collimator causes magnification of the image generated as the body part is moved further away from the collimator. However, the

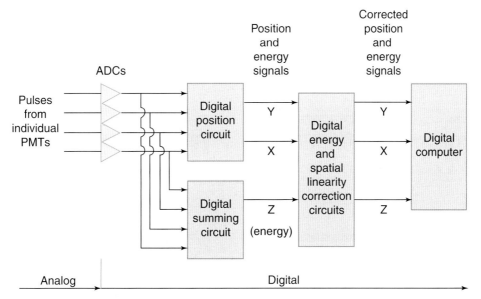

FIG. 9.24 ● **The diagram of the electronics typically involved in a modern scintillation camera.** ADC, analog-to-digital converter; PMT, photomultiplier tube. Reprinted with permission from Bushberg JT, Seibert JA, Leidholdt EM, Boone JM. *Essential Physics of Medical Imaging*. 3rd ed. Philadelphia, PA: Wolters Kluwer Health/Lippincott Williams & Wilkins; 2012.

FOV decreases with increasing distance. In contrast to a converging collimator, a diverging collimator comprises of multiple holes coming to a focal point behind the camera. The diverging collimator generates an image in which magnification is increased as the body part is moved closer toward the camera. Both the converging and diverging collimators are rarely employed in every day practice (Figure 9.25).

Image Formation

Owing to the isotropic emission of radioisotopes, a number of photons pass through the patient without interacting, scatter within the patient, or are absorbed within the patient. Of the photons that escape from the patient, some are not detected because they are emitted away from the gamma camera. Of the photons emitted in the direction of the image receptor, the collimators absorb a high percentage. As such, a small number of the total emitted photons have trajectories that are measured. Thus, over 99% of emitted photons go undetected. The photons that pass in between the septa of the collimator also have variable outcomes. The photons reaching the crystal are either absorbed, scattered, or pass through the crystal without interacting.

Depending on the interactions of the photons, the spatial resolution and image contrast can be degraded. For instance, photons scattered in the patient interacting with the crystal, photons infiltrating the collimator septa, and photons scattering within the crystal all lead to increased background noise and degradation of the image. To counteract this, the discrimination circuits function to reduce the loss of resolution and contrast by rejecting photons undergoing these interactions.

Because photons are emitted isotropically from a patient, collimation is necessary to develop a useful projection image. It is not possible to differentiate primary photons from scattered photons by their emitted directions. The collimators reduce about the same percentage of both primary and scattered photons. They do not reduce the number of counts due to scatter alone. As a result, the only way to distinguish primary photons from scattered photons is by energy because scattering reduces photon energy. Therefore, energy discrimination is utilized to minimize the fraction of counts caused by scattered photons.

Effects of Scatter

Attenuation of photons in the patient, incorporation of scattered photons, patient motion, and degradation of spatial resolution with patient distance from the collimator all contribute to noisy projection images. The degree of attenuation of photons in the patient can be summarized by the length of tissue traversed and the densities of the tissues between a point in the patient and a corresponding point on the gamma camera. More specifically, photons from structures deeper in the patient are more attenuated because they have to travel farther to the patient surface than do photons originating closer to the camera face. Furthermore, attenuation has a greater impact on lower energy photons than do higher energy photons. By adjusting the pulse height discrimination, the number of scattered photons contributing to the final image can be reduced. However, having a greater energy window will permit most of the photopeak and allow a greater amount of scattered photons to contribute to the image.

Computers, Whole-Body Scanning, and SPECT

Digital computer systems coupled to scintillation cameras allow acquisition, processing, and projection of digital images as well as control movement of the camera heads. Large-area cameras can be utilized for whole-body scanning and can even rotate around a stationary patient versus moving the patient table relative to a stationary scintillation camera. Large-area camera heads have the capability to scan each side of a patient in a single pass, which saves time and generates greater quality images. In addition, modern multielement scintillation cameras can rotate automatically around the patient and acquire images from different projections.

Optimizing for High-Quality Images

By adjusting various parameters, higher quality images can be acquired. A sufficient number of counts must be obtained to prevent quantum mottle from obscuring lesions. Imaging time should be adjusted so that an adequate number of counts are obtained, but not long enough where patient motion degrades the image quality. The table pitch or camera speed should be optimized to obtain sufficient image statistics. By employing higher resolution collimators, spatial resolution can be improved. Minimizing the collimator-to-patient distance can also improve the spatial resolution. In addition, narrower energy spectra may help reduce scatter from contributing to the image. Jewelry and metallic objects worn by patients can contribute to artifacts on the images. These artifacts can be reduced by eliminating metal objects from entering the FOV.

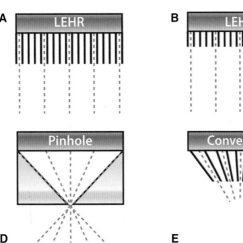

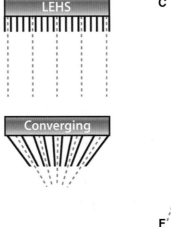

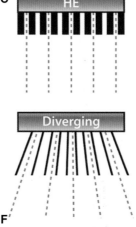

FIG. 9.25 ● Six types of collimators used with gamma cameras: low-energy high-resolution (LEHR [A]), low-energy high-sensitivity (LEHS [B]), high-energy (HE [C]), pinhole (D), converging (F), and diverging (F). LEHR, LEHS, and HE all use parallel holes. Reprinted with permission from Huda W. *Review of Radiologic Physics*. 3rd ed. Philadelphia, PA: Wolters Kluwer Health/Lippincott Williams & Wilkins; 2010.

Digital images by scintillation camera

In nuclear medicine, a digital image comprises a rectangular collection of numbers, with each element in the image representing a single number called a pixel. The pixel represents the number of counts detected from a specific location in a patient. Typically, image formats are 64 × 64 or 128 × 128 pixels consistent with the low spatial resolution of scintillation cameras. Whole-body images, which are stored in larger formats, are generally 256 × 1024 pixels.

Data Acquisition Modes

For nuclear medicine, frame mode and list mode are two types of data acquisition modes.

- **Frame mode acquisition**
  Before acquisition of the image, the pixels are reset to zero. During acquisition, detection of a single X- or gamma ray corresponds to a pair of X- and Y-position signals received from the gamma camera. The pair of values is assigned to a single pixel in the image. The pixel value represents the number of counts obtained and assigned to that particular pixel. The number of position signal pairs obtained will determine the image formed (Figure 9.26).

  Static, dynamic, and gated imaging data are three types of frame mode acquisitions. Static acquisition is a single image obtained for a specified time interval or until a sufficient number of counts are obtained to develop an image. Dynamic acquisitions are a sequential series of images obtained for a specified time interval per image.

  Gated acquisitions are performed when certain dynamic processes occur too rapidly for a sufficient number of counts to be obtained to accurately depict the process. In gated acquisitions, a repetitive physiologic process acts as the impetus to begin acquiring the series sequentially. A common example is myocardial perfusion studies. During gated acquisition of a cardiac study, an electrocardiogram monitor detects a QRS complex which prompts the sequential image acquisition (Figure 9.27).

- **List-mode acquisition**
  By contrast, list-mode acquisition stores the X- and Y-position coordinate data in a list rather than in the image. Timing components are also included in the list. After obtaining an acquisition, the list-mode data are transformed into a projection image. The major advantage of list-mode data acquisition is that the data can be manipulated to form an image. However, list-mode data requires more memory to acquire, and takes more time to process to generate an image (Figure 9.28).

Image Processing in Nuclear Medicine

Computers in nuclear medicine allow further processing of the raw imaging data to provide more useful information to aid the clinician. Given here are a few examples of image processing techniques used in nuclear medicine:

- **Image subtraction**
  For instance, by utilizing image subtraction techniques, the pixel counts in one image are subtracted from the pixel counts in another image. Subtracted images resulting in negative values are reverted to zero. The final image demonstrates the difference in activity from the two different time acquisition periods.
- **Regions of interest and time-activity curves**
  A region of interest is a closed area drawn on an image to indicate activity. The counts within the defined area of interest are summed to represent activity corresponding to a selected area

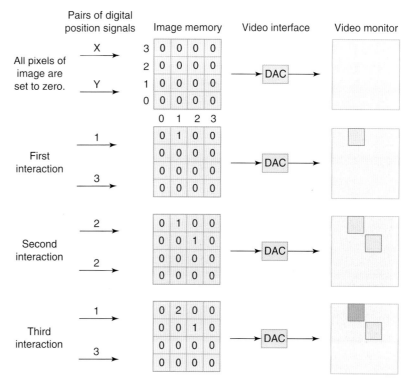

FIG. 9.26 ● **The acquisition of an image in frame mode.** DAC, digital-to-analog converter. Reprinted with permission from Bushberg JT, Seibert JA, Leidholdt EM, Boone JM. *Essential Physics of Medical Imaging.* 3rd ed. Philadelphia, PA: Wolters Kluwer Health/Lippincott Williams & Wilkins; 2012.

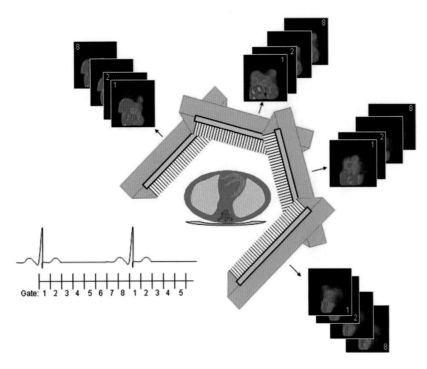

FIG. 9.27 ● **The electrocardiography-gated acquisition of projection images for a myocardial perfusion single photon emission computed tomography study.** In this example, the cardiac cycle is divided into eight phase bins. Reprinted with permission from Garcia, MJ. *NonInvasive Cardiovascular Imaging: A Multimodality Approach.* 1st ed. Philadelphia, PA: Wolters Kluwer Health/Lippincott Williams & Wilkins; 2011.

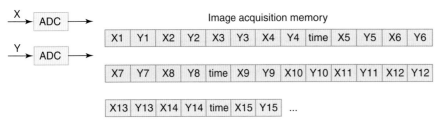

FIG. 9.28 ● **The acquisition of images in list mode.** ADC, analog-to-digital converter. Reprinted with permission from Bushberg JT, Seibert JA, Leidholdt EM, Boone JM. *Essential Physics of Medical Imaging.* 3rd ed. Philadelphia, PA: Wolters Kluwer Health/ Lippincott Williams & Wilkins; 2012.

of the patient. Time-activity curves are derived from dynamic or gated imaging sequences. To obtain a time-activity curve, a region of interest is drawn on each of the sequential images of a dynamic or gated study. The sum of all the counts in each region of interest is plotted corresponding to the image in the series. The final function curve represents the change in activity as a function of time (Figure 9.29).

● **Spatial filtering**

Imaging studies in nuclear medicine have an inherent coarse and grainy appearance because of the acquisition process. Smoothing is a postprocessing type of spatial filtering designed to reduce the quantum mottle. However, the spatial resolution of the image can be degraded by smoothing. Too much smoothing can result in rendering the images nondiagnostic.

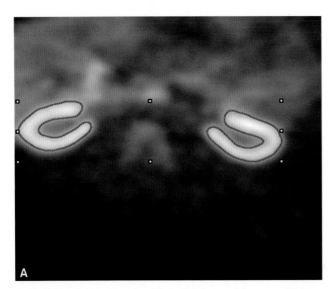

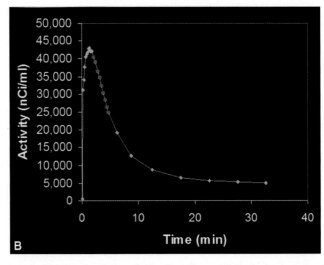

FIG. 9.29 ● Region of interest (A) and its time-activity curve (B) for a renal study. Reprinted with permission from Saremi F. *Perfusion Imaging in Clinical Practice.* Philadelphia, PA: Wolters Kluwer; 2015.

NUCLEAR IMAGING: EMISSION TOMOGRAPHY

In nuclear medicine, projection imaging depicts the 3D radiopharmaceutical activity distribution in a patient in a 2D format. The disadvantage of such a projection is that activity at varying depths in a patient overlap. To circumvent this, tomographic imaging demonstrates the activity distribution in a single cross section of the patient.

Tomographic imaging comprises either conventional tomography or computed tomography. In conventional tomography, overlapping structures are blurred and contribute to an image, resulting in reduced contrast and added noise to the image. Conversely, in computed tomography, overlapping structures are not blurred together. In computed tomography, a series of projection images are acquired in an arc greater than 180° about the patient. The end result is then processed by an algorithm to form images representing the cross sectional area of the patient. PET and SPECT are forms of computed tomography.

Single Photon Emission Computed Tomography

Design and principles of operation

SPECT produces transverse images that demonstrate the distribution of X- or gamma ray–emitting radiopharmaceuticals in patients. Standard planar projection images in SPECT are acquired in an arc greater than 180° (most cardiac SPECT) or 360° (most noncardiac SPECT) about the patient. Although the data can be acquired by any collimated imaging device, most SPECT systems use one or more scintillation camera heads that rotate about the patient. The acquired data sets are then processed using either filtered back projection or an iterative reconstruction method or a combination of both to reconstruct the final images.

Image acquisition

Imaging acquisition is typically performed with a single detector or dual detector, or sometimes with a triple detector system. During image acquisition, the SPECT system rotates about the patient. The most common method of acquiring data is accomplished with a step-and-shoot protocol. In this protocol, the SPECT system rotates to a preprogrammed angle and stops in a particular location to acquire data for a specified amount of time. The system then stops acquiring data and moves to the next preprogrammed angle to acquire data for a specified amount of time. This acquisition process is repeated until the rotational arc is completed. Alternatively, the SPECT system may acquire data while moving continuously (Figure 9.30).

In SPECT imaging acquisition, attenuation of the photons from activity in half of the patient opposite the camera head results in substantial spatial resolution degradation. As such, for most noncardiac studies, the projection images are acquired over a complete revolution (360°) about the patient.

Older generations of SPECT systems consisted of camera heads that revolved in a circular orbit around the patient while acquiring data. SPECT imaging of the brain employing circular orbits results in adequate images. However, there is a loss of spatial resolution in body imaging because the circular orbit results in varying distances of the camera head away from the surface of the body. Modern SPECT systems employ noncircular orbits called body contouring that maintains close proximity of the gamma heads to the surface of the body throughout the acquisition. In certain SPECT systems, the technologist determines the noncircular orbit by placing the camera head in specific positions close to the patient at several angles, from which the camera's computer determines the orbit. In addition, some systems automatically perform body contouring by utilizing sensors on the camera heads to maintain their proximity to the patient at each preprogrammed angle (Figure 9.31).

Transverse image reconstruction

Following acquisition, the data are processed and corrected for nonuniformities as well as for center-of-rotation misalignments. After this processing, transverse image reconstruction is performed utilizing filtered back projection and/or iterative reconstruction methods.

Reconstruction algorithms using filtered back projection technique are relatively fast and efficient. However, the attenuation of photons, inclusion of Compton scattered photons, and degradation of spatial resolution with increasing distance from the collimator make filtered back projection techniques less than ideal.

In SPECT imaging reconstruction, iterative reconstruction algorithms are also being utilized. Under this algorithm, the radiopharmaceutical activity distribution is predicted. The projection images are subsequently calculated from the predicted activity distribution. For each iteration, the calculated projection images are compared with the actual projection images, and the predicted activity distribution is accordingly adjusted. Multiple iterations are performed with successive adjustments until the calculated projection images are similar to the actual projection images (Figure 9.32).

Compared to filtered back projection, iterative reconstruction methods take more time to compute. However, by incorporating the point spread function of the scintillation camera into the iterative reconstruction algorithm, the iterative process may generate higher quality tomographic images than does filtered back projection. The point spread function mathematically accounts for the decreasing spatial resolution with distance from the camera face. It can also be customized to account for the effect of photon scattering in the patient and for the effects of attenuation.

Attenuation correction in SPECT

Owing to attenuation, fewer counts are produced from X- or gamma rays deeper within a patient than does radioactivity more superficially within the patient closer to the gamma camera. Thus, transverse image slices produced from a phantom with a uniform activity distribution will demonstrate a gradual decrease in activity toward the center (Figure 9.33).

One of the most widely employed methods for attenuation correction is the Chang method. The Chang method assumes a constant attenuation coefficient throughout the patient. However, this method can overcompensate or undercompensate for attenuation. Before any attenuation correction methods are employed, they should be stringently tested using phantoms before implementation in clinical studies. Another downside is that when attenuation is not uniform in a patient, such as in the thorax, the correction methods cannot compensate appropriately for the nonuniform attenuation.

Manufacturers offer SPECT cameras with sealed radioactive sources to measure the attenuation through the patient. The sealed radioactive sources can be used to acquire transmission data from different projections about the patient. Following acquisition, the projection data are reconstructed to provide maps of tissue attenuation characteristics for transverse sections of the patient, much like CT images. The attenuation maps are then incorporated into the iterative reconstruction process to provide attenuation-corrected SPECT images.

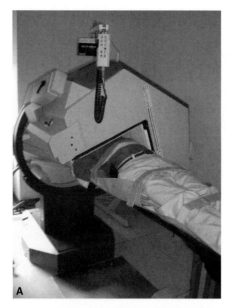

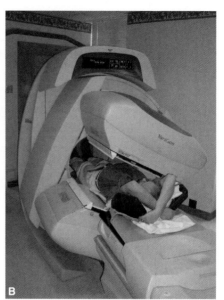

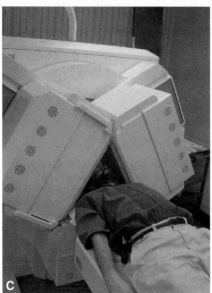

FIG. 9.30 ● **Examples of single photon emission computed tomography cameras:** (A) dual-head camera in 90° configuration; (B) dual-head camera in 180° configuration; and (C) triple-head camera. Reprinted with permission from von Schulthess GK. *Molecular Anatomic Imaging.* 3rd ed. Philadelphia, PA: Wolters Kluwer; 2016.

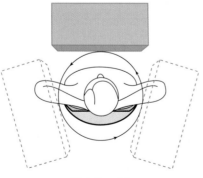

Circular orbit

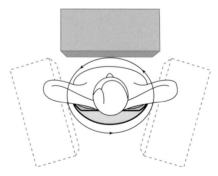

Body contouring orbit

FIG. 9.31 ● **Two types of orbit gamma cameras typically follow in acquisition of projection images for a single photon emission computed tomography study: the circular orbit and the body contouring orbit.** Following the body contouring orbit, the gamma camera is placed as close as practically allowed to maximize the spatial resolution of the acquired images. Reprinted with permission from Bushberg JT, Seibert JA, Leidholdt EM, Boone JM. *Essential Physics of Medical Imaging.* 3rd ed. Philadelphia, PA: Wolters Kluwer Health/Lippincott Williams & Wilkins; 2012.

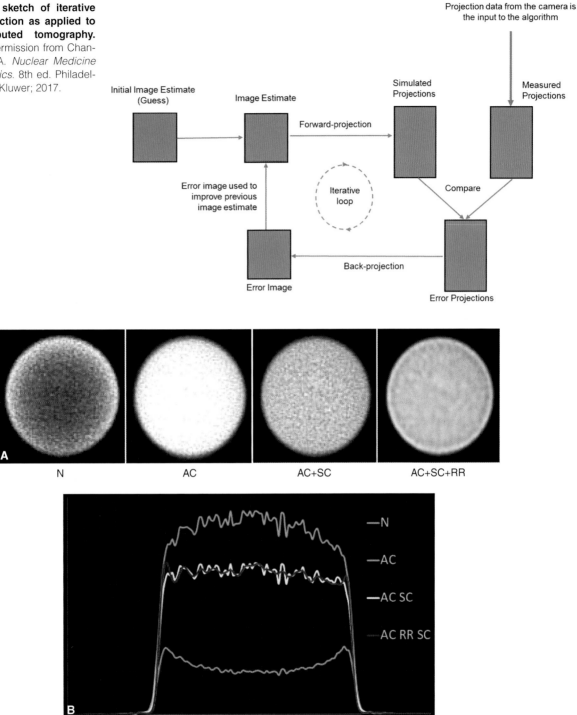

FIG. 9.32 ● A sketch of iterative image reconstruction as applied to emission computed tomography. Reprinted with permission from Chandra R, Rahmim A. *Nuclear Medicine Physics: The Basics.* 8th ed. Philadelphia, PA: Wolters Kluwer; 2017.

Projection data from the camera is the input to the algorithm

Initial Image Estimate (Guess)

Image Estimate

Simulated Projections

Measured Projections

Forward-projection

Error image used to improve previous image estimate

Iterative loop

Compare

Back-projection

Error Image

Error Projections

N   AC   AC+SC   AC+SC+RR

—N
—AC
—AC SC
AC RR SC

FIG. 9.33 ● Illustration of different corrections in single photon emission computed tomography image reconstruction of a phantom with uniform activity distribution (A) and the comparison of plots of signal through the center of the phantom horizontally (B). An iterative reconstruction algorithm is applied here with no correction (N), attenuation correction (AC), addition of scatter correction (AC + SC), and final addition of resolution recovery (AC + SC + RR). Reprinted with permission from Chandra R, Rahmim A. *Nuclear Medicine Physics: The Basics.* 8th ed. Philadelphia, PA: Wolters Kluwer; 2017.

Transmission data are typically acquired concurrently with the emission projection data, because acquiring the two types of data separately can result in significant misregistration in the spatial alignment of the two data sets as well as substantially increase the total imaging time. The radionuclide chosen for the transmission measurements generally has a primary gamma-ray emission that differs considerably in energy from that of the radiopharmaceutical chosen. The separate energy windows are required to differentiate the photons emitted by the transmission source from those emitted by the radiopharmaceutical. However, scattering of the higher energy photons in the patient and in the detector results in cross-talk at the lower energy window.

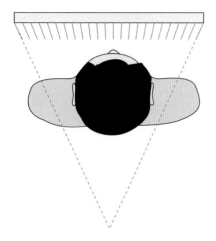
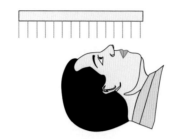

FIG. 9.34 ● **Illustration of a fan-beam collimator, whose holes lined by lead septa are parallel in the axial direction and converging in the transaxial plane.** Reprinted with permission from Bushberg JT, Seibert JA, Leidholdt EM, Boone JM. *Essential Physics of Medical Imaging*. 3rd ed. Philadelphia, PA: Wolters Kluwer Health/ Lippincott Williams & Wilkins; 2012.

Generation of coronal, sagittal, and oblique images

The pixels comprising the transverse image slices may be restructured to produce coronal and sagittal images. In cardiac imaging, oblique images oriented either parallel or perpendicular to the long axis of the left ventricle are often reconstructed.

Collimators for SPECT

Parallel-hole collimators are widely utilized in SPECT imaging. In addition, more specialized collimators, such as the fan-beam collimator, were developed for SPECT imaging. The fan-beam collimator is both a converging and parallel-hole collimator. More specifically, in the *y*-direction, the collimator employs a parallel-hole design so that each row of pixels in a projection image corresponds to a transaxial slice of the patient. In the *x*-direction, the collimator employs a converging design, which results in superior spatial resolution and efficiency characteristics compared to a parallel-hole collimator. The fan-beam collimator is typically used for brain SPECT because the FOV decreases with distance from the collimator as a result of the converging collimator design. Thus, the fan-beam collimator is not routinely used for body SPECT because portions of the body would be excluded from the FOV. This can result in artifacts called truncation artifacts (Figure 9.34).

Multihead SPECT cameras

Manufacturers have designed SPECT systems with dual and triple scintillation camera heads that rotate about the patient to circumvent the limitations of collimation and acquisition time. Multiple camera heads allows for the use of higher resolution collimators for a given level of quantum mottle in the images compared to a single-camera head system.

Multihead SPECT cameras are available in a variety of configurations. Double-head cameras may come in a 90° head configuration or have opposed heads in a 180° head configuration. Double-head, variable-angle cameras are resourceful because they are capable of head and body SPECT as well as whole-body planar scans with the heads in the 180° configuration. Cardiac SPECT can also be performed with the heads in a 90° configuration. Triple-head, fixed-angle cameras are useful for head and body SPECT, and not sufficient for whole-body planar scans because of the limited width of the crystals.

Positron emission tomography

PET is the production of images that portray the distribution of a positron-emitting radionuclide in a patient. A vast majority of PET systems in use today are combined with CT scanners with a single bed passing through the bores of each system.

In a PET system, rings of detectors are built into the bore of the scanner. A PET system relies on the use of ACD as opposed to collimation to generate projection images of the radioactivity distribution in a patient. As the data are gathered by the PET system, the computer processes the information and reconstructs the transverse images in much the same way as the SPECT system does. Modern PET scanners allow for multiple slices to be acquired simultaneously. The primary use of PET is mainly due to the radiopharmaceutical fluorine-18 fluorodeoxyglucose (FDG). FDG is a glucose analog used to help the clinician differentiate malignant neoplasms from more benign lesions, staging malignancy in patients, and monitoring treatment response, among other applications. A few additional positron-emitting radiopharmaceuticals are approved for clinical use and several others are under development or clinical investigation (Figure 9.35).

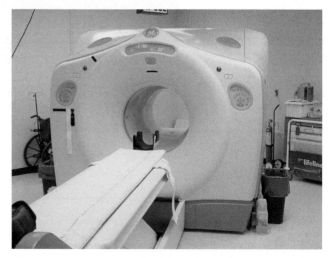

FIG. 9.35 ● **A modern PET-CT scanner.** Reprinted with permission from Braverman LE, Cooper D. *Werner & Ingbar's the Thyroid*. 10th ed. Philadelphia, PA: Wolters Kluwer Health/Lippincott Williams & Wilkins; 2012.

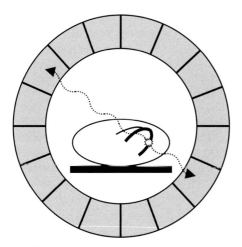

FIG. 9.36 ● **Schematic representation of annihilation coincidence detection by positron emission tomography (PET) imaging.** When a PET radiotracer decays, it emits a positron, which travels a short distance before interacting with an electron, resulting in their mutual annihilation. The annihilation event produces two 511 keV photons traveling in diametrically opposed directions. PET imaging, through the detection of two photons "in coincidence" (arriving at opposite detectors at about the same time), identifies true annihilation events and localizes them to the volume between the two detectors. Reprinted with permission from Griffin BP, Kapadia SR, Rimmerman CM. *Cleveland Clinic Cardiology Board Review.* 2nd ed. Philadelphia, PA: Wolters Kluwer Health/Lippincott Williams & Wilkins; 2012.

Annihilation coincidence detection

Positron emission is a form of radioactive transformation. Emitted positrons dissipate most of their kinetic energy by causing ionization and excitation. After most of the kinetic energy is dissipated, the positron interacts with a local electron by means of annihilation. The masses of both the electron and positron are then converted into two 511 keV photons, which are emitted in opposing directions.

If the photons from an annihilation event, without scatter, interact with the detectors in the PET system, then the annihilation event occurred in a line connecting the two interactions. Using a process called ACD, the electronic circuitry of the PET computer system identifies pairs of interactions occurring within a specified time interval. From the line connecting the interactions, the scanner then localizes in space where the interaction occurred (Figure 9.36).

True, random, and scatter coincidences

A true coincidence is the interaction with the detectors of emissions resulting from a single annihilation within a specified time interval. A random coincidence happens when emissions from different annihilations interact with the detectors in the same specified time interval. A random coincidence is also called an accidental or chance coincidence. A scatter coincidence occurs when a single photon or both photons from a single annihilation event are scattered, and then both scattered photons are detected. Random and scatter coincidences result in misinterpretation of coincidences because they are assigned to lines of response (LORs) that do not correspond to the actual locations of the annihilations. Thus, they contribute to sources of noise, which reduces image contrast and increases statistical noise.

Detection of interactions

Detectors in modern commercial PET systems use scintillation crystals coupled to PMTs. The signals generated from the interactions within the PMTs are processed using pulse mode. In pulse mode, the signals from each interaction are processed independently from those of other interactions. The energy signal aids in energy discrimination to minimize the misplaced events due to scatter. The time signal aids in coincidence detection and time-of-flight determination (Figure 9.37).

In older generations of PET scanners, each scintillation crystal was coupled to a single PMT. Modern PET scanners are designed with larger crystals coupled to a number of PMTs. In these newer generations of PET scanners, a crystal is divided into segments by slits. In this manner, each segment can be considered as a detector element. The relative amounts of energy of the signals from the PMTs are then used to locate the position of the interaction in the crystal (Figure 9.38).

The scintillation crystal chosen must possess certain characteristics to maximize the counting efficiency and to minimize dead-time count losses at high interaction rates. The scintillation crystal must also emit light rapidly enough to allow true coincident interactions from being distinguished from random coincidences. In addition, high conversion efficiency allows more precise event localization in the detector elements along with better energy discrimination.

Older PET systems employed crystals of BGO. Owing to its density and average atomic number, BGO is quite efficient in detecting 511 keV annihilation photons. However, BGO emits light relatively slowly, which results in dead-time count losses and

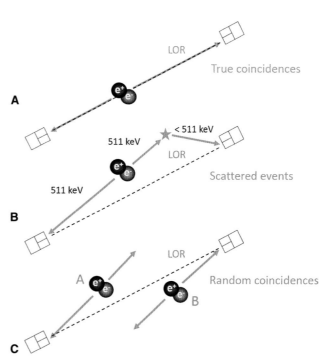

FIG. 9.37 ● Schematic representation of different types of coincidence events that may be detected in positron emission tomography image acquisition, including true events (A), scattered events (B), and random coincidences (C). LOR, line of response. Reprinted with permission from von Schulthess GK. *Molecular Anatomic Imaging.* 3rd ed. Philadelphia, PA: Wolters Kluwer; 2016.

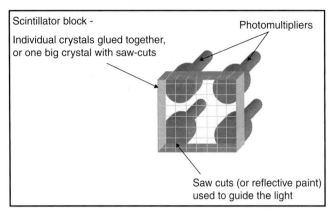

FIG. 9.38 ● **The block detector design used on positron emission tomography scanners.** Reprinted with permission from Brant WE, Helms CA. *Fundamentals of Diagnostic Radiology*. 3rd ed. Philadelphia, PA: Lippincott Williams & Wilkins; 2007.

random coincidences at high interaction rates. More advanced PET systems are designed with inorganic scintillators that emit light more quickly than does BGO. Examples include LSO, LYSO, and GSO, all of which are activated with cerium. These newer scintillators emit light much faster compared to BGO, which results in better performance at high interaction rates, reduction in dead-time effects, and discrimination between true and random coincidences.

The energy signals from the detector elements are analyzed and processed by the energy discrimination circuits of the PET system. The energy discrimination circuits can reject registered events in which the deposited energy varies substantially from 511 keV to minimize the effect of photon scattering and the Compton effect in the patient. An energy discrimination window can be set with a range that includes the photopeak. The range can be adjusted so that only the photopeak is included with rejection of scatter, or adjusted so that the range can incorporate a portion of the Compton continuum.

Following analysis by the energy discrimination circuits, the specified time intervals of the interactions are used for coincidence detection. After a coincidence is detected, the system determines a line in space connecting the two interactions, called a line of response (LOR). The computer stores the data of all the coincidences detected along each LOR. Upon completion of the acquisition, images are generated of the radionuclide distribution in the patient in much the same way as SPECT.

Timing of interactions and detection of coincidences

To detect coincidences, the exact timing of individual interactions in the detector elements must be evaluated by the timing circuits. A coincidence is recorded when the time signals from two detector elements occur within a specified time interval called the time window. The time window for a PET system designed with BGO detectors is about 12 ns. In general, the time window for a PET system designed with LSO detectors is about 4.5 ns due to the rapid emission of light.

True versus random coincidences

The rate of random coincidences between any pair of detectors is determined by the equation: $R_{random} = \tau S_1 S_2$. In this equation, τ is the coincidence time window and S_1 and S_2 are the singles

rates. The time window is the specified time interval during which a pair of interactions in different detector elements is measured as a coincidence. The ratio of true to random coincidences increases as the radioactivity increases in the patient and decreases as the time window is reduced. However, the time window must be long enough to accommodate the difference in arrival times of the photons from annihilations occurring in the periphery of the scanner's FOV. Moreover, the time window can be no shorter than length of time it takes for an unscattered photon to travel the longest distance through the FOV. The choice of scintillation material also influences the time window. Scintillation materials that emit light rapidly allow for a shorter time window, and consequently, improved differentiation between true and random coincidences.

Scatter coincidences

A scatter coincidence is one in which an annihilation occurs and one or both of the photons are scattered in the patient and both are then detected. The number of scatter coincidences is dependent on the amount of tissue available for scattering to occur. Because scatter coincidences are classified as true coincidences, reducing the radioactivity administered, shortening the time window, or employing a scintillator with more rapid light emission does not substantially decrease the scatter coincidence fraction. In addition, corrections for random coincidences does not account for scatter coincidences. By adjusting the energy discrimination circuit, a fraction of the scatter coincidences can be rejected. However, using a narrow energy window centered on the photopeak often results in rejecting a number of annihilation photons that have not actually scattered in the patient. The number of scatter coincidences may be decreased by 2D data acquisition and axial septa.

2D and 3D data acquisition

In 2D PET acquisition, data is gathered in the form of slices where coincidences are detected within each ring or a couple adjacent rings of detector elements. In 2D acquisition, PET scanners are designed with axial septa, typically made of tungsten. These axial septa, or thin annular collimators, reduce the radioactivity outside a transaxial slice from reaching the detector ring for that particular slice being acquired. In this design, the number of scatter coincidences is substantially reduced. In addition, most photons from outside the slice being acquired are absorbed by the axial septa.

To improve sensitivity in 2D data acquisitions, adjacent detector rings may be added together to reconstruct slices. Data from a pair of adjacent detector rings can also be included in the reconstruction of a slice between the two rings to improve sensitivity. The disadvantage to incorporating the data from multiple adjacent detector rings is that the axial spatial resolution is decreased.

In 3D PET acquisition, coincidences are gathered between any combinations of detector rings. Axial septa are not employed. Consequently, the number of true coincidences detected is higher compared to 2D acquisition. Under this technique, a smaller dose of radioactivity may be administered to the patient. However, with 3D data acquisition, the greater number of interactions detected means that a higher number of random and scatter coincidences are counted in the data. This also increases the dead-time count losses.

Advanced PET systems are designed with retractable axial septa that allow the scanner the versatility to perform either 2D or 3D acquisitions (Figure 9.39).

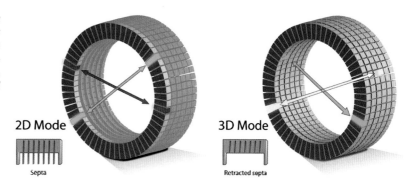

2D Mode   3D Mode

Septa   Retracted septa

Transverse image reconstruction

Following acquisition of the PET data, the data for each LOR are corrected for scatter coincidences, random coincidences, dead-time count losses, and attenuation. Upon completion of these corrections, image reconstruction is performed. For 2D data acquisition, image reconstruction algorithms employ filtered back projection and/or iterative reconstruction methods, similar to those in SPECT imaging. For 3D data acquisition, 3D analytical and iterative reconstruction methods are necessary. During reconstruction of PET images, the correction for nonuniform attenuation can be applied to the projection data before reconstruction. By contrast, for reconstruction of SPECT images, the correction for nonuniform attenuation is incorporated into the reconstruction process.

Time-of-flight determination

Mathematically it is possible to measure the difference between the times of the interactions in the detectors of a pair of annihilation photons. By doing so, the exact point on a line between the two interactions where an annihilation occurred could be determined. However, current PET scintillators are not capable of discerning with extreme precision the exact location on a line where an annihilation occurred. Newer fast scintillators, such as LSO and LYSO, aid in the determination of the location of annihilation within a number of centimeters. This data may be used in the image reconstruction process to improve the signal-to-noise ratio.

CHAPTER SELF-ASSESSMENT QUESTIONS

1. Which of the following is *NOT* true regarding gas-filled detectors?
   A. Ionization survey meters and dose calibrators typically operate in current mode.
   B. GM survey meters typically operate in pulse mode.
   C. Both ionization survey meters and GM survey meters are used for low-level radiation contamination surveys.
   D. Dose calibrators are typically filled with pressurized noble gas to increase sensitivity.

2. What properties would an ideal scintillator have for the detection of gamma photons?
   A. It should be transparent to its own emitted light.
   B. It converts gamma radiation into detectable light photon efficiently.
   C. The amount of light should be proportional to radiation energy.
   D. All of these

3. Which of the following causes the most degradation of spatial resolution of a SPECT scan?
   A. Using a 64 × 64 acquisition matrix (compared to 128 × 128)
   B. Using a camera with a half inch scintillator crystal (compared to 3/8 inch)
   C. Using an ultrahigh resolution collimator (compared to general purpose ones)
   D. Using a noncircular orbit that conforms to the patient's body contour (compared to circular)

4. Which of the following does *NOT* improve sensitivity of a PET scan?
   A. 3D acquisition mode
   B. Larger bore size
   C. More detector rings
   D. Thicker scintillator crystal

Answers to Chapter Self-Assessment Questions

1. C   GM survey meters are more sensitive than ionization survey meters and therefore more useful in detecting some quantities of radioactivity as encountered in low-level contamination surveys.

2. D   Ideal scintillators are expected to have all listed characteristics.

3. A   Thinner crystal, ultrahigh resolution collimator, and an orbit that places gamma as close as possible to the anatomy all contribute to improved spatial resolution. A larger pixel size leads to poorer spatial resolution.

4. B   3D scan (compared to 2D scan), more detector rings, and thicker crystal all result in more annihilation coincidence events being detected. Larger bore size may allow more events escape the detectors and cause a decrease in efficiency.

Radiation Biology and Safety

Joshua Adam Tarrence, DO

LEARNING OBJECTIVES

1. Understand the ways ionizing radiation interacts with molecules and cells in organic tissue.
2. Be able to describe the ways ionizing radiation exposure can cause harm to humans.
3. Understand the relationship between radiation exposure and carcinogenesis.
4. Be familiar with the various dose-response curves.
5. Understand the principles behind radiation safety and their implementation.
6. Know how radiation exposure is monitored and regulated.
7. Recognize the expected organ system responses and whole-body responses to radiation injury based on dose.

INTRODUCTION

Radiation energy allows for many of the conveniences enjoyed by modern society, not least of which is advanced medical imaging for the diagnosis of disease. However, most understand to a certain degree that radiation carries with it the potential for harmful effects. The study of the effects of radiation on the human body has closely accompanied the study of radiation as an imaging modality from the earliest stages. As such, it is imperative for one working in the field of medical imaging or in medicine in general to be familiar with the potentially harmful effects radiation can have on the human body and how the potential for harm can be kept to the lowest level possible.

This chapter consists of two main sections: *radiation biology* and *radiation safety*. *Radiation biology* examines the mechanisms through which radiation interacts with the human body down to the molecular level and the implications those mechanisms have on analyzing, treating, and preventing the body's response to radiation exposure. This is followed by a review of radiation as a carcinogen, a hereditary risk factor, and a potentially harmful agent in utero. *Radiation safety* details how radiation exposure is measured and the preventative measure implemented to ensure that patient and personnel exposure to harmful amounts of radiation is avoided. This is followed by a brief review of radiation regulatory bodies and exposure limits, radiation exposure emergencies, and special considerations for radiation exposure in female pregnant patients.

RADIATION BIOLOGY

The response to radiation exposure is not uniform across different biologic systems or even across time in the same biologic system. Factors that determine how a biologic system reacts to radiation include variables in the radiation source and in the biologic

system itself. Variables related to the radiation source include the absorbed dose, the dose rate, and the type of radiation. Variables related to the irradiated biologic system include factors that are inherent to the system and factors related to the conditions in the cells at the time of radiation exposure.

Stochastic effects and deterministic effects

There are two categories of effects of radiation exposure on biologic tissues: *stochastic effects* and *deterministic effects*. Stochastic effects have an increased risk of occurring with an increase in dose. However, the severity of disease, once disease is present, it not affected by dose. For example, a substantial exposure to ionizing radiation can increase the risk of certain types of cancer, such as thyroid cancer. In the stochastic effect model, theoretically the radiation only needs to affect a very small number of cells to create the potential for cancer growth. Therefore, as the dose increases, so does the opportunity of damage to cells and, as a result, the risk of cancer increases. However, once a cancer has been caused by the radiation exposure (thyroid cancer in this case), the severity of the cancer is not dependent on the dose of the radiation exposure. Although unproven, this model of increasing risk of disease with increasing dose and no dose under which the risk will be zero is the model on which the modern approach to radiation protection is based. Because the risk increases and decreases with the dose in this model, the current approach of "ALARA" (as low as reasonably achievable) seeks to decrease the risk of radiation-induced disease as much as possible by always using the lowest possible dose.

In contrast, deterministic effects are those of which the *severity* increases with an increase in dose. Deterministic effects have an approximate threshold dose, under which the risk of the effect occurring is essentially zero. For example, if a patient receives an X-ray of her hand, there is essentially no chance of her receiving skin damage from the single radiograph under standard methodology. If the same patient were to undergo fluoroscopy on her hand, for a procedure for instance, and were to receive a much higher dose of radiation to that skin surface area, she would eventually experience skin and tissue damage after a certain dose is reached and the damage would increase as the dose increases.

Interaction of low energy electrons with tissue

The known physical effects of radiation on tissues are the result of chemical changes in biomolecules, and these changes are brought about by a series of serial excitations and the resulting release of kinetic energy following a single ionizing event. When X-ray or gamma rays come into contact with tissues, energetic free electrons are released. The kinetic energy of these electrons is in turn dissipated by excitation, ionization, and heat. As the energy is released, it will interact with and excite surrounding electrons in a rapid and random fashion, exciting a large number of secondary, low-energy electrons in its path. This is known as secondary ionization. For example, a single electron with an energy of 30 keV set in motion by absorption of an X-ray or gamma-ray photon may produce over 1000 secondary electrons of lower energy. The secondary electrons, known as *delta rays*, may then each cause their own set of ionizations in the tissues, resulting in a chain of ionization events. Eventually, as energy is lost during these reactions, the electrons will be excited below the threshold of excitation of liquid water (7.4 eV), leaving them in a so-called *subexcitation* state. These electrons then release their energies in the form of rotation, vibration, and collision events with surrounding water molecules.

The low-energy electrons set in motion by the initial ionizing event will form shorter tracks off of the path of the sentinel electron and will each result in three additional ionizing events on average. These secondary tracks along the path of the sentinel electron path are known as *spurs*. Approximately 95% of the energy deposited in tissues by X-rays and gamma rays is estimated to occur in spurs.[1] Additionally, longer secondary tracks that occur less frequently along the sentinel path and deposit more energy are known as *blobs*. The higher energy released along the path of blobs results in more ionization events along their paths on average. The areas around spurs and blobs experience a high concentration of reactive chemical species, which increases the opportunity for molecular damage in these locations. Should such a cluster of ionizations occur near deoxyribonucleic acid (DNA), there is the potential for several, closely grouped areas of damage to occur in the DNA. Such groups of multiple damage sites are more difficult for the cell to repair correctly.[2,3] This type of damage can be referred to as *clustered damage*, *complex damage*, or *multiply damaged sites*. This form of clustered damage is characteristic of ionizing radiation-induced damage to DNA, but the functional changes to molecules, cells, tissues, and organs brought about by this damage cannot be distinguished from those caused by other types of damage. Although these types of ionizing radiation-induced damage are more difficult for the cell to repair, the cell remains very efficient in correcting the damage or killing and replacing the cell. Only a fraction of the energy deposited into irradiated tissues brings about any chemical changes, and the effects of these changes may never be made apparent or may declare themselves at any time ranging from minutes to years.

Interactions of free radicals with tissue

Biologic changes in irradiated tissues can occur *directly* or *indirectly*. Direct damage occurs when macromolecules such as DNA, RNA, or proteins are ionized by an ionizing particle or photon passing nearby. Indirect damage is caused by chemically reactive species that are the result of radiation interactions with other molecules, usually water. Radiation interaction with water produces several types of reactive chemical species. When water is contacted by radiation, it is first ionized to form H_2O^+ and e^-. Immediately the e^- thermalizes and becomes hydrated and is surrounded by water molecules to form an aqueous electron (e_{aq}^-). The e_{aq}^- subsequently reacts with another water molecule and forms a negative water ion H_2O^-. The H_2O^+ and H_2O^- ions are unstable and quickly react with water to form another ion and a free radicle

$$H_2O^+ + H_2O \rightarrow H_3O^+ + \cdot OH \text{ (hydroxyl radical)}$$

$$H_2O^- \rightarrow OH^- + H \cdot \text{ (hydrogen radical)}$$

The majority of biologic damage caused by radiation in medical imaging is caused by free radicals. Free radicals are atoms or molecules with unpaired orbital electrons. Hydrogen and hydroxyl radicals can also be created, among other pathways, through radiation-induced excitation and disassociation of a molecule of water. The resulting H^+ and OH^- ions have extremely short half-lives and typically do not cause a significant amount of biologic damage. They also tend to recombine to form water, also limiting their interactions with other nearby biologic molecules. Once free radicals have formed, they can undergo reactions with other free radicals to form nonreactive molecules such as water and no biologic damage occurs. Additionally, a free radical can undergo a reaction with a free radical of the same type to form other molecules such as hydrogen peroxide. Hydrogen peroxide can cause damage to a cell, but the majority of damage caused by linear energy transfer (LET) radiation does not involve hydrogen peroxide. Instead, the majority of indirect damage caused by X-rays and gamma rays is the result of hydroxyl radicals reacting with biologic molecules such as DNA. The potential for harmful effects by free radicals is increased in the presence of oxygen, because oxygen acts as a stabilizer of the free radicals and makes it less likely that they will combine to form nonharmful molecules such as water or molecular hydrogen. Oxygen can also combine with a hydrogen radical to form highly reactive oxygen species such as the hydroperoxyl radical ($HO_2\cdot$). Free radicals can act as strong oxidizing or reducing agents when they combine directly with macromolecules. Although free radicals have short half-lives, they can diffuse sufficiently far in the cell to cause damage in locations away from their origin. Approximately two-third of total damage caused by medical imaging radiation is caused by the indirect effects of free radicals.

Relative biologic effectiveness

The biologic effects of radiation depend on several factors, including dose, dose rate, tissues being irradiated, and so on. An additional factor is the *linear energy transfer* (LET). LET refers to the energy deposition of an ionizing particle per unit distance of the material it transverses. Experiments are performed to determine the relative effectiveness of different types of radiation and their LETs by comparing the dose required to produce the same biologic effect as a particular dose of a reference form of radiation. The term *relative biologic effectiveness* (RBE) refers to the relationship of the effectiveness of the test radiation to the reference radiation

$$RBE = \frac{\text{Dose of 250 kV X-rays required for certain effect}}{\text{Dose of test radiation required for same effect}}$$

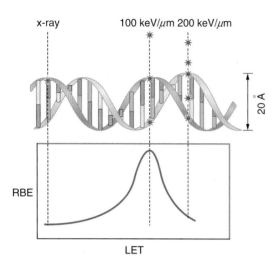

FIG. 10.1 ● **The relative biologic effectiveness (RBE) of a given radiation generally increases with the linear energy transfer (LET) of the radiation.** However, beyond ~100 keV/mm, radiation becomes less efficient and further increase in LET results in wasted dose. Reprinted with permission from Hall EJ, Giaccia AJ. *Radiobiology for the Radiologist.* 8th ed. Philadelphia, PA: Wolters Kluwer; 2018.

RBE is initially proportional to LET. The increase in the RBE with increasing LET (Figure 10.1) is thought to be due to the increased specific ionization (ionization density) associated with high-LET radiation, which results in more cellular damage. RBE is directly proportional to LET until approximately 100 keV/μm in tissue, beyond which the RBE *decreases* with increasing LET (Figure 10.1). This can be explained by the *overkill* or *wasted dose* effect. Overkill refers to the deposition of radiation energy in tissues beyond the levels necessary to produce maximum biologic effects.

Molecular and cellular responses to radiation

DNA damage and repair

Ionizing energy deposition in tissues results in chemical and subsequent structural changes in molecules. These structural changes include hydrogen bond breakage, molecular degradation or breakage, and intermolecular and intramolecular cross-linking. These processes occurring in DNA molecules may result in single-strand breaks (SSBs) or double-strand breaks (DSBs) in the DNA, base loss, base changes, or cross-links between DNA strands or between DNA and proteins. SSBs in DNA are usually rejoined with high repair fidelity. DSBs that are incompletely or incorrectly repaired may lead to activation of oncogenes or inactivation of tumor suppressor genes, which is the basis of carcinogenesis. Such changes can also result in loss of heterozygosity.

The low-LET radiation used in medical imaging is capable of causing DSBs, but is more likely to produce SSBs, which are more likely to be correctly repaired. However, the low-energy secondary electrons produced along the course of the path of initial ionizing radiations, as discussed earlier in the chapter, increases the chances that complex damage including SSBs and DSBs as well as base damage will occur near one another. These areas of complex damage prove much more difficult to repair correctly and may lead to permanent damage.[2,4]

The loss or damage of a base is termed a mutation. Some mutations can cause physical changes to a chromosome. When a chromosome is damaged before DNA replication, it is termed a

chromosome aberration. Damage occurring in a chromosome after DNA replication is termed a chromatid aberration. Chromatid aberrations result in only one daughter cell being affected as long as only one of the chromatids of a pair is damaged. This is not true of chromosome aberrations. Chromosomal aberrations occur spontaneously to a certain extent. Quantifying chromosomal aberrations in human lymphocytes is even used as a means of estimating a dose of radiation received after an accidental exposure by comparing the number of aberrations against the expected background number of aberrations. The extent of genetic damage transmitted with chromosomal aberrations depends on factors such as the type of cell, the types and number of genes deleted, and the lesion occurring in either a somatic or gametic cell.

DNA is constantly undergoing damage and repair even in the absence of radiation. The cell is normally quite capable of repairing the damage to avoid mutations. When DNA is damaged, there are cellular responses that either repair the damage or allow the cell to cope in spite of the damage. There are checkpoints in the reproductive pathway of a cell that will either arrest the cell cycle while the DNA damage is repaired or will initiate apoptosis if the damage cannot be repaired and is harmful enough to the cell.

There are many types of DNA repair, including SSB repair, DSB repair, cross-link repair, direct nucleotide repair, nucleotide excision repair, and short- and long-patch base excision repair. Homologous recombination repair (Figure 10.2), which involves exchanges with homologous DNA strands from sister chromatids, preserves DNA fidelity. However, most DSBs are repaired by nonhomologous end-joining, which involves the ends of the broken strands being joined together (Figure 10.2). This method of repair is prone to errors, but most DSBs are repaired correctly.

There is strong cohesion between the ends of chromatin material, and during these repairs, interchromosomal and intrachromosomal recombination can occur. In approximately 50% of these instances of double-strand misrepair, a translocation occurs. Translocations are large-scale rearrangements of chromosomes, and they may change the phenotype of the cell dramatically without resulting in cell death.

Cellular response to radiation

Radiation exposure initiates a number of cellular responses, depending of the type of cell, the stage of the cell cycle during the exposure, the dose of the radiation exposure, and so on. The cell may respond by dying (apoptosis), delaying reproduction, failing to reproduce, delaying expression of the genome, DNA mutation, phenotypic transformation, or bystander effects (damaging neighboring unirradiated cells). Cells may also become altered to be more radioresistant, termed an adaptive response.

One marker of the biologic effects of radiation exposure is reproductive integrity. Irradiated cells in culture may not show physical changes for a long time, but reproductive failure will eventually occur. This allows the radiosensitivity of a particular cell line to be determined by irradiating individual cells in vitro and counting the number of colonies that arise from that known number of irradiated cells. This method may also be used to determine the biologic effectiveness of different types of radiation as well as the effects of environmental condition on the radiation effects.

Cell survival curves are a plot of the loss of ability of a cell to reproduce as a function of the cell's exposure to radiation (Figure 10.3). The shape of a cell survival curve is an indication of the cell line radiosensitivity. There is a "shoulder" before the semilogarithmic plot of the cell survival curve, dependent on D_q. D_q is a measure of sublethal damage, an entity based on the concept

FIG. 10.2 ● **Two main DNA double-strand break damage repair mechanisms.** Homologous recombination uses an identical DNA strand as template for precise repair. Non-homologous end joining (NHEJ), in comparison, is more prone to errors in repair. Reprinted with permission from Halperin EC, Wazer DE, Perez CA, Brady LW. *Perez & Brady's Principles and Practice of Radiation Oncology.* 7th ed. Philadelphia, PA: Wolters Kluwer; 2018.

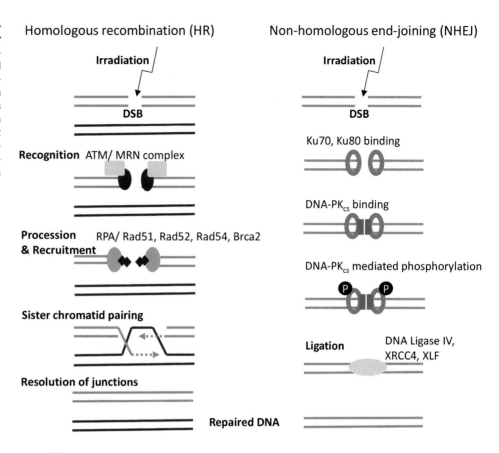

that when certain radiation doses are split into fractions, more than one exposure to the radiation is required to kill the cell and that the cell is capable of repairing the damage between fractions of the dose.

An additional method of describing cell survival is the linear quadratic (LQ) model. This model is used more commonly than the model described earlier because it fits most experimental data on human cell lines and is more useful in explaining fractionation effects in late-responding versus early-responding tissues for radiotherapy. The LQ model is expressed by the following equation:

$$SF(D) = e^{-\alpha D + \beta D^2}$$

where D is the dose (in Gy), α is the coefficient of cell killing proportional to dose, and β is the coefficient of cell killing proportional to the square of the dose. The α and β constants can be used to predict dose-response of certain tissues. The linear portion of the survival curve (α) represents cell killing by individual radioactive particle tracts without interaction, making it independent of dose rate. Conversely, the quadratic (β) portion of the curve represents cell killing as a result of interacting particles. The linear portion of the curve (α) dominates in high-LET radiation and the quadratic portion (β) dominates in low-LET radiation. When a radiation dose causes equal linear and quadratic cell killing, this is termed the α/β ratio. The α/β ratio is a measure of certain tissues' sensitivity to radiation dose fractionation. Early-responding tissues such as bone marrow have a larger α/β ratio, meaning the tissues have less ability to repair damage in between doses. Thus, fractionating the dose in these tissues would have less effect than in those which are late-responding tissues with a lower α/β ratio. A lower α/β ratio would indicate the tissues are more capable of repair in between dose fractions and thus fractionating the dose would decrease lasting damage in these tissues.

Tissue radiosensitivity

As discussed earlier, there are many factors that must be considered when determining radiation dose and its effect on tissues. However, there are many factors apart from the dose of radiation itself, which affect the response of tissues to a certain dose of radiation. These can be classified as conditional or inherent factors.

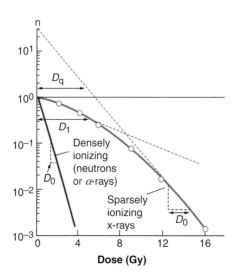

FIG. 10.3 ● **Typical cell survival curve characterized by the initial slope D_1, the final slopt D_0, and a parameter related to the width of the shoulder, D_q.** Reprinted with permission from Hall EJ, Giaccia AJ. *Radiobiology for the Radiologist.* 8th ed. Philadelphia, PA: Wolters Kluwer; 2018.

Conditional factors exist before or during an irradiation even, whereas inherent factors are the physical characteristics of the irradiated cells themselves.

Conditional Factors

The effects of radiation are partly determined by the dose rate and fractionation of the dose. Changes in the rate at which low-LET radiation is delivered has been shown to affect the degree of chromosomal aberrations, reproductive delay, and cell death in the irradiated tissues. High-dose rates are generally more effective in causing biologic damage due to the lower potential for radiation damage repair to take place (Figure 10.4).

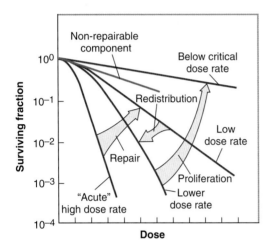

FIG. 10.4 ● **Different cell survival curves as a result of different dose rate.** The observed dose-rate effect results from repair of sublethal damage, redistribution in the cycle and cell proliferation. Reprinted with permission from Hall EJ, Giaccia AJ. *Radiobiology for the Radiologist.* 8th ed. Philadelphia, PA: Wolters Kluwer; 2018.

Such a phenomenon is not observed with high-LET radiation due to the increased potential for clustered damage to occur and the lower potential for DNA repair at baseline. Fractionation of a given dose over time also decreases the potential for radiation-induced biologic damage, with the intervals between doses allowing for repair mechanisms in the healthy tissues to repair sublethal damage. This concept is important in radiotherapy due to the ability of noncancerous tissues to be repaired when therapeutic radiation doses are fractionated.

The presence of oxygen increases damage caused by low-LET radiation because it prevents the recombination of free radicals and the formation of harmless chemical species. Oxygen also inhibits repair of damage caused by free radicals. Increasing the oxygen concentration at the time of irradiation has been shown to lead to increased killing of otherwise resistant cells in some tumors. The oxygen enhancement ratio (OER) is an expression of the effectiveness of radiation to cause damage at different oxygen tensions. The OER is defined as the dose of radiation required to produce a given response in the absence of oxygen divided by the dose required to produce the same response in the presence of oxygen. The OER for low-LET radiation in mammalian cells is usually between 2 and 3. OER is lower for high-LET radiation because its damage is not dependent on free radicals.

Inherent Factors

Cells have inherent properties that determine their relative radiosensitivity. Cells that are rapidly dividing will continue to undergo mitosis for a long period of time, and are undifferentiated and typically more radiosensitive. A more detailed classification scheme of cells and their relative radiosensitivity is included below. An exception to these general rules is lymphocytes, which are very radiosensitive despite possessing characteristics of radioresistant cells (Table 10.1). In addition to these characteristics, the phase of reproduction the cell is found in during irradiation greatly affects its radiosensitivity. Cells are most sensitive in the M-phase (mitosis) as well as the time between the S-phase and mitosis (G_2) (Figure 10.5).

Table 10.1 CLASSIFICATION OF CELLULAR RADIOSENSITIVITY

Cell Type	Characteristics	Examples	Radiosensitivity
VIM	Rapidly dividing, undifferentiated, do not differentiate between divisions	Type A spermatogonia, erythroblasts, crypt cells of intestines, basal cells of epidermis	Most radiosensitive
DIM	Actively dividing, more differentiated than VIMs, differentiate between divisions	Intermediate spermatogonia, myelocytes	Relatively radiosensitive
MCT	Irregularly dividing; more differentiated than VIMs or DIMs	Endothelial cells, fibroblasts	Intermediate in radiosensitivity
RPM	Do not normally divide but retain capability of division, differentiated	Parenchymal cells of the liver and adrenal glands, lymphocytes,[a] bone, muscle cells	Relatively radioresistant
FPM	Do not divide; differentiated	Some nerve cells Erythrocytes Spermatozoa	Most radioresistant

[a]Lymphocytes, although classified as relatively radioresistant by their characteristics, are in fact very radiosensitive.
Abbreviations: DIM, differentiating intermitotic; FPM, fixed postmitotic; MCT, multipotential connective tissue; RPM, reverting postmitotic; VIM, vegetative intermitotic.
Rubin P, Casarett GW. Clinical radiation pathology as applied to curative radiotherapy. *Clin Pathol Radiat.* 1968;22:767–768. Reprint of Table 20.1 with permission from Bushberg JT, Seibert JA, Leidholdt Jr EM, Boone JM. *The Essential Physics of Medical Imaging.* 3rd ed. Philadelphia, PA: Lippincott Williams and Wilkins; 2011.

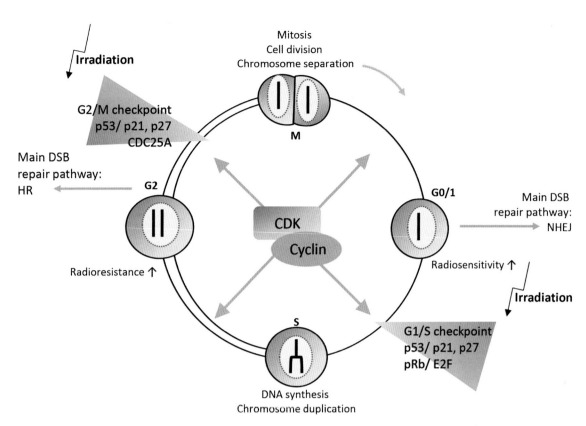

FIG. 10.5 ● **Phases of a cell's reproductive cycle and checkpoints.** Different phases of a cell's cycle have different susceptibilities to radiation damage. Checkpoints are critical control points in the cycle that have built-in stop signals that may halt the cell cycle. Reprinted with permission from Halperin EC, Wazer DE, Perez CA, Brady LW. *Perez & Brady's Principles and Practice of Radiation Oncology.* 7th ed. Philadelphia, PA: Wolters Kluwer; 2018.

Additional responses to radiation have been observed in vitro, which are not completely understood. For example, there is evidence of an adaptive response that results in decreased effectiveness of a subsequent dose of radiation following exposure of the affected material to an initial dose. Additionally, there is a so-called "bystander effect" with which effects in nearby, non-irradiated cells are observed when certain nearby cells are irradiated. Finally, genomic instability has been observed in vitro, which refers to a phenomenon involving delayed lethal mutations in irradiated cells, possibly due to errors in DNA repair. While these phenomena raise interesting questions about possible other factors affecting radiosensitivity and response to radiation, they are still incompletely understood and their observed effects are typically limited to experimental environments.

Organ system responses to radiation

In addition to analyzing responses to radiation on the molecular and cellular level, the response of organ systems to radiation is also of interest, namely the functional and morphologic changes observed in the organ system as a whole. When analyzing organ responses to radiation, there is a latent period between the exposure and the observed effects, which typically decreases in length as dose increases. Higher dose also decreases the amount of time required for the full physiologic effects caused by the dose to occur. Additionally, threshold doses do exist in some cases under which no observable effects will occur.

Repair and regeneration

When damage to an organ system occurs as a result of radiation exposure, cellular regeneration and repair occur to heal the damage. Regeneration is replacement of damaged cells by the same type of cells. Repair is the replacement of the damaged cells by fibrotic tissue and the functionality of the organ system is reduced or lost. Whether repair or regeneration occurs and how much repair or regeneration occurs depends on the dose of radiation, the type and amount of tissue irradiated, and the capacity of the irradiated tissues to repair or regenerate. When a radiation dose is fractionated, it allows regeneration to occur in between fractions while also allowing for reoxygenation of tumor cells (increasing the potential for biologic damage in the cells upon subsequent exposures) and redistribution of irradiated cells into more sensitive phases of the cell cycle thus increasing effectiveness of radiotherapy.

Specific organ system responses

There are specific and characteristic physiologic responses that have been observed in vivo in certain organ systems in the human body. These will be described in the following paragraphs.

Skin

Skin damage is the most common tissue reaction resulting from high-dose image-guided procedures. The degree of damage to skin by ionizing radiation (also termed the cutaneous radiation syndrome) depends on the dose, quality, and quantity of the radiation as well as the location and extent of exposure to the radiation. Damage ranges from mild erythema to chronic necrosis based on these factors.

Often, there are no immediate symptoms of skin damage caused by radiation exposure. The earliest symptoms such as pruritus and erythema can be delayed up to months following the exposure. When the skin is exposed to damaging levels of radiation, there is an oxidative stress placed on the tissues resulting in a series of inflammatory responses, reduction/impairment of stem cells, changes to endothelial cells, and apoptosis and necrosis of epidermal cells. These reactions are deterministic, meaning there is a threshold dose of approximately 1 Gy that must be reached before effects are observed. As doses increase, there may be eventual loss of mitotic activity of the germinal cells of the hair follicles, sebaceous glands, basal layer, and intimal cells of the microvasculature.

Following an acute dose ≥2 Gy of low-LET radiation, early transient erythema may occur. This consists of a generalized erythema that subsequently fades and is thought to be the result of release of vasoactive amines, resulting in increased vascular permeability. A secondary erythema, termed main erythema, can appear as early as 2 weeks after initial exposure to a high dose of radiation or after repeated exposures to lower doses. This response reaches its peak around the third week following exposure, with edema, erythema, and tenderness of the skin. Main erythema is thought to be the result of the release of proteolytic enzymes from damaged basal cells of the epithelium as well as a reflection of the loss of those epithelial cells. Several pathways of vascular damage are also upregulated as a result of the presence of radiation-induced free radicals. Finally, late erythema may be seen 8 to 52 weeks after exposure and is a result of dermal ischemia, which causes a bluish color of the skin. Temporary hair loss is associated with doses of 3 to 6 Gy, occurring approximately 3 weeks following exposure. Regrowth typically begins approximately 2 months later.

Following moderately large doses (20 Gy single dose or 40 Gy over 4 weeks), acute radiation dermatitis and moist desquamation occur. This is characterized by edema, inflammation, vascular damage, dermal hypoplasia, and permanent hair loss. Moist desquamation is a predictor of future development of telangiectasia. Reepithelialization will occur within 6 to 8 weeks if the vasculature and germinal epithelium are not too severely damaged. The skin will return to normal in 2 to 3 months. If vascular or germinal layer damage is too extensive, the skin will undergo healing but may remain atrophic with altered pigmentation. The skin in this state is easily damaged by physical trauma and is prone to recurrent infections and lesions, including necrotic ulcerations. Following repeated low-level exposures of 10 to 20 mGy per day with the total dose close to 20 Gy, chronic radiation dermatitis can develop. This causes hypertrophy or atrophy of the skin and places it at increased risk of skin neoplasms, especially squamous cell carcinoma (Figure 10.6).

Reproductive Organs

The gonads are very radiosensitive. Radiosensitivity of the cell populations found in the male testes ranges from very sensitive (spermatogonia) to relatively radioresistant (mature spermatozoa). Radiation effects on the male reproductive system include decreased fertility, temporary sterility, and permanent sterility.[5] Reduced fertility secondary to decreased sperm count and motility can occur following doses of 150 mGy. These effects typically occur after 6 weeks. Doses of 500 mGy can produce temporary sterility, with the duration ranging from 1 to 3.5 years based on dose. Chronic exposures to 20 to 50 mGy per week with total doses exceeding 2.5 to 3 Gy can produce permanent sterility. Exposures related to medical imaging are not likely to exceed 100 mGy and are thus unlikely to affect the testes.

The ova within ovarian follicles are radiosensitive. Small and large (mature) follicles are relatively more radioresistant than intermediate follicles. A period of reduced fertility can be seen after an exposure of 1.5 Gy after an initial period of fertility preservation due to the presence of mature follicles. Fertility will eventually return to normal as long as the exposure is not high enough to kill the small, relatively radioresistant primordial follicles. Doses resulting in permanent sterility are age-dependent, with higher doses (~10 Gy) needed to sterilize a prepubescent female than in premenopausal women over age 40 (~2-3 Gy).

Eyes

Radiation can damage or kill cells in the lens of the eye; however, there is no system for the body to remove these cells from the lens. Sufficient accumulation of these damaged cells may lead to cataracts. Cataracts caused by radiation exposure begin forming in the anterior subcapsular region and travel posteriorly, unlike senile cataracts that usually develop in the anterior pole of the lens. The posterior subcapsular cataracts can impair vision by causing a "halo effect" around lights at night even at minor levels of cataract formation. The formation of cataracts was previously viewed as deterministic. There was thought to be a threshold dose under which the formation of cataracts will not occur. Recent data have indicated that if a threshold does exist, it is likely much lower than originally thought. There is some thought that the formation of cataracts is actually better represented by a stochastic model. The International Commission on Radiological Protection (ICRP) has recently changed recommendations for occupational exposure limits from 150 mSv per year to 20 mSv per year averaged over 5 years (with no year exceeding 50 mSv).

Whole-body response to radiation

As discussed previously, the various tissues of the body vary in their relative radiosensitivities, and an acute exposure to radiation results in more cellular damage than exposure to the same dose of radiation delivered over a protracted period of time. In addition to the localized effects on certain tissues following radiation exposure discussed above, there is a series of observed responses by the body to an acute exposure of a large portion of the body to a high radiation dose. This is known as the acute radiation syndrome (ARS). The ARS is distinct form of localized radiation injuries such as skin ulceration consisting of a group of hematopoietic, gastrointestinal (GI), and neurovascular syndromes occurring in stages over the course of hours to weeks following a radiation exposure event as a result of the differing radiosensitivities of the irradiated tissues.

Following an adequately high exposure, the sequence of events occurring in the body follows a predictable course. The typical sequence of events consists of prodromal illness, latent illness, manifest illness, and recovery (if the dose is not fatal). Prodromal symptoms can occur within minutes of exposure with a high exposure dose. Prodromal symptoms include nausea, vomiting, diarrhea, fever, anorexia, lethargy, headache, and altered mental status. As the dose increases, the severity of the effects increases and the latency of the onset of symptoms decreases. The latent period follows the prodromal period and may last for up to 4 weeks for exposures less than 1 Gy. Higher exposures result in a shorter latent period. The manifest illness stage represents organ tissue damage and its clinical manifestations. This stage may last for 2 to 4 weeks and is characterized by immune system compromise due to damage to the hematopoietic system. For this reason, treatment of ARS should be started within 6 to 8 weeks of the initial exposure, before significant immunocompromise, to increase chances of recovery. Survival of the manifest illness stage is a good predictor of recovery but the patient remains at risk of future cancers.

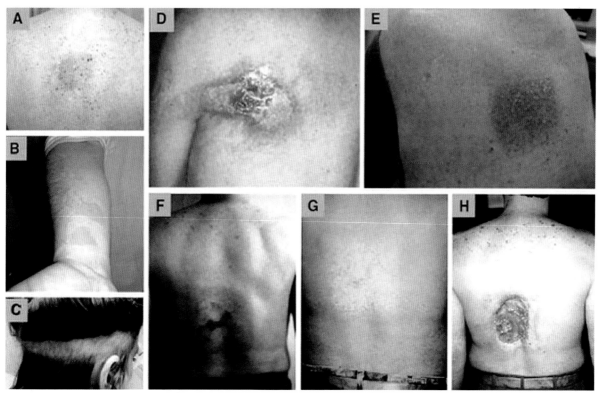

FIG. 10.6 ● **Examples of radiation-induced effects on skin.** A, National Cancer Institute (NCI) skin toxicity grade 1: Two fluoroscopically guided procedures were performed through overlapping skin ports in a 65-year-old man. Note enhanced reaction in the overlap zone. The first procedure was performed 6 weeks before and the second procedure was performed 2 weeks before the photograph was obtained (Reprinted from Balter S, Hopewell JW, Miller DL, et al. Fluoroscopically guided interventional procedures: a review of radiation effects on patients' skin and hair. *Radiology.* 2010;254(2):326–341. Copyright © 2010 Radiological Society of North America. With permission). B, Radionuclide skin contamination. Slight erythema after accidental contamination by F-18 fluorodeoxyglucose (https://rpop.iaea.org/rpop/rpop/content/informationfor/healthprofessionals/5_interventionalcardiology/phaseserythema.htm, Accessed July 11, 2011). C, Epilation following unnecessarily high-dose CT perfusion scan. (Photo courtesy of New York Times: The Radiation Boom After Stroke Scans, Patients Face Serious Health Risks by Walt Bogdanich Published: July 31, 2010.) D, NCI skin toxicity grade 3 (Copyright © The Regents of the University of California, Davis campus. Originally published in Dermatology Online Journal. All Rights Reserved. Used with permission.). Chronic radiodermatitis after interventional cardiac catheterization. Grade 3 is classified as moist desquamation in areas other than skinfolds and creases. Note the increased severity of reaction in an area of radiation field overlap (From Henry FA, Maender JL, Shen Y, et al. Fluoroscopy-induced chronic radiation dermatitis: a report of three cases. *Dermatol Online J.* 2009;15(1):3. Copyright © 2009 The Regents of the University of California, Davis campus. Originally published in Dermatology Online Journal. All Rights Reserved. Used with permission. E, Dry desquamation (poikiloderma) at 1 month in a patient receiving approximately 11 Gy calculated peak skin dose (From Chambers C, Fetterly K, Holzer R, et al. Radiation safety program for the cardiac catheterization laboratory. *Catheter Cardiovasc Interv.* 2011;77:546–556. Copyright © 2011 Wiley & Liss, Inc. Reprinted by permission of John Wiley & Sons, Inc). F-H, NCI skin toxicity grade 4. A 40-year-old male who underwent multiple coronary angiography and angioplasty procedures. The photographs show the time sequence of a major radiation injury (From FDA. *Radiation-Induced Skin Injuries from Fluoroscopy.* Rockville, MD: U.S. Food and Drug Administration; 1995. http://www.fda.gov/Radiation-EmittingProducts/RadiationEmittingProductsandProcedures/MedicalImaging/MedicalX-Rays/ucm116682.htm. Accessed February 1, 2011). F, Six to eight weeks postexposure (prolonged erythema with mauve central area, suggestive of ischemia). The injury was described as "turning red about 1 month after the procedure and peeling a week later." By 6 weeks, it had the appearance of a second-degree burn; (G) 16 to 21 weeks postexposure (depigmented skin with central area of necrosis); and (H) 18 to 21 months postexposure (deep necrosis with atrophic borders). Skin breakdown continued over the following months with progressive necrosis. The injury eventually required a skin graft. Although the magnitude of the skin dose received by this patient is not known, from the nature of the injury it is probable that the dose exceeded 20 Gy. This sequence is available on the FDA Web site (From FDA. *Radiation-Induced Skin Injuries from Fluoroscopy.* Rockville, MD: U.S. Food and Drug Administration; 1995. http://www.fda.gov/Radiation-EmittingProducts/RadiationEmittingProductsandProcedures/MedicalImaging/MedicalX-Rays/ucm116682.htm. Accessed February 1, 2011.). https://ncrponline.org/publications/reports/ncrp-report-168/. Reprinted with permission from Bushberg JT, Seibert JA, Leidholdt EM, Boone JM. *The Essential Physics of Medical Imaging.* 3rd ed. Philadelphia, PA: Wolters Kluwer Health/Lippincott Williams & Wilkins; 2011.

Hematopoietic syndrome

Whereas mature hematopoietic cells in circulation are radioresistant (with the exception lymphocytes), hematopoietic stem cells are very radiosensitive. Because the majority of active bone marrow is in the spine, posterior ribs, and pelvis, posterior-approach radiation exposures result in the most damage to the hematopoietic system. The hematopoietic syndrome is the primary clinical effect that occurs following exposures of 0.5 to 10 Gy. Doses greater than 8 Gy are almost always fatal. Recovery is usually possible with doses less than 2 Gy. The dose expected to kill 50% of an exposed population (the $LD_{50/60}$) is 3.5 to 4.5 Gy to the bone marrow for humans. Intensive therapies including transfusions, antibiotics, and hematopoietic-stimulating factors may raise this as high as 8 Gy.

Prodromal symptoms of hematopoietic syndrome include nausea, vomiting, diarrhea, and headache and can occur within a few hours after exposure. Early appearance of symptoms and severe diarrhea in the first 2 days may indicate a fatal dose.

Hematopoietic prodromal and latent periods may last for weeks. An initial rise in neutrophils may be observed, which is thought to be related to stress response. As damage to stem cells reduces their number, their ability to replace circulating blood cells is impaired. As the circulating blood cells eventually die by senescence, the lack of ability to replace these cells leads to generalized pancytopenia. Physical manifestations peak at 3 to 4 weeks after exposure and include hemorrhage, infections, anemia, and impaired healing.

GI syndrome

The physical manifestations of the GI syndrome are often the most immediate and severe consequences of acute high-dose radiation exposure. It is the GI syndrome that usually causes death after an exposure of greater than 12 Gy, with lethality reaching close to 100%. Damage, however, begins at lower doses (2-10 Gy) and is responsible for many of the prodromal symptoms that occur. Death occurs within 3 to 10 days without medical attention and within 2 weeks with intensive care. Physical manifestations include nausea, vomiting, cramps, and watery diarrhea. These acute symptoms are followed by a shorter latent period and the manifest illness stage 5 to 7 days later. Damage to the intestinal mucosa limits reproductive ability of the crypt cells and they eventually die and slough. The breakdown of the mucosal lining allows antigens, bacteria, and digestive enzymes in the bowel lumen to enter the intestinal wall and leads to mucositis. This, in turn, impairs ability to absorb nutrients and electrolytes and allows intestinal flora to enter systemic circulation. As the bone marrow changes are leading to a simultaneous leukopenia, the resulting infectious complications can be devastating. In additions to these infections and the malabsorption, manifestations of the GI syndrome include ulceration and hemorrhage of the mucosa, alteration of enteric flora, depletion of gut lymphoid tissue, and disturbance of motility.

Neurovascular syndrome

Doses of greater than 50 Gy result in neurovascular syndrome and quickly lead to death. The neuromuscular syndrome is characterized by cardiovascular shock and loss of serum and electrolytes into extravascular tissues. Edema, increased intracranial pressure, and cerebral anoxia ensue, eventually resulting in death before significant physical manifestations of damage to other organs and tissues. The prodromal stage may include a burning sensation of the skin within minutes, with subsequent nausea, vomiting, confusion, ataxia, and disorientation within an hour of exposure. A very short (4-6 hour) latent period leads to a manifest illness stage in which the prodromal symptoms return with greater severity, along with the development of tremors, convulsions, respiratory distress, coma, and eventually death.

Cancer effects of radiation — carcinogenesis

In contrast to the effects of radiation exposure that become apparent within hours to days, some effects of radiation exposure are delayed by years or decades. The most important delayed effect of radiation exposure is the development of cancer. Cancer remains the second most likely cause of death in the United States after cardiovascular disease, and although the total incidence of cancer varies little between worldwide populations, environmental exposures do play a large role in the incidence of certain types of cancers in certain areas. Radiation is a relatively weak carcinogen at low doses. The low doses typically encountered during diagnostic imaging do not produce detectable effects. However, moderate doses of radiation do result in well-documented effects.

Cancer development

The development of a cancer consists of a series of stages, which include initiation, promotion, and progression. During the initiation stage, a somatic mutation occurs, which is misrepaired. These mutations can be caused by a variety of carcinogens, including radiation. During promotion, the resulting preneoplastic cell (containing the misrepaired mutation) is stimulated to divide by a promoter agent. A promoter agent does not lead to cancer by itself, but promotes another cell containing the original mutation. An example would be estrogen, which does not cause cancer but can promote the formation of breast cancer in certain settings. During progression, the final stage of cancer development, the transformed cell produces phenotypic clones. One phenotype will eventually acquire the ability to evade host defenses, leading to tumor development and possibly metastasis. Radiation is unique in that, unlike many other carcinogens, it may act both as an initiator and a promoter and may also aid progression by causing host immunosuppression.

Factors affecting radiation-included cancer risk

As discussed, the development of radiation-induced cancers depends on both physical and biologic factors. Physical factors include radiation quality, dose, and rate. There is a great deal of ongoing research regarding the biologic factors and how they affect carcinogenesis. Some of these biologic factors include age, gender, and tumor type.

Radiation Quality

Damage from high-LET radiation is more extensive and less likely to be correctly repaired compared with that of low-LET radiation. As a result, for a given exposure, the probability of developing cancer caused by radiation is higher for high-LET radiation than for low-LET radiation. For certain biologic endpoints, such as production of dicentrics in human lymphocytes, low-energy photons are actually more efficient than high-energy photons. This is thought to be due to the higher LET of secondary, lower-energy electrons and the complex DNA damage that results at the end of the secondary electrons' paths. Although these differences between low- and high-energy radiation are experimentally and theoretically valid, the differences have not revealed themselves in epidemiologic data.

Dose Rate and Fractionation

The effectiveness of radiation-induced damage to cells is decreased with dose fractionation, which allows the cell time to repair damage in between fractions. Although experimental data support the increased probability of cellular repair and the decreased incidence of carcinogenesis in some cases, dose rate may not influence cancer risk with the low doses associated with diagnostic imaging and occupational exposures.

Age, Gender, Tumor Type, and Latency

Certain differences in carcinogenesis have been observed based on some simple biologic characteristics. For certain cancers, such as ovarian cancer, exposure at an early age is more likely to result in cancer development than exposure later in life. In general, females are 40% more likely to develop cancer after whole-body exposure due to the increased formation of breast, ovarian, and lung cancer in women and the decreased risk of radiogenic carcinogenesis in the testes and prostate of men. For certain cancers such as liver cancer, the risk is much lower (50%) for females compared with males. Following exposure, latency to cancer development varies widely, from 2 to 3 years for leukemia to 5 to 40 years for solid tumors.

Genetic factors

It is widely known that mutations in certain genes increase the risk of development of certain cancers. For example, women with the *BRCA1* or *BRCA2* genes and a family history of multiple cases of breast cancer carry an increased lifetime risk of breast cancer development that is approximately five times higher than in the general population. Ataxia-telangiectasia, a rare recessive genetic disorder, is another example. Patients with this condition have the ataxia-telangiectasia mutation and are at increased risk of developing leukemia and lymphoma and more sensitive to ionizing radiation due to dysfunctional DNA repair mechanisms.

Dose-response model

Although scientific data and observations indicate that there is a small increase in cancer risk as a result of the levels of ionizing radiation used in diagnostic procedures, no one can agree on how small the risk increase actually is. Even though there is general agreement that cancer risk increases with doses above 100 to 150 mSv, it is very difficult to detect small increases in cancer risk from lower exposures. This is due to the fact that radiation is a relatively weak carcinogen and the natural incidence of many cancers is already high. The latent period is also quite long for many cancers. These factors lead to significant difficulty in associating cancer development with these low levels of radiation exposure. Additionally, very large irradiated populations are needed to detect small increases in cancer risk, and populations and resources for such large studies are often not available.

Despite these limitations, scientists have developed dose-response models to characterize the risk of cancer development related to radiation exposure. The three shapes that have been described are the linear nonthreshold (LNT), linear quadratic (LQ), and threshold curves (Figure 10.7). The LQ curve demonstrates lower effectiveness of radiation at lower doses with the effectiveness increasing as dose increases. The effectiveness of the radiation eventually flattens out, which reflects doses with significant cell killing. The threshold curve is supported by some epidemiologic evidence regarding cancers in certain tissues, but the evidence supporting this

model is not sufficient for use in assessing cancer risk from radiation exposure. Alternatively, the current recommendation of radiation exposure as low as reasonable achievable (ALARA) is favored.

The BEIR VII report published in 2006 includes the lifetime attributable risk of site-specific cancer incidence due to radiation exposure (Table 10.2). Using these data, the increased risk of cancer due to radiation exposure can be estimated for persons of a specific age undergoing a known level of radiation exposure. From this information, it is clear that the same radiation exposure will produce a higher increase in cancer risk in a child versus an adult. Additionally, as discussed earlier, the risk also increases for females more than males, although the difference between these risk levels decreases with age.

Cancer risks for certain organs/tissues
Leukemia

The incidence of leukemia in the general U.S. population is approximately 1 in 10 000 per year. Genetics play a large role in the development of leukemia and can increase this risk dramatically. Although rare in the general population, leukemia is one of the most frequently observed radiation-induced cancers. Increases in all types of leukemia have been observed in human and animal populations following radiation exposure, with the exception of chronic lymphocytic leukemia and viral-induced leukemia. Increased incidence of leukemia was evident in the atom bomb survivors within a few years of detonation. Evidence from these survivors and from other exposed cohorts indicates that excess leukemia cases can be detected as early as 1 to 2 years after exposure and peak around 12 years. The increased incidence is partially dependent on age, with shorter latency and expression periods with exposure at younger ages.

Thyroid

The preferred BEIR VII model for thyroid cancer is based on pooled analyses of the Life Span Study data and medically irradiated cohorts. There is a significant gender difference for thyroid cancer development in both the general population (spontaneous) and in irradiated populations, thought to be two to three times higher for women than for men. There is also increased risk for people of Jewish or North African ancestry. A rapid decrease in radiogenic cancer risk is observed with age, and most studies do not support an increased risk of thyroid cancer due to radiation exposure in adulthood.

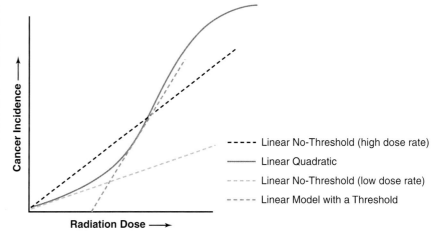

FIG. 10.7 ● Possible dose-response relationship for radiation-induced cancer. National Research Council. Health Risks from Exposure to Low Levels of Ionizing Radiation: BEIR VII, Phase 2. DOI https://doi.org/10.17226/11340. Adapted and reprinted with permission from the National Academy of Sciences, Courtesy of the National Academies Press, Washington, DC; 2006. Reprint of Figure 20.27 with permission from Bushberg JT, Seibert JA, Leidholdt EM, Boone JM. *The Essential Physics of Medical Imaging.* 3rd ed. Philadelphia, PA: Wolters Kluwer Health/Lippincott Williams & Wilkins; 2012.

Table 10.2 **LIFETIME ATTRIBUTABLE RISK OF SITE-SPECIFIC CANCER INCIDENCE**

Number of Cases Per 100 000 Persons Exposed to a Single Dose of 0.1 Gy

Cancer Site	Age at Exposure (y)										
	0	5	10	15	20	30	40	50	SO	70	80
Men											
Stomach	76	65	55	46	40	28	27	25	20	14	7
Colon	336	285	241	204	173	125	122	113	94	65	30
Liver	61	50	43	36	30	22	21	19	14	8	3
Lung	314	261	216	180	149	105	104	101	89	65	34
Prostate	93	80	67	57	48	35	35	33	26	14	5
Bladder	209	177	150	127	108	79	79	76	66	47	23
Other	1123	672	503	394	312	198	172	140	98	57	23
Thyroid	115	76	50	33	21	9	3	1	0.3	0.1	0.0
All solid	2326	1667	1325	1076	881	602	564	507	407	270	126
Leukemia	237	149	120	105	96	84	84	84	82	73	48
All cancers	2563	1816	1445	1182	977	686	648	591	489	343	174
Women											
Stomach	101	85	72	61	52	36	35	32	27	19	11
Colon	220	187	158	134	114	82	79	73	62	45	23
Liver	28	23	20	16	14	10	10	9	7	5	2
Lung	733	608	504	417	346	242	240	230	201	147	77
Breast	1171	914	712	553	429	253	141	70	31	12	4
Uterus	50	42	36	30	26	18	16	13	9	5	2
Ovary	104	87	73	60	50	34	31	25	18	11	5
Bladder	212	180	152	129	109	79	78	74	64	47	24
Other	1339	719	523	409	323	207	181	148	109	68	30
Thyroid	634	419	275	178	113	41	14	4	1	0.3	0.0
All solid	4592	3265	2525	1988	1575	1002	824	678	529	358	177
Leukemia	135	112	86	76	71	63	62	62	57	51	37
All cancers	4777	3377	2611	2064	1646	1065	886	740	586	409	214

Adapted from BEIR VII Table 12 D-1. BEIR. Health risks from exposure to law levels of ionizing radiation: BEIR VII, Phase 2. Committee to Assess Health Risks from Exposure to Low Levels of Ionizing Radiation, Board of Radiation Effects Research, Division on Earth and Life Studies, National Research Council of the National Academies. Washington, DC: The National Academies Press, 2006. Reprint of Table 20.14 with permission from Bushberg JT, Seibert JA, Leidholdt Jr EM, Boone JM. *The Essential Physics of Medical Imaging.* 3rd ed. Philadelphia, PA: Lippincott Williams and Wilkins; 2011.

The most common radiogenic thyroid cancer is well-differentiated papillary thyroid adenocarcinoma. Follicular forms of thyroid cancers are the second most common radiogenic thyroid cancer. The dose-response data for radiogenic thyroid cancer fit a linear pattern. Latency for benign nodules is approximately 5 to 35 years, and latency for thyroid malignancies is approximately 10 to 35 years. External radiation to the thyroid is generally more effective than internally deposited radionuclides at producing thyroid cancer. Besides cancer, other effects from thyroid radiation are possible, including thyroiditis and hypothyroidism. These effects follow a threshold pattern with estimated thresholds of 2 Gy for external radiation and 50 Gy for low-dose internal radiation. Doses of 200 to 300 Gy from radioactive iodine may cause thyroiditis and sore throat and higher doses may cause thyroid ablation. The dose to the thyroid from radioiodine therapy is usually 1000 time greater than for other organs due to the ability of the thyroid to concentrate iodine. The high thyroid dose per unit activity administered is the reason for concern for thyroid cancer following radioiodine exposure, especially in children.

Breast

There has been much debate recently over the appropriate use of mammography in screening for breast cancer. Breast cancer is the most common cancer in females, and although this alone makes screening a major priority, certainly the formation of cancer secondary to ionizing radiation from diagnostic and/or screening procedures must be avoided. The BEIR VII committee, analyzing atomic bomb survivors and medically exposed persons, determined that the breast cancer risk for low-LET radiation fits a linear dose-response model, with doubling of the natural incidence of breast cancer with a dose of approximately 800 mGy. Fractionation of dose reduces the cancer risk. The latent period is 10 to 40 years, with longer latencies observed in younger women. Unlike some other cancers, such as leukemia, there is no identifiable window of expression and the risk remains throughout the life of the exposed individual. The lifetime attributable risk of developing breast cancer is dependent on age, with approximately 13 times higher risk for those exposed at age 5 than those exposed at age 50.[6] Improvements in mammography have reduced the dose to the breast during screening and diagnostic mammography.

Noncancer radiation effects

Increased risk of certain noncancer diseases such as cardiovascular disease has been demonstrated in some radiotherapy patient populations. Increased risk of cardiovascular disease has also been observed in atom bomb survivors. No statistically significant increase in risk of cardiovascular disease has been demonstrated at radiation doses under 0.5 Sv. There has been no direct evidence of an increase in risk of cardiovascular disease or other noncancer diseases associated with low-dose radiation exposures associated with occupational exposure and diagnostic imaging.

In utero effects

The developing embryo is extremely sensitive to ionizing radiation exposure, and the effects of exposure on the embryo depend on the total dose, the dose rate, the radiation quality, and the stage of development during which the exposure occurs. The gestational period can be divided into three periods: the preimplantation period, the organogenesis period, and the fetal growth period. Preimplantation begins when the sperm and egg unite and continues until the zygote implants in the uterine wall (day 9). While the conceptus is very sensitive during this stage, the risk posed to the conceptus from radiation exposure less than 100 mGy is very low. During this period, the embryo exhibits an all-or-none response to radiation exposure, meaning there is unlikely to be any additional radiation-induced risk of congenital abnormalities should the exposure prove to be nonlethal. This is thought to be due to the fact that the few number of cells in this stage are undifferentiated and that damage to one of these cells during this period would be overcome by differentiation of the additional cells later in development. The cells are also very capable in terms of repair during this time and exist in a relatively hypoxia state, reducing the effects of free radicals. Similarly, however, if a cell were to sustain some chromosomal aberrations or misrepaired chromosomal damage during this time, the eventual manifestation throughout the majority of cell progeny would lead to effects that are usually lethal.

The majority of embryonic malformations occur during the organogenesis period (weeks 2-8 after conception). Since different organ systems begin to form at different times during this period, not every organ system is at equal risk during the entire organogenesis period. The term critical period refers to the time when radiation exposure poses the highest risk of causing malformation in that organ system and it usually coincides with the period of peak differentiation of the system. The central nervous system (CNS) is the only organ system that has demonstrated an association between malformations and radiation exposure less than 250 mGy. No cases of radiation-induced malformations caused by in utero irradiation have been observed without accompanying CNS abnormalities or growth retardation.

The fetal growth stage begins after day 50 when organogenesis ends and continues until term. Occurrence of radiation-induced prenatal death and congenital abnormalities is negligible in this period unless exposures are very high. Damage during this period may not manifest until later in life as behavioral disturbances or low IQ. There is evidence to suggest that in utero radiation exposure acts a carcinogen, increasing the lifetime risk of cancer in exposed individuals. Although there are arguments for and against this, the increased risk to the exposed individual, if real, remains extremely low. For example, if a fetus received twice the U.S. regulatory agencies' maximally allowed dose of 0.5 mSv in 1 month, the probability of developing cancer in childhood as a result of the exposure would be approximately 1 in 1600. There is relatively more risk to the fetus from in utero exposure to radionuclides under certain conditions. The best example is radioiodine, which rapidly crosses the placenta and is concentrated in the fetal thyroid around week 11 to 12 postconception. The ability of the fetal thyroid to concentrate iodine increases progressively after week 22 and eventually exceeds that of the mother. Should the mother receive a high enough dose, the result could be fetal hypothyroidism or thyroid ablation.

RADIATION SAFETY

Sources of radiation exposure

Approximately half of the average annual per capita effective dose from exposure to ionizing radiation in the United States (Figure 10.8) came from naturally occurring sources. An additional 2% came from additional sources such as consumer products, consumer activities, and occupational exposure.

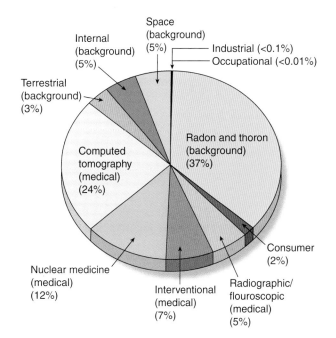

All exposure categories
Total S and E_{us} (percent), 2006

FIG. 10.8 ● **Percentage contribution of various sources of radiation to the average annual per capita effective dose in the United States.** Data based on Report 160 by National Council of Radiation Protection and Measurements (NCRP). Reprinted with permission from Orth D. *Essentials of Radiologic Science.* 2nd ed. Philadelphia, PA: Wolters Kluwer; 2017.

Naturally occurring sources

Naturally occurring sources of radiation include cosmic rays, cosmogenic radionuclides, and primordial radionuclides and their decay products. Although primary cosmic rays consist of highly penetrating high-energy particulate radiation (of which ~80% is high-energy protons), collisions with the earth's atmosphere produces secondary particulate radiations and electromagnetic radiation. Cosmic radiation produces an average per capita effective dose of approximately 0.33 mSv per year, accounting for approximately 11% of natural background radiation. The exposure is not uniform, and there is more exposure at higher altitudes and near the earth's poles. Primordial radionuclides are radioactive materials that have been present on earth since its formation. Some of these materials have half-lives similar to the age of the earth itself, and their decay products serve as a major source of terrestrial radiation exposure. The dose to the population from primordial radionuclides comes from external exposure, inhalation, and incorporation into the body itself. The most significant source of inhalation exposure is radon 222 and its decay products. Radon gas emanates from the soil and quickly disperses. Because it is restricted by structures, the concentration of radon gas is usually higher indoors. Most of the dose from inhalation is deposited in the tracheobronchial tree. In the United States, exposure to radon gas accounts for approximately 68% of naturally occurring background radiation.

Medical sources

As mentioned, nearly half of the average annual effective dose in the United States from all sources comes from medical use of radiation, predominantly diagnostic radiology. Nuclear medicine contributes an additional, albeit smaller, source of medical exposure. The current average annual effective dose to the U.S. population from medical use is approximately 3 mSv, and this is increased from 0.53 mSv in 1980. Increased use of computed tomography (CT) and nuclear medicine imaging account, at least partially, for this increase. CT and nuclear medicine imaging account for only approximately 22% of all medical imaging utilizing radiation, but account for approximately 75% of the collective effective dose. CT of the abdomen and pelvis and Tc-99m and Tl-201 myocardial perfusion imaging together account for more than half of the effective dose to the population from medical imaging. Conventional radiographic and noninterventional fluoroscopic procedures, which account for approximately 74% of total imaging procedures, contribute only 11% of the collective effective dose.

Other sources

Additional sources of radiation exposure include consumer products and occupational exposures. The most important consumer product source of radiation exposure is tobacco products. The alpha-emitting radionuclides Pb-210 and Po-210 have been measured in both tobacco leaves and cigarette smoke. Estimates indicate that a smoker of one pack of cigarettes a day increases the annual effective dose by approximately 0.36 mSv. The average annual effective dose of the entire U.S. population from tobacco is approximately 0.045 mSv. Additional sources include building materials containing primordial radionuclides (uranium, thorium, radium, potassium), air travel (which increases cosmic ray exposure), and several other sources that contribute very minimal additional dose (fertilizers, combustible fuels, optical lenses, etc).

Occupational exposure is another important area of concern, primarily for those in the fields of medicine, aviation, nuclear power, the military, and the department of energy. Those who are occupationally exposed usually receive low exposures, and the average annual per capita effective dose for those exposed was 1.1 mSv. The average annual effective dose to medical personnel in 2006 was 0.75 mSv.[7] Those performing fluoroscopic procedures receive the highest exposures, with partial body exposures typically in the range of 5 to 15 mSv per year as measured by the dosimeter worn outside the lead apron. After adjustments for lead shielding, these values are typically reduced by a factor of 3 or more.

Radiation monitoring

The potentially harmful effects of radiation necessitate adequate shielding from the majority of the radiation that some workers work with or near, and there is an associated need for accurate measurement of the amount of radiation exposure to those workers. In the fields of radiology and nuclear medicine, personnel dosimeters are used for monitoring and recording radiation doses to individual workers. There are three main types of personnel dosimeters: film badges, dosimeters that use storage phosphors (eg, thermoluminescent dosimeters), and pocket dosimeters.

Film badges

Film badges contain small, sealed radiosensitive film packets. The packets are usually encased in plastic with a clip allowing for clipping to clothing. When radiation contacts the film, it causes darkening of the film when developed. The amount of darkening increases with increasing absorbed dose and measurement is done with a densitometer. Due to the makeup of the film, the dose to the film is not equal to the dose to the tissues of the body. For this reason, several metal filters are placed over the film and the relative optical densities of the film under the metal filters are used to approximate the energy range of the radiation and determine the dose to tissues. There is usually an area of the film not covered by any materials and directly exposed to radiation. This is used to detect medium- and high-energy beta radiation that would be attenuated by the overlying materials otherwise.

Film badges are usually designed to record doses ranging from approximately 100 µSv to 15 Sv for photons and 500 µSv to 10 Sv for beta radiation. The badges' film is usually replaced on a monthly basis, allowing the previous month's dose to be calculated from the film once it is processed.

Thermoluminescent and optically stimulated luminescent dosimeters

Thermoluminescent dosimeters (TLDs) contain storage phosphors in which a fraction of the electrons become trapped in an excited state once they are excited by ionizing radiation. The excited electrons can be released by heating or exposure to light, and they emit light as they return to lower energy states. Measurement of the amount of light emitted can be used to determine the radiation dose to the phosphors. TLDs are somewhat more expensive than film badges but they are reusable and can collect data for up to 6 months before being returned to the supplier for analysis. The most common material used for personal dosimeter TLDs is lithium fluoride (LiF). The atomic number of LiF is close to that of tissues, which means that, over a wide energy range, the dose to the LiF chip is close to the dose to the tissues. LiF TLDs are capable of measuring doses of approximately 100 µSv to 10 Sv. Whereas the film inside film badge dosimeters can be stored for permanent record, the LiF chip loses the deposited energy when it is heated to read the exposure and a permanent record is not possible. Finger ring TLDs are commonly used as extremity dosimeters in nuclear medicine.

Optically stimulated luminance (OSL) dosimeters are an alternative to TLDs that use laser light instead of heat to release the trapped electrons and allow the required light emission. OSL dosimeters can be read several times and the filter pattern can be produced to differentiate between static (instantaneous) and dynamic (normal) exposure. OSL dosimeters use materials with a higher atomic number than tissues, and so a series of filters are used over the material to estimate the dose to tissues similar to the method used with film badges. OSL dosimeters can detect a wide range of doses and allow for measurement of doses over a prolonged period of time similar to TLDs.

Direct-ion storage dosimeters

Direct-ion storage dosimeters involve a nonvolatile analog memory cell surrounded by a gas-filled ion chamber. Initially, X-ray and gamma-ray photons interact with the wall materials. The secondary electrons then ionize the gas of the chamber. The resulting positive ions are collected on a negative electrode, which results in a reduction in voltage that is proportional to the dose received by the dosimeter. The dosimeter can be plugged into a USB port on a computer, and certain algorithms can be used to determine deep, shallow, and lens of the eye doses. Advantages of this type of dosimeter include broad dose-response range (0.01 mSv to 5 Sv), unlimited real-time dose reading accessible to the end-user, online management, and elimination of the logistical considerations that must go into the use of dosimeters that are collected and distributed by the supplier every month or after several months. However, these dosimeters are costlier than other options, they cannot measure beta radiation and they depend on the user to upload information.

Pocket dosimeters

One problem with the dosimeters that have been discussed to this point is the fact that they cannot be read in real time. Pocket dosimeters allow for real-time reading of exposure in a small and easy-to-use form factor about the size of a ballpoint pen. Both analog and digital versions of pocket dosimeters are available. The analog versions typically detect exposures ranging from 0 to 200 mR. The analog pocket dosimeters are sensitive to external forces and may give incorrect readings if bumped or dropped. Digital pocket dosimeters are solid-state and detect doses ranging from 10 µSv to 100 mSv.

Wearing dosimeters

Dosimeters are typically worn on the portion of the torso that is most sensitive to radiation or that is expected to receive the most dose. It is typical for those working around radiation in a medical setting to wear a dosimeter near the waist or chest. Those exposed during fluoroscopy usually wear a dosimeter near the collar level in front of the lead apron to measure the dose to the thyroid and the lens of the eye, as the majority of the rest of the body is shielded by a lead apron. Other users of fluoroscopy may wear one dosimeter outside the apron at the collar and another inside the apron on the torso. A pregnant radiation worker may wear an additional dosimeter behind the apron at the waist to assess fetal dose. The National Council on Radiation Protection and Measurements (NCRP) provides equations for estimating the effective dose and effective dose equivalent for staff wearing protective lead aprons using collar-level dosimeters outside the apron or using a combination of a collar-level dosimeter outside the apron and a waist- or chest-level dosimeter inside the apron.

Dosimeter pitfalls

Several major human factors limit the accuracy and effectiveness of dosimeters in terms of measuring exposure. Some workers forget to wear the dosimeters or accidentally leave them in the radiation field when not being worn. Others position the dosimeters incorrectly on the body. Most dosimeters are susceptible to physical damage or are small enough to be lost. Still, when used properly, dosimeters are able to provide an approximation of an individual's true exposure.

Radiation detection

Aside from dosimeters designed to measure dose to an individual, portable radiation detection instruments are also used in radiology and nuclear medicine to detect the presence of radioactivity in various places. Most of the applications of portable radiation detectors in radiology and nuclear medicine use Geiger-Mueller (GM) survey meters or portable ionization survey meters.

GM survey meter

GM survey instruments detect the presence and semiquantitatively estimate the intensity of radiation fields. The measurements are usually in counts per minute (cpm) instead of mR/h because the condition in which the exposure occurs is not standardized. These instruments are commonly used to detect radioactive contamination in nuclear medicine. For this purpose, a survey meter is typically coupled with a certain type of GM probe called a "pancake" probe. The thin-window "pancake" probe can detect alpha, beta, X-, and gamma radiations. However, although the detectors are very sensitive to charged particulate radiations with sufficient energy to penetrate the window, they are much less sensitive to X- and gamma radiations. Some GM instruments will become saturated in the presence of very high doses and will read zero, which can lead to significant overexposures if not recognized. GM survey instruments are best suited for low-level contamination detection.

Portable ionization chamber survey meter

When accurate measurements of radiation exposure rates are required, portable ionization chamber survey meters are used. These devices are used in a variety of applications, including assessing radiation fields near radionuclide therapy patients and surveying radioactive material packages. Some ion chambers are filled with ambient air, whereas some are sealed. Sealed chambers can be pressurized to increase sensitivity. Factors such as photon energy, exposure rate, magnetic field, and orientation (as well as temperature and atmospheric pressure for those open to ambient air) can influence measurements. However, the effects are minimal in conditions typical of medical imaging environments. Most of these devices must be allowed to warm up and stabilize before they can give accurate measurements. They respond slowly to rapid increases in exposure and therefore serve as poor portable detectors of low-level contamination.

Radiation control and radiation protection
Methods

The three principal methods used to minimize X-ray radiation exposure include reduction in exposure time, increase in distance, and the use of shielding. In handling radioactive material, contamination control is also a major consideration for radiation control and radiation protection.

Time

Logic dictates that decreasing the amount of time spent near a source of radiation will reduce the overall exposure. Because not all sources of radiation produce constant exposure rates, it is important to keep in mind the type of radiation source in question and to employ tailored practices depending on the source in order to effectively reduce exposures. For example, because X-ray machines typically produce a high amount of radiation in a short period of time, exposure reduction through simply not activating the machine while others are near the radiation source is a very effective method of exposure reduction. For those using fluoroscopy, proficiency in the procedure will allow the operator to reduce the total time personnel are exposed to radiation.

Distance

Another straightforward concept is that exposure is reduced as distance from the radiation source is increased. In this case, the inverse square law applies, meaning that, as the distance from the radiation source doubles, the radiation exposure is reduced by a factor of 4. This relationship is only valid for point sources (sources whose dimensions are small compared with the distance from the source) and would not necessarily apply in a situation such as a patient injected with a radionuclide. Distance is the main exposure control method employed by technologists while performing nuclear medicine imaging on patients because shielding is often not practical. For this reason, it is necessary for imaging rooms in nuclear medicine to be designed to allow the needed distance between the patient and the technologist.

Shielding

Shielding of patients, staff, and the public is widely used in diagnostic radiology. The various types and locations of shielding must be tailored based on the photon energy, intensity, and geometry of the radiation sources in order to be effective. Shielding is commonly installed in the walls, floor, or ceiling of a room, especially those used for medical imaging. Additionally, shielding can be placed around storage containers for radioactive materials, around individual components of medical imaging machinery, and even around workers in diagnostic imaging.

Shielding materials in medical imaging need to be able to shield from the photon energies of X-rays (up to 140 keV), gamma rays from radionuclides (up to 365 keV), or annihilation photons used in positron emission tomography (up to 511 keV). A material with a high atomic number will allow for photoelectric absorption and will result in less mass required for shielding than for a material of lower atomic number. For this reason, lead is commonly used for shielding because of its high atomic number, density, and relatively low cost. Placing shielding material closer to a radiation source, while not reducing the required thickness of the shield, does reduce the total required mass of the shield by reducing the area of shielding.

Shielding design for X-ray radiation

Shielding of rooms containing X-ray machines is designed to limit radiation exposures to employees and members of the public to acceptable levels. There are several factors that must be considered when designing medical imaging environments and installing appropriate shielding. Exposures to staff and the public must be kept below accepted exposure limits and must adhere to the ALARA principle. NCRP Report No. 147, Structural Shielding Design for Medical X-ray Imaging Facilities, outlines methods and technical information for the design of shielding for diagnostic and interventional X-ray rooms. The quantity recommended for shielding design calculations is air karma (K) and the recommended unit is the Gy. Effective dose (E) is the recommended radiation protection quantity for the limitation of exposure to people and is defined as the sum of the weighted equivalent doses to specific organs or tissues. Areas protected by shielding are classified as *controlled* or *uncontrolled* areas. Controlled areas are usually in the immediate vicinity of the medical imaging equipment, where radiologists, technologists, and other workers are trained in the use of radiation. Individual exposures are usually monitored in these areas, and they are under supervision of a person responsible for radiation protection. Uncontrolled areas are typically other areas in the hospital or imaging center (offices, etc). Shielding design goals (P) are amounts of air kerma delivered over a specified time at a stated reference point (usually beyond a barrier) and are used in designing and evaluating radiation protection barriers. Different shielding design goals are used for controlled and uncontrolled areas, and recommendations are found in NCRP Report No. 147.

Sources of Exposure

There are three sources of exposure that must be considered when designing adequate shielding for a diagnostic or interventional X-ray room: primary radiation, scattered radiation, and leakage radiation. Primary radiation is the radiation passing through the open area defined by the collimator of the X-ray source. Scatter radiation is a result of the interaction of the primary radiation with the patient, which causes some of the X-rays to be redirected. Leakage is the radiation that escapes from the X-ray tube housing but is not a part of the primary radiation (Figure 10.9).

Primary Radiation	Scattered Radiation	Leakage Radiation

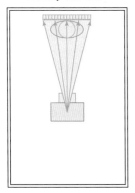 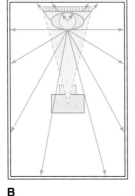 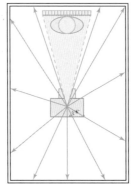

A **B** **C**

FIG. 10.9 ● The sources of exposure in a diagnostic X-ray room. A, Primary radiation emanating from the focal spot. B, Scattered radiation emanating from the patient. C, Leakage radiation emanating from the X-ray tube housing (other than the collimated primary radiation). Reprinted with permission from Bushberg JT, Seibert JA, Leidholdt EM, Boone JM. *The Essential Physics of Medical Imaging.* 3rd ed. Philadelphia, PA: Wolters Kluwer Health/Lippincott Williams & Wilkins; 2012.

Types of facilities

General-purpose radiographic installations produce intermittent exposures with tube potentials of 50 to 150 kV. Large portions of the exposures will be directed toward the floor or an image receptor in most cases. Barriers that intercept the primary beam are considered primary barriers. There must be a protected control area for the technologist, with a shielded window and some way for the technologist to speak directly to the patient. The switch to activate the X-ray tube should be placed in a location that makes it impossible for the technologist to activate it while standing outside of the protected area.

Fluoroscopic imaging systems operate in the range of 60 to 120 kV. The image receptor is also designed to be a primary barrier, so only secondary radiation barriers have to be considered in the design and implementation of shielding. If a fluoroscopic and radiographic combined unit is installed, the considerations above also apply.

Interventional facilities include angiography and vascular interventional, neuroangiography, and cardiovascular and electrophysiology imaging suites. Similar to fluoroscopic rooms, these suites have walls, floors, and ceilings that are considered secondary barriers. These rooms often require more shielding than conventional fluoroscopy rooms because there are often multiple radiation sources that may be used for long periods of time during prolonged procedures.

Dedicated chest radiography installations have X-ray tubes that are directed toward an image receptor on a particular barrier at all times. The image receptor's height from the floor can be adjusted, so the wall behind the receptor is considered a primary barrier. All other areas of the room are secondary barriers.

Mammography suites operate in the low range of 25 to 35 kV, and the breast support device serves as a primary barrier for incident radiation. The radiation barriers serve as secondary barriers only, and often all that is needed in these suites is a second layer of gypsum wallboard and metal doors due to the low energies used. Mammography machines have lead acrylic barriers to protect the control area.

CT uses collimated X-ray beams intercepted by the patient and the detector array. Only secondary radiation reaches the barriers. Operation is in the range of 80 to 140 kV, with 120 kV used for most scans. Secondary scatter radiation is higher along the axis of the table than in the direction of the gantry. Assuming isotropic scatter distribution, however, allows for conservative estimates of shielding needs and creates flexibility for future scanner installations.

Mobile radiography and fluoroscopy systems come with unique challenges for protection. For portable radiographs, the main methods of protection are keeping the beam directed away from nearby individuals and maintaining a distance from the radiation source. For portable fluoroscopy, anyone within 2 m of the patient should wear protective lead aprons and mobile shielding should be placed between the patient and personnel if available.

Bone mineral densitometry systems use well-collimated beams with low intensity and low scatter. These systems do not typically require structural shielding, but the control console should be as far away as possible to reduce exposure to the technologist.

Shielding Materials

In order to reduce radiation exposures below acceptable limits, an attenuating material must be placed between the radiation source and the area to be protected. Lead is the most common material used because of its relatively low cost and high attenuation properties. In structural shielding applications, commercially available sheets of lead are typically glued to another material such as gypsum wallboard and installed on studs. Where two sheets meet, they must overlap to ensure adequate shielding without gaps. Other shielding materials used in construction of medical facilities include gypsum wallboard itself, concrete, glass, leaded glass, and leaded acrylic. Gypsum wallboard (sheetrock) is most commonly used for wall construction in medical facilities at 5/8 in thickness, which is adequate to attenuate low X-ray energies such as those produced in mammography. When sheetrock is used for shielding purposes, an extra layer is required due to the internal nonuniformity of the material. Concrete, commonly used in walls, floors, and roofs, requires the density to be known in order to determine the thickness needed for certain levels of attenuation. When transparent shielding materials are desired, glass, leaded glass, and leaded acrylic can be used. Ordinary glass is capable of low levels of attenuation, which increases when multiple sheets are laminated together. Leaded glass and leaded acrylic are used more commonly for shielding purposes and come with specifications for various equivalent lead thicknesses.

Computing Shielding Requirements

The shielding design goals for controlled and uncontrolled areas are 0.1 and 0.02 mGy/wk, respectively. The distance between the source of radiation and the barrier protecting the sensitive organs of a person in the area must be chosen. These points of closest approach are assumed to be 0.3 m for a wall, 1.7 m above the floor, and at least 0.5 m above the floor of the room above for transmission through the ceiling.

The occupancy factor (T) is defined as the average fraction of time that the maximally exposed individual (usually employees of the facility) is present while the X-ray beam is activated. Barrier attenuation must lower radiation to the level of P/T.

Workload (W) is defined as the time integral of the X-ray tube current, given in milliampere-minutes over a 1-week time period (mA-min/wk). The NCRP Report No. 147 describes a normalized average workload per patient (W_{norm}) depending on the type of examination being performed. The total workload (W_{tot}) is the product of W_{norm} and the average number of patient per week (N).

Workload distribution is described in the NCRP Report No. 147 as the function of the kV spread over a range of operating potentials depending on the type of radiographic examination. Workload distributions are specific to a given radiological installation. The distribution of workload as a function of kV is more important than the magnitude of the workload in terms of shielding design, because shielding materials' attenuation properties depend mainly on kV.

Use factor (U) is the fraction of the primary beam workload that is directed toward a given primary barrier. Use factor depends on the type of radiographic room and the equipment orientation. In a dedicated chest radiography room, eg, the $U = 1$ for the chest receptor wall because the X-ray beam is always directed toward the receptor located on the wall. In a general radiographic room, the U must be estimated based on the types of procedures being performed and the amount of time the X-ray beam spends in different orientations and positions. In fluoroscopy and mammography rooms, the primary beam is stopped at the image receptor assembly, and the U should be zero.

The primary barrier attenuates the primary beam to the shielding design goal. The unshielded primary air kerma at the protected point per week must be considered and is dependent on the average number of patients per week, the use factor for the barrier, the air kerma per patient at 1 m, and the distance to the point. The secondary barrier attenuates the unshielded secondary air kerma (caused by leakage and scatter) to the shielding design goal. Any wall that is not considered a primary barrier is a secondary barrier. The same factors influencing primary air kerma also influence the secondary air kerma.

Shielding for CT

The detector array in a CT scanner gantry acts as the primary radiation barrier. Therefore, all walls in the scanner room are considered secondary barriers. The scatter from the scanner is highly directional and greatest along the scanner axis. Scattered radiation from CT scanners is highly penetrating because of the 120 to 140 kV and highly filtered beam typically used. There are three methods used to determine the shielding requirements for CT scanner rooms: one based on $CTDI_{vol}$, another based on dose length product (DLP) values, and the third based on the measured scatter distribution isodose maps provided by the manufacturer.

PET/CT and SPECT/CT Shielding

For shielding installations in nuclear medicine facilities using PET/CT, shielding must be considered for the room containing the PET/CT scanner as well as for the room where patients rest after the administration of radiopharmaceutical and before imaging. The type and amount of shielding required depend on the patient workload, the amount of radioactivity administered to each patient, the areas surrounding the PET/CT scanner rooms and uptake rooms, and the distance to, and occupancy of, these surrounding areas. As a result of the high energies of annihilation photons, required shielding thicknesses, can be very large. Strategies such as placing the rooms together in the same place and placing them on the bottom floor in the corner of the building can reduce the amount of shielding required. Additionally, rooms with low occupancy such as storage rooms can be placed around these areas to further reduce the shielding requirement. PET/CT and SPECT/CT facilities shielding must also protect against the radiation produced by the X-ray CT system. In most cases, the thick shielding for annihilation photons is more than adequate for this purpose. SPECT rooms are not usually shielded, and SPECT/CT rooms are typically shielded for the CT scanner if needed.

Radiation protection for diagnostic and interventional applications

Personnel protection

In most cases during medical imaging, medical staff are not allowed in the room during the production of X-rays and they are protected by the structural shielding installed in the room. However, physicians and assisting staff do remain in the room for fluoroscopic and CT-guided procedures. In these situations, it is important for those in the room to understand the radiation exposure pattern in the room and use appropriate protective methods to reduce exposure. Stray radiation varies in intensity based on location as illustrated in Figure 10.10. Understanding this spatial distribution of stray radiation allows those in the room to reposition themselves and movable shielding fixtures to reduce exposure.

Protective aprons are worn by all personnel in the room during operation of an X-ray tube. Although many materials are available, lead is the most commonly used material. These lead aprons are typically made of a flexible rubber material with lead equivalent thickness of 0.25 to 0.50 mm. Although many styles are available, most protect the anterior torso and the proximal lower extremities. The 0.25-mm aprons typically attenuate more than 90% of the scatter radiation incident upon them at standard X-ray energies. Thyroid shields of similar design are often added to attenuate radiation to the thyroid gland. Leaded glasses are sometimes worn to protect the eyes. Leaded glasses typically attenuate 30% to 70% of incident X-rays depending on the amount of lead used. Finally, mobile radiation barriers are sometimes mounted to the ceiling or table in rooms where high-workload angiographic or interventional procedures are performed. These devices are moved between the place where the primary beam intercepts the patient and the personnel in the room. Leaded glass or leaded acrylic shields allow for a transparent shield that is more effective than lead at attenuating the incident radiation.

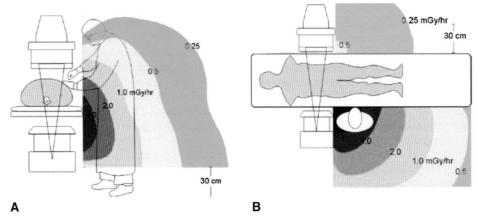

A   **B**

FIG. 10.10 ● **Dose rates from scattered radiation during fluoroscopy, with the X-ray beam in PA (A) and lateral (B) orientations.** These diagrams show the decrease in dose rate with distance from the location where the X-ray beam enters the patient. When the X-ray tube is beneath the patient (A), the highest scatter intensity is to the lower part of the operator's body. When the X-ray beam has a lateral angulation (B), the scatter intensity is much less on the side of the patient toward the image receptor. From National Council on Radiation Protection and Measurements. Radiation dose management for fluoroscopically guided interventional medical procedures. NCRP Report No. 168. National Council on Radiation Protection and Measurements, Bethesda, MD, 2010. Reprinted with permission from Bushberg JT, Seibert JA, Leidholdt EM, Boone JM. *The Essential Physics of Medical Imaging.* 3rd ed. Philadelphia, PA: Wolters Kluwer Health/Lippincott Williams & Wilkins; 2012.

Patient protection

While exposing patients to radiation is necessary in medical imaging, care must be taken to keep exposures at safe levels. This is primarily achieved by only performing medically necessary examinations and by ensuring that doses from examinations are no larger than necessary.

Tube Voltage and Beam Filtration

In diagnostic imaging, it is necessary to balance the quality of the image with the dose to the patient. Increasing kV will result in more transmission of X-rays through the patient. Increasing kV also increases exposure; however, there is accompanying reduction in the mAs of the beam to produce a similar signal to the image receptor that will actually result in a reduction of incident exposure to the patient. Although this would be beneficial in terms of image quality and dose to the patient, there is an associated reduction in image contrast due to the higher effective energy of the X-ray beam. This tradeoff is acceptable to a certain extent, and patient exposure can often be reduced by increasing the kV of the beam and decreasing the mAs. In angiography and CT angiography, where visualization of contrast material is desired over that of soft tissues, lower kV with greater beam filtration can improve the contrast to noise ratio and lower the dose to the patient.

Filtration of the X-ray beam allows for selective attenuation of low-energy X-rays that would otherwise be absorbed by the patient and increase dose without contributing to the image. As a beam is filtered, it becomes "hardened," meaning the average photon energy increases and the patient dose decreases. Excessive beam hardening, however, will reduce contrast. Filtration is necessary in fluoroscopy to reduce the risk of skin injury in prolonged procedures.

Field Area and Organ Shielding

Collimation involves restricting the field size to the necessary area of interest and is integral to dose reduction. Dose to the patient is reduced by decreasing the volume of tissue in the beam while also decreasing the amount of scatter (decreasing radiation to adjacent organs). Collimation also improves contrast and signal to noise ratio since scatter radiation incident upon the receptor is also reduced.

Radiosensitive organs not being directly imaged should be shielded from the X-ray beam. Organs typically shielded include the gonads, breasts in young females, and the lenses of the eyes.

Dose to the patient is also reduced as the distance from the radiation source to the patient increases. This is due to the reduced entrance dose (based on the inverse square law) as well as lower exposure due to tube leakage and reduced beam divergence resulting in lower volume of the tissues being irradiated.

Image Receptors

Film screen image receptors require different numbers of X-ray photons to adequately darken the film based on the speed of the receptor. Higher speed receptors require less exposure to produce the same optical density as lower-speed receptors, which also reduce patient exposure as a result. There is, however, an accompanying decrease in spatial resolution, which limits the effectiveness of using fast receptors as a dose-reduction method.

Fluoroscopy

Fluoroscopy is responsible for some of the highest patient exposures in medical imaging. While the energies and pulsed-exposure methods used are designed to limit exposure to patients, the sheer length of some procedures can lead to significant patient doses. Severe skin injuries have been reported as a result of X-ray exposure during prolonged fluoroscopic procedures. These injuries may not manifest for weeks or months after the procedure. Although large radiation doses are sometimes unavoidable due to the nature of the procedure being performed, it is necessary to implement dose-reduction techniques in every procedure. Modern fluoroscopes display the cumulative air kerma at a reference point, the kerma-area product or dose-area product, and the fluoroscopy time. Studies have shown that the kerma-area product or dose-area product are better correlates for peak skin dose than total fluoro time.[8,9]

Computed Tomography

In CT, many of the parameters that determine patient dose, including the kV and mA, the time per X-ray tube rotation, the detector table motion pitch, and the beam filter, are selected by the scanner operator. These parameters are typically specified in protocols that the technologist selects based on the patient and indication and then adjusts the individual parameters of the protocol if needed. For instance, the kV and mAs can sometimes be adjusted down for thinner patients, decreasing the dose without a significant sacrifice in image quality. Modern CT scanners are able to modulate tube current as a function of tube rotation angle and axial position on the patient to compensate for variations in attenuation along the beam path through the patient. Automatic tube current modulation can also be performed based on the scout image or on the amount of radiation transmitted during the scan. Automatic current modulation is effective in reducing patient dose while preserving image quality.

Modern scanners typically display $CDTI_{vol}$ or DLP to indicate patient dose. These values are displayed before and after each scan and can be transmitted via picture archiving and communication system. Some scanners have the ability to alert the technologist when the expected dose for a pending scan is expected to exceed a certain threshold. When an alert is encountered, the technologist must try to resolve the alert by reviewing the acquisition parameters for errors. If no errors are identifiable and the alert persists, the technologist must obtain approval by the radiologist before continuing.

Optimizing CT protocols is necessary for adequate CT dose control. There are many parameters that must be taken into account in this process. For example, one must consider whether high spatial resolution is necessary, as thin slices with higher noise require higher mA. The portion of the body being examined must also be considered, as certain areas with more inherent contrast such as the lungs and bones require less dose. There are many more factors to consider when developing CT protocols, which are beyond the scope of this chapter. However, all address the balance between adequate images for use in diagnosis and the cumulative dose to the patient.

Other considerations

Additional reductions in the population dose can be achieved by reducing the number of screening exams, which only rarely detect disease. Ubiquitous medical imaging procedures as part of a protocol (such as a presurgical chest X-ray for all patients) are not particularly useful in the absence of considerations of the individual patient and her or his risk factors for disease. Similarly, age should be a consideration and a decision point. For example, screening mammograms have been proven to be an effective and beneficial screening tool, but they should be limited to women over a certain age (typically 40) to avoid unnecessary exposure to younger individuals with a very low risk of disease. Of course, these guidelines should be tailored based on the individual patient, the history, and the relevant risk factors (eg, family history of breast cancer).

Every imaging institution should monitor how many examinations must be repeated and the technical competency of the technologists performing the examinations. Errors in technique result in nondiagnostic examinations and may necessitate repeating certain examinations, thus increasing exposures. In addition, poor technique by a technologist may result in inappropriately high doses to patients undergoing routine exams. Care should be taken by the quality control personnel of the imaging center to ensure equipment is kept up-to-date in terms of software updates and equipment repairs and that image processing is uniform and adequate.

Reference levels refer to a value of a metric of dose delivered to a patient or a phantom, which is used in quality assurance programs to identify doses to patients that are excessive or to identify protocols or equipment that may be delivering excessive doses to patients. Dose values above the reference level are subjected to investigation. Reference levels are typically derived from study of dose values across many different imaging systems and imaging institutions. Reference values are usually set so that three-fourth of the data set measurements fall below the reference level value.

Radiation protection for Nuclear Medicine

Procedures performed in nuclear medicine tend to result in low exposures for long periods of time. In contrast to other forms of medical imaging, however, the decay of radioactive materials must be considered when implementing exposure control with nuclear medicine patients. Minimizing the time spent around radiation sources in nuclear medicine requires a *thorough* knowledge of the steps and procedures involved in certain nuclear medicine preparations practices and imaging examinations. Planning ahead, having all the necessary equipment at hand, and practicing steps in advance will minimize the time spent in actually handling the radioactive material. Unshielded sources of radiation must be handled by tongs or other handling devices to increase the distance from the source to the hand.

Various types and forms of shielding are used in nuclear medicine to reduce exposures. Syringe shields are used to reduce the exposure to personnel during preparation and administration of radioactive materials. A combination of lead, leaded glass, and leaded acrylic shields are used in radiopharmaceutical preparation areas. The personnel preparing the radiopharmaceuticals are required to wear personal protective equipment, including a lab coat and disposable gloves as well as ring TLD dosimeters and body dosimeters. Conventional lead aprons used in diagnostic radiology attenuate too little medium-energy photons to prove useful in nuclear medicine.

Precautions must be taken to avoid contamination during the handling of radioactive materials, and there are standard practices to reduce the risks of contamination similar to those used to reduce the risk of contamination in surgical fields. In the case of large radioactive spills, first aid considerations take precedence over contamination control measures. Following this, personnel decontamination takes precedence over decontamination of facilities.

Reduction of exposure to the patient in nuclear medicine is primarily accomplished by limiting radioactive material administration to only those treatments and examinations medically

necessary and by using safety assurance practices to ensure the correct patient receives the correct dose and substance. For those undergoing radionuclide therapy, careful instructions must be given to ensure the patient does not expose others to radiation through direct contact or contamination. In some cases, the patient may even be hospitalized as a protective measure.

The amount of radioactive waste produced is an important consideration in the use of radioactive materials. Many radionuclides have half-lives that are short enough to allow the material to be held until it decays. Standard practices include holding the material for 10 half-lives and then surveying the material for any radioactivity. If there is no detectable radioactivity, the substance is then discarded as nonradioactive waste. It is acceptable for small amounts of water-soluble radioactive material to be discarded in the sewer system within certain regulatory limits. Radioactive human waste products from radiopharmaceutical administration are exempt from these regulations.

Regulatory requirements
Agencies and advisory bodies

There are a number of regulatory agencies at the state and national levels that regulate the use of radioactive materials in medicine. The U.S. Nuclear Regulatory Commission regulates special nuclear material (plutonium and uranium enriched in the isotopes U-233 and U-235), source material (thorium, uranium, and their ores), and by-product material used in the commercial nuclear power industry, research, medicine, and a variety of other commercial activities. The Atomic Energy Act of 1954 established the Atomic Energy Commission whose regulatory arm currently exists as the NRC. In addition, the Food and Drug Administration (FDA) regulates the manufacture of radiopharmaceuticals and the manufacturing of medical imaging equipment. Besides these regulatory agencies, there are a number of advisory organizations that review literature and issue recommendations but do not carry the force of law. The two most prominent advisory boards are the NCRP and the ICRP.

Exposure limits

There are differences between internal and external exposure due to the fact that internal exposures continue to provide a dose to the patient after ingestion or inhalation until the substance is eliminated by radioactive decay or biologic elimination. The committed dose equivalent ($H_{50,T}$) is the dose equivalent to a tissue or organ over the 50 years following the ingestion or inhalation of radioactivity. The committed effective dose equivalent is a weighted average of the committed dose equivalents to the various tissues and organs of the body.

The NRC provides dose-limit regulations designed to limit the risks of stochastic effects and deterministic effects. To limit risk of stochastic effects, the limit for the sum of internal and external doses to the entire body may not exceed 0.05 Sv. To prevent deterministic effects, the sum of the external dose and committed dose equivalent to any organ except the lens of the eye cannot exceed 0.5 Sv. The dose limit to the lens of the eye is 0.15 Sv in 1 year. The dose to a fetus of a radiation worker may not exceed 5 mSv over the 9-month gestational period.

Appropriate use of radiation on pregnant patients

Occasionally, the need to perform a medical imaging procedure on a pregnant patient may arise, typically in the setting of trauma or emergent medical conditions. When the emergent need to irradiate a pregnant female arises for the sake of medical imaging or radionuclide administration, careful consideration must be given to the amount of radiation exposure to the embryo and fetus. The beginning point is determining the pregnancy status of the patient, which should be done for any female of childbearing age, usually regarded as age 12 to 50. For most examinations, the technologist may simply ask the patient if she could be pregnant and about last menstruation. For examinations that would result in high doses to a fetus (>100 mSv) such as possibly prolonged fluoroscopic procedures and multiphase CT, a pregnancy test should be obtained within 72 hours before the examination, except in the case of emergency or when pregnancy is not possible such as with history of hysterectomy. Pregnancy tests should always be obtained before radiopharmaceutical administration. In certain situations, in which the benefits of medical imaging are thought to outweigh the risks of exposure to the fetus, the risks and benefits should be explained to the patient and informed consent should be obtained before continuing with the examination. In these cases, every precaution should be taken to shield the fetus from radiation within the limits of producing a diagnostic examination.

Should it be discovered after an examination or treatment with radiation that the exposed patient is pregnant, then fetal age at the time of exposure, dose to the embryo or fetus, and potential effects on the embryo or fetus should be estimated. The patient is then counseled by a physician with this information at hand, and occasionally the decision on whether to intervene or terminate the pregnancy must be made. No medical intervention to the pregnancy should be considered for doses under 100 mSv. For higher doses, the decision for medical intervention or termination should be guided by the fetal age and individual circumstances of the exposure, the patient, and the pregnancy.

References

1. Hall EJ, Giaccia AJ. *Radiobiology for the Radiologist.* 7th ed. Philadelphia, PA: Lippincott Williams and Wilkins; 2012.
2. Goodhead DT. Initial events in the cellular effects of ionizing radiations: clustered damage in DNA. *Int J Radiat Biol.* 1994;65:7–17.
3. Ward JF. DNA damage produced by ionizing radiation in mammalian cells: Identities, mechanisms of formation, and repairability. *Prog Nucleic Acid Res Mol Biol.* 1988;35:95–125.
4. Goodhead DT. Spatial and temporal distribution of energy. *Health Phys.* 1988;55:231–240.
5. Clifton DK, Bremner WJ. The effect of testicular x-irradiation on 6872 spermatogenesis in man. A comparison with the mouse. *J Androl.* 1983;4:387–392.
6. BEIR. Health Risks from Exposure to Low Levels of Ionizing Radiation: BEIR VII, Phase 2. Committee to Assess Health Risks from Exposure to Low Levels of Ionizing Radiation, Board of Radiation Effects Research, Division on Earth and Life Studies, National Research Council of the National Academies. Washington, DC: The National Academies Press; 2006.
7. National Council on Radiation Protection and Measurements. Ionizing radiation exposure of the population of the United States. NCRP Report No. 160. National Council on Radiation Protection and Measurements, Bethesda, MD; 2009.
8. Fletcher DW, Miller DL, Balter S, Taylor MA. Comparison of four techniques to estimate radiation dose to skin during angiographic and interventional radiology procedures. *J Vasc Interv Radiol.* 2002;13:391–397.
9. Miller DL, Balter S, Cole PE, et al. Radiation doses in interventional radiology procedures: the RAD-IR study: part II: skin dose. *J Vasc Interv Radiol.* 2003;14:977–990.

CHAPTER SELF-ASSESSMENT QUESTIONS

1. The majority of biologic damage caused by ionizing radiation can be contributed to

   A. ionization of DNA, RNA, and proteins, which is indirect damage.
   B. the creation of free radicals, which is direct damage.
   C. the creation of free radicals, which is indirect damage.
   D. ionization of DNA, RNA, and proteins, which is direct damage.

2. A fluoroscopic technologist receives a radiation dose of 0.01 mSv during a fluoroscopic procedure. All things being equal, what would the technologist's approximate radiation dose have been if he doubled his distance from the radiation source?

   A. 0.001 mSv
   B. 0.025 mSv
   C. 0.04 mSv
   D. 0.0025 mSv

3. Which of the following is *not* true regarding radiation biology and radiation safety?

   A. There are mainly two types of biologic effects of radiation exposure: stochastic and deterministic.
   B. Among the different stages of fetal development, the risks of prenatal death and congenital anomalies are at their highest during the fetal growth stage.

   C. Three sources of exposure are considered in X-ray shielding design: primary radiation, scattered radiation, and leakage radiation.
   D. According to NRC's requirement, the total effective dose equivalent to the whole body (TEDE) of a radiation worker may not exceed 50 mSv in a year.

Answers to Chapter Self-Assessment Questions

1. C   Biologic damage by ionization radiation is made in an indirect way; it creates free radical through interaction with water molecules, and these free radicals then incur damage to DNA, RNA, and other molecules.

2. D   Assuming that radiation is emitted from a point source, radiation dose is inversely proportional to the square of the distance from the source. If the distance doubles, radiation dose should fall to ¼=25% of its original value.

3. B   The occurrence of prenatal death and congenital anomalies is negligible unless there is exceptionally high radiation exposure. Risks of both are typically much higher in earlier stages of fetal development.

Self-Assessment Exam

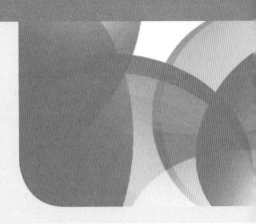

1. Which of the following is NOT true regarding radiation?

    A. When there is a vacancy created in one of the inner shells of an atom, an outer-shell electron may fill the vacancy accompanied by the release of energy in the form of either characteristic X-rays or Auger electrons.

    B. For the same amount of radiation dose, protons cause more biologic damage to tissue than do X-ray photons because of their higher LET (linear energy transfer).

    C. All stable nuclei have equal numbers of protons and neutrons; otherwise they would undergo radioactive decay.

    D. When electrons interact with a certain material, the probability of Bremsstrahlung X-ray emission increases with the atomic number of the material.

2. For a tungsten atom with the following binding energies, K-shell = 70 keV, L-shell = 12 keV, and M-shell = 3 keV, characteristic X-rays of which of the following different energies (in keV) could be emitted by a 100-keV electron striking a tungsten target?

    A. 100, 70, 30

    B. 97, 88, 30

    C. 70, 12, 3

    D. 67, 58, 9

    E. 30, 18, 15

3. The contrast in an image as perceived by the observer is determined by:

    A. Subject contrast

    B. Displayed contrast

    C. Detected contrast

    D. All of the above

4. Which of the following is NOT true regarding X-ray interactions?

    A. Compton scattering and the photoelectric effect are two primary interactions for diagnostic X-rays.

    B. The photoelectric effect is more pronounced with materials of low effective atomic number.

    C. The energy of the X-ray photon remains unchanged in Rayleigh scattering.

    D. The probability of the photoelectric effect generally decreases with the energy of the X-ray photons, but sharply increases right at the K-edge.

5. The photon interaction most responsible for the high soft-tissue contrast in mammography with 15- to 30-keV X-rays is:

    A. Compton scattering

    B. Coherent scattering

    C. Photoelectric effect

    D. Pair production

    E. Photonuclear disintegration

6. Which of the following is true regarding X-ray production?

    A. The discrete energy peaks of characteristic X-ray photons are the same for different anode materials.

    B. The closer a high-speed electron gets to the atomic nucleus, the lower energy the resulting bremsstrahlung radiation has.

    C. Materials with higher atomic numbers are preferred for the anode because of their high attenuation coefficients.

    D. When high-speed electrons interact with the anode, the majority of the kinetic energy of these electrons is lost via heat.

7. Which of the following is NOT true regarding X-ray tubes?

    A. The anode heel effect becomes more pronounced with a smaller anode angle.

    B. X-ray tubes typically can operate at higher power when the large focal spot is selected.

    C. The effective focal spot size is constant across the radiation field.

    D. Thicker filter results in higher effective energy of the produced X-ray beam.

8. Which of the following is NOT true regarding an X-ray tube for medical imaging?

    A. It typically provides two or more focal spots.

    B. X-ray tubes with rotating anode are primarily used in radiography.

    C. Tungsten is commonly used as the target material.

    D. The majority of the input electrical energy is converted into X-ray photons.

9. Which of the following is true regarding the use of antiscatter grids in radiography?

    A. When available on the system, the grid should be used at all times to reduce scatter.

    B. The use of grid is an effective way of radiation dose reduction.

    C. The grid needs to be placed at its intended distance and well centered during its use.

    D. The use of grid is beneficial in imaging of hands and wrists.

10. Which of the following is NOT true regarding radiographic image quality?

    A. Short exposure time can be used to reduce motion-caused blur on image.

    B. Spatial resolution is the same everywhere on the image.

    C. Automatic exposure control keeps image noise constant regardless of object size.

    D. Changes in kVp (all other parameters unchanged) affect both image contrast and image noise.

11. Which of the following is NOT true regarding comparisons between II-based and FPD-based fluoroscopy?

    A. FPD-based systems support magnification modes, whereas II-based systems do not.
    B. FPD-based systems give more room around patient than II-based systems.
    C. FPD-based systems are less affected by geometric distortions than II-based systems.
    D. Both FPD- and II-based systems have ABC or are equivalent to ensure constant signal level on image receptor.

12. Which of the following is NOT true regarding mammographic X-ray tubes using tungsten as anode target material?

    A. Tungsten targets are often used on digital mammography systems.
    B. Tungsten targets produce X-ray spectra with higher mean energies than do molybdenum or rhodium targets.
    C. Tungsten targets allow the tubes to operate at higher power than do molybdenum or rhodium targets.
    D. Tungsten targets are less affected by heel effects than are molybdenum or rhodium targets.

13. Which of the following is NOT true regarding the magnification mode in mammography?

    A. Magnification mode has a smaller field of view than the normal mode.
    B. Magnification mode has poor image contrast because antiscatter grid is NOT used.
    C. Magnification mode has improved spatial resolution compared to normal mode.
    D. Magnification mode uses the small focal spot.

14. Which one of the following is NOT true regarding breast compression in mammography?

    A. It brings more tissues near the chest wall into the field of view.
    B. It reduces overlapping of breast tissues and improves image contrast.
    C. It leads to substantial increases in radiation dose compared to no compression.
    D. It reduces the chances of motion caused by image blur.

15. Which of the following scenarios would NOT benefit from the use of kVp lower than 120?

    A. Abdomen CT of a 3-year-old child
    B. Abdomen-pelvis CT of an obese patient
    C. Brain perfusion CT
    D. Abdominal CT angiography of an undersized patient for whom iodine contrast volume needs to be reduced because of impaired kidney function

16. Which of the following is NOT true regarding bow-tie filters in CT?

    A. It is made in the shape of a "bow-tie," that is, thin in the middle and thicker at the ends, to account for the oval shape of body in general.
    B. It narrows the range of signal levels detected by the detector and thus improves image contrast.
    C. It cuts down unnecessary radiation dose to tissues at the periphery of the body.
    D. It eliminates scattered photons from signals on the detector.

17. Which of the following is NOT true regarding dual-energy CT?

    A. It allows quantification of iodine quantification by separating signal contributions from water and iodine.
    B. It allows synthesis of CT images acquired with monochromatic X-ray beams, which may be used to reduce beam hardening artifacts.
    C. It allows characterization of kidney stones of different types by material differentiation.
    D. It allows for substantial reduction in radiation dose.

18. Which of the follow is NOT true regarding radiation dose in CT?

    A. Increase in mA alone leads to increase in both CTDIvol and DLP.
    B. Increase in longitudinal scan coverage alone leads to increase in DLP.
    C. Increase in helical pitch leads to increase in both CTDIvol and DLP.
    D. With the same CTDIvol, scans of an undersized patient have higher SSDE than do scans of oversized patients.

19. Gradients are turned on to perform _____ in an MR sequence.

    A. slice selection
    B. spatial encoding
    C. diffusion weighting
    D. All of these

20. Field inhomogeneity can cause _____artifacts, which is _____ when magnet field is higher.

    A. distortion, improved
    B. aliasing, worse
    C. distortion, worse
    D. aliasing, improved

21. Contrast-enhanced MRA injects Gd-based contrast agents to ___ T1 of blood. To limit the acquisition window in arterial phase, _____ sequence is usually used.

    A. increase, SE
    B. decrease, SE
    C. increase, GE
    D. decrease, GE

22. SNR of image can be improved by _____.

    A. higher bandwidth
    B. higher spatial resolution
    C. higher magnet field strength
    D. higher gradient strength

23. Echo planar imaging is most commonly used in _____.

    A. diffusion imaging
    B. BOLD imaging
    C. vascular imaging
    D. A and B
    E. A, B, and C

24. Which of the following is NOT true regarding spatial resolution of ultrasound images?

    A. Axial resolution worsens with an increase in the number of cycles emitted per pulse by the transducer.
    B. Axial resolution worsens with an increase in the frequency of the ultrasound wave.
    C. Lateral resolution varies with tissue depth.
    D. Lateral resolution at different depths may be kept constant by using multiple transmit/receive focal zones.

25. Which of the following leads to lower frame rate of real-time ultrasound images?

    A. Decreased depth of the field of view
    B. Decreased angle of the field of view
    C. Decreased number of lines across the field of view
    D. The use of more transmit/receive focal zones

26. Which of the following increases the maximum blood velocity that can be measured by pulsed Doppler ultrasound and therefore reduces aliasing artifacts?

    A. Higher pulse repetition frequency (PRF)
    B. Lower frequency of the ultrasound beam
    C. Higher frequency of the ultrasound beam
    D. Larger angle between the ultrasound beam and the axis of the blood vessel

27. A patient undergoing FDG PET/CT scanning is concerned about possible side effects of radiation from the scan. Which of the following effects could be seen as a result of radiation from this scan?

    A. Skin erythema (redness)
    B. Epilation (hair loss)
    C. Nausea
    D. Cancer induction

28. Which of the following measures is intended to correlate with stochastic risk?

    A. Activity
    B. Absorbed dose
    C. Effective dose
    D. Equivalent dose

29. Which of the following is true for most cyclotron-produced radionuclides used in nuclear medicine?

    A. They are proton deficient and undergo beta-plus decay.
    B. They are neutron deficient and undergo beta-plus decay.
    C. They are neutron deficient and undergo beta-minus decay.
    D. They are neutron deficient and undergo alpha decay.

30. What would be the result of eluting a Mo-99/^{99m}Tc generator every 8 hours, compared with once per day?

    A. Higher activity of ^{99m}Tc pertechnetate for each elution
    B. Lower activity of ^{99m}Tc pertechnetate for each elution, but higher total activity yield for the day
    C. Generator life decreased by two-thirds
    D. Decrease in the half-life of Mo-99 by two-thirds

31. Which of the following is NOT true regarding gas-filled detectors?

    A. Ionization survey meters and dose calibrators typically operate in current mode.
    B. GM survey meters typically operate in pulse mode.
    C. Both ionization survey meters and GM survey meters are used for low-level radiation contamination surveys.
    D. Dose calibrators are typically filled with pressurized noble gas to increase sensitivity.

32. What properties would an ideal scintillator have for the detection of gamma photons?

    A. It should be transparent to its own emitted light.
    B. It converts gamma radiation into detectable light photon efficiently.
    C. The amount of light should be proportional to radiation energy.
    D. All of these.

33. Which of the following causes the most degradation of spatial resolution of a SPECT scan?

    A. Using a 64 × 64 acquisition matrix (compared to 128 × 128)
    B. Using a camera with a half-inch scintillator crystal (compared to 3/8 inch)
    C. Using an ultrahigh resolution collimator (compared to general purpose ones)
    D. Using a noncircular orbit that conforms to the patient's body contour (compared to circular)

34. Which of the following does NOT improve sensitivity of a PET scan?

    A. 3D acquisition mode
    B. Larger bore size
    C. More detector rings
    D. Thicker scintillator crystal

35. The majority of biologic damage caused by ionizing radiation can be contributed to:

    A. Ionization of DNA, RNA, and proteins, which is indirect damage
    B. The creation of free radicals, which is direct damage
    C. The creation of free radicals, which is indirect damage
    D. Ionization of DNA, RNA, and proteins, which is direct damage

36. A fluoroscopic technologist receives a radiation dose of 0.01 mSv during a fluoroscopic procedure. All things being equal, what would the technologist's approximate radiation dose have been if he doubled his distance from the radiation source?

    A. 0.001 mSv
    B. 0.025 mSv
    C. 0.04 mSv
    D. 0.0025 mSv

37. Which of the following is NOT true regarding radiation biology and radiation safety?

    A. There are mainly two types of biologic effects of radiation exposure: stochastic and deterministic.
    B. Among the different stages of fetal development, the risks of prenatal death and congenital anomalies are at their highest during the fetal growth stage.
    C. Three sources of exposure are considered in X-ray shielding design: primary radiation, scattered radiation, and leakage radiation.
    D. According to NRC's requirement, the total effective dose equivalent to the whole body (TEDE) of a radiation worker may not exceed 50 mSv in a year.

Answers to Self-Assessment Questions

1. C When the atomic number is low, the ratio between the numbers of neutrons and protons of a nucleus is close to 1. But as the atomic number increases, the ratio begins to increase until it approaches about 1.5 for the heaviest nuclei.

2. D After the 100-keV electron knocks a K-shell electron out of its orbit, filling of the K-shell vacancy by an M-shell electron, filling of the K-shell vacancy by an L-shell electron, and filling of the L-shell vacancy by an M-shell electron lead to emitted X-ray photons at 70 keV − 3 keV = 67 keV, 70 keV − 12 keV = 58 keV, and 12 keV − 3 keV = 9 keV, respectively.

3. D All the three factors from A to C affect the perceived image contrast.

4. B The photoelectric effect is more pronounced for higher Z elements.

5. C Interactions of 15- to 30-keV X-ray photons are dominated by photoelectric effect. Both Compton scattering and coherent scattering have substantially fewer interactions within the range. Pair production and photonuclear disintegration occur only at much higher photon energies.

6. D Photon energies of characteristic X-ray are strongly dependent on the type of anode material. When the high-speed electron gets closer to the nucleus, there is more energy loss from the electron and therefore the resulting bremsstrahlung radiation has higher energy.

7. C The effective focal spot size varies across the radiation field. Along the cathode–anode direction, the effective focal spot size is typically larger on the cathode side.

8. D The majority of the input electrical energy is converted into heat.

9. C Since antiscatter grids remove both scattered and primary photons, the use of antiscatter grids involves trade-off between image quality improvement and dose penalty. Typically, an increase in radiation dose is necessary for the desired image quality (compared with when there is no scatter). Their use in imaging of small-sized anatomy is not well justified because the amount of scatter is relatively insignificant.

10. B Spatial resolution varies with the location in the field. The projected focal spot size, a major factor affecting spatial resolution, is not the same everywhere in the field (typically smaller near the anode).

11. A Magnification modes are supported on both FPD- and II-based systems.

12. D Tungsten targets are less affected by heel effects than are molybdenum or rhodium targets.

13. B Magnification mode has poor image contrast because antiscatter grid is not used.

14. C It leads to substantial increases in radiation dose compared to no compression.

15. B Abdomen-pelvis CT of an obese patient.

16. D Bow-tie filters help to mitigate scatter caused by artifacts; they, however, do not eliminate scatter.

17. D The benefits of dual-energy CT do not include substantial reduction in radiation dose. Its clinical use today is typically with equivalent radiation dose to that used by traditional CT.

18. C CTDIvol and DLP are inversely proportional to helical pitch.

19. D Gradient fields can be applied for all listed purposes.

20. C Spatial encoding in MRI is done by superimposing gradient fields on the ideally homogeneous static field. Inhomogeneity in the static field will be confused with the effect from the superimposed gradient fields and lead to signals being misplaced during reconstruction, eventually causing image distortion. Homogeneity is generally more difficult to achieve in higher strength magnetic field.

21. D The use of gadolinium as MRI contrast is primarily based on its T1 shortening effect. Gradient echo pulse sequences are usually used to acquire the arterial phase because of its fast speed.

22. C Both higher bandwidth and higher spatial resolution are associated with increased noise, and therefore lower SNR. SNR is not dependent on gradient strength.

23. D Faster acquisition time of EPI has made it a valuable tool in applications like diffusion imaging and functional imaging. Poor SNR, low spatial resolution, and artifacts have limited the use of EPI in vascular imaging and many other applications.

24. B Axial resolution is determined by the spatial pulse length (SPL), which is equal to the product of the number of cycles emitted per pulse by the transducer and the wavelength. Increased frequency of the ultrasound wave leads to decreased wavelength and therefore poorer axial resolution.

25. D The frame rate is inversely proportional to the time spent acquiring each frame. Decreases in the depth and the angle of the field of view and the number of lines across the field of view all result in shorter acquisition per frame. More focal zones lead to longer acquisition per frame and therefore lower frame rate.

26. C The maximum blood velocity that can be measured by pulsed Doppler ultrasound follows $V_{\max} = \dfrac{c \times PRF}{4 f_0 \cos\theta}$, where c is the speed of ultrasound in tissue, f_0 is the frequency of the ultrasound beam, PRF is the pulse repetition frequency, and is the angle between the ultrasound beam and the axis of the blood vessel. Higher frequency of the ultrasound beam actually results in an decrease in the maximum blood velocity that can be accurately measured by pulsed Doppler ultrasound.

27. D Cancer induction. By the linear no-threshold model, there is no radiation dose free from stochastic effects such as the (low) risk of cancer induction. The doses received in diagnostic studies such as FDG PET/CT are ordinarily below the thresholds for deterministic effects (tissue reactions) such as erythema, epilation, and sterility.

28. C Effective dose. The stochastic risk of a radiation exposure is, in part, related to the amount and types of radiation involved, the distribution in the organs of the body, and the radiation sensitivity of organs. These factors are reflected in the effective dose. Effective dose can be a useful gauge of risk for the purposes of radiation protection; however, it is important to note that it is not useful for determining risk for individual patients.

29. B They are neutron deficient and undergo beta-plus decay. Medical cyclotrons bombard stable target material with protons, producing neutron-deficient radioisotopes that decay by beta-plus decay (positron emission) or electron capture. Most radionuclides used in PET imaging are cyclotron produced.

30. B Lower activity of ^{99m}Tc pertechnetate for each elution, but higher total activity yield for the day. Figure 8.21 shows that at 8 hours, ^{99m}Tc has regenerated to more than half the activity that would be obtained at 24 hours. The sum of the activities for the three 8-hour elutions will be greater than that of a single elution obtained at 24 hours.

31. C GM survey meters are more sensitive than ionization survey meters and therefore more useful in detecting some quantities of radioactivity as encountered in low-level contamination surveys.

32. D   Ideal scintillators are expected to have all listed characteristics.

33. A   Thinner crystal, ultrahigh resolution collimator, and an orbit that places gamma as close as possible to the anatomy all contribute to improved spatial resolution. A larger pixel size leads to poorer spatial resolution.

34. B   3D scan (compared to 2D scan), more detector rings, and thicker crystal all result in more annihilation coincidence events being detected. Larger bore size may allow more events escape the detectors and cause a decrease in efficiency.

35. C   Biologic damage by ionization radiation is made in an indirect way; it creates free radical through interaction with water molecules, and these free radicals then incur damage to DNA, RNA, and other molecules.

36. D   Assuming that radiation is emitted from a point source, radiation dose is inversely proportional to the square of the distance from the source. If the distance doubles, radiation dose should fall to ¼ = 25% of its original value.

37. B   The occurrence of prenatal death and congenital anomalies is negligible unless there is exceptionally high radiation exposure. Risks of both are typically much higher in earlier stages of fetal development.

INDEX